THE BEST-EVER
BOOK OF
BEAUTY

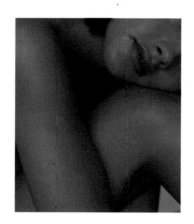

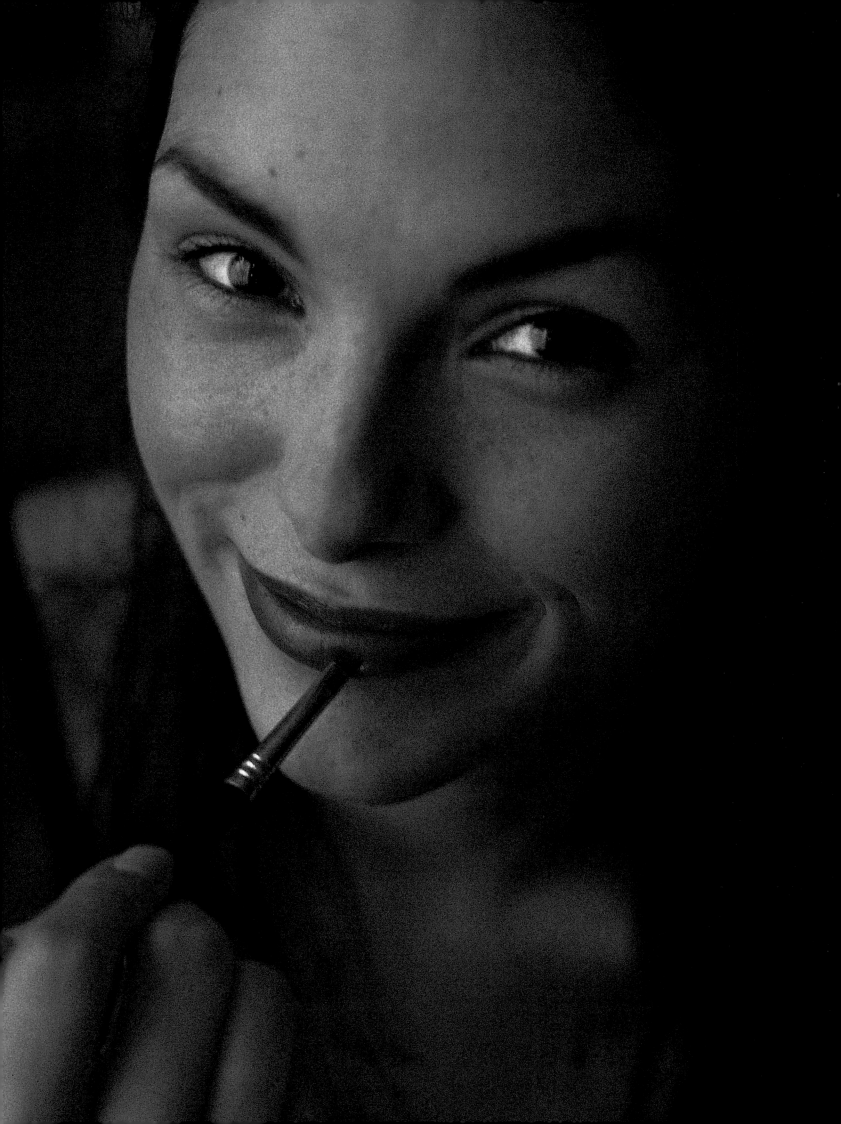

THE BEST-EVER
BOOK OF
BEAUTY

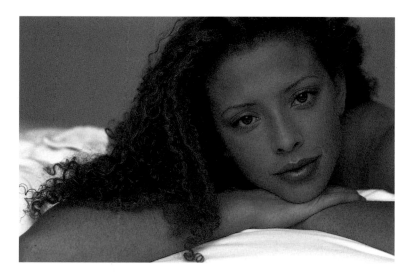

MAKE-UP • SKINCARE • FITNESS • DIET
HAIRCARE • DETOX • CLEANSING
NAILCARE • TONING

Consultant editor: HELENA SUNNYDALE

HERMES
HOUSE

This edition is published by Hermes House
an imprint of Anness Publishing Ltd
Hermes House, 88–89 Blackfriars Road, London SE1 8HA
tel. 020 7401 2077; fax 020 7633 9499;
www.hermeshouse.com; www.annesspublishing.com

Anness Publishing has a new picture agency outlet for images for
publishing, promotions or advertising. Please visit our website
www.practicalpictures.com for more information.

Publisher: Joanna Lorenz
Editorial Director: Helen Sudell
Project Editors: Sylvie Wooton, Casey Horton, Debra Mayhew
Skincare and make-up written by Sally Norton, *Haircare and styling*
written by Jacki Wadeson, *Keeping Fit and healthy eating* written by
Kate Shapland, and *Introducing Pilates* written by Emily Kelly.
Photography: Nick Cole, Alistair Hughes, Simon Bottomley and
Christine Hanscomb
Designer: Design Principals
Make-up: Debbi Finlow, Vanessa Haines, Liz Kitchiner and Paul Miller
Additional Make-up: Bettina Graham
Hair: Debbie Finlow and Kathleen Bray, assisted by Wendy M.B. Cook
Exercise Adviser: Dean Hodgkin
Exercise and Diet Consultant: Dr Naomi Lewis
Illustrators: Samantha Elmhurst (p104) Cherril Parris (hair),
David Cook (pilates)
Models: Amanda, Christiana, Carley, Laura, Emily, Frieda, Hannah,
Juliet, Sarah, Zonna, Cheryl, Jane, Joanna and Stacey

Sections of this book were previously published as *The Ultimate
Beauty Book* and *Commonsense Pilates*

Contents

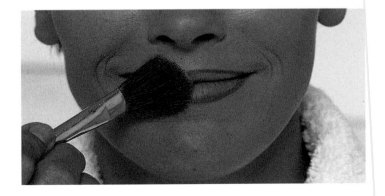

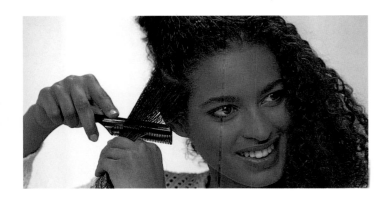

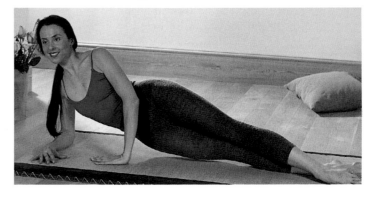

Introduction

This book covers every aspect of women's health and beauty, head to toe, inside and out. Beauty – looking good, feeling great and making the best of all your physical features – is an important part of improving every aspect of a woman's life. This book has simple, basic routines and habits that contribute to complete well-being, including healthy exercise, therapeutic treatments, regenerating remedies, soothing relaxation techniques, detoxifying diets and massages, as well as extras that contribute new and special dimensions to your appearance, including make-up skills, expert hairstyling and work-outs that will shape and tone your body.

skincare and make-up

While your actual skin type is determined by your genes, there is plenty you can do daily to ensure it always looks as good as possible. Understanding how your skin functions will help you to understand its special needs. In the skincare section, you can find out how to care for your own specific skin type. You can't neglect your complexion for months or years, then make

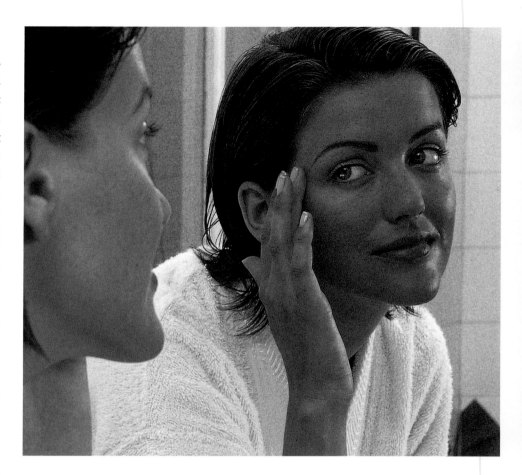

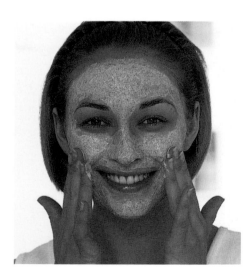

△ A facial scrub removes dead skin cells, stimulates the circulation and brings fresh oxygenated blood to the surface, leaving the skin clean and soft.

up for it with expensive and intensive attention in the short term. Regularly spending time and care on your skin is a great investment – it's never too early or too late to follow a good skincare regime – and the results will last a lifetime.

Skincare is all about making sure your skin is in good shape – clear, soft and supple – and then keeping it that way through good habits, sensible cleansing and using skincare products in the right way. The bodycare section will also show you how to freshen, tone, pamper and maintain your whole body from top to toe – from bathroom essentials to natural pampering treats – to help you achieve natural, beautiful, hassle-free skin.

The key to successful make-up is to understand how to enhance your features using the best cosmetic fomulations and colours around. This doesn't mean spending a small fortune on the latest season's colours and promotions. Instead, it means analysing what will work for you, your colouring and

△ The single biggest cause of skin ageing is sunlight. So it is important to choose a moisturizer that contains an effective sunscreen.

your lifestyle, then making your purchases. If you research the best of the products, brush up your application techniques and give yourself time to experiment, you can find the perfect look for you. And, once you have mastered the basics, you can solve your own particular beauty problems and try out some inspirational make-up ideas.

Every woman can use make-up to enhance her looks, but the secret is understanding your own beauty needs. This section provides fresh and inspiring ideas to help you find a look to suit you.

haircare and styling

Beautiful, silky, shining hair makes you feel fantastic, it reflects well-being and has a natural beauty of its own. Hair can also be a versatile fashion accessory, and can be coloured, curled, dressed up or smoothed

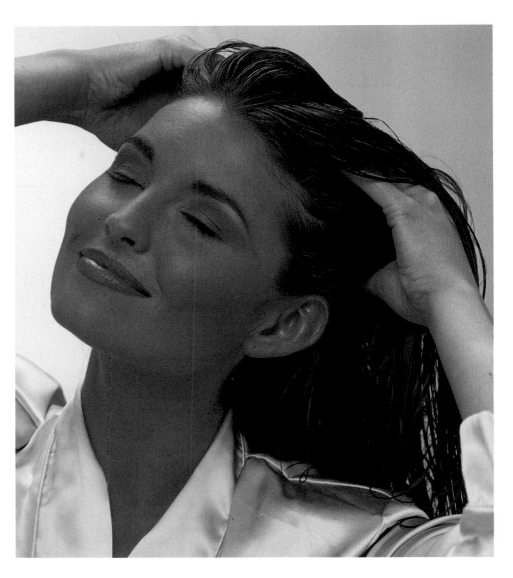

▷ Individual hair types need individual treatments: adopt a personal routine to keep your hair at its best. A massage with warm olive oil is ideal for a dry, tight scalp.

down – all in a matter of minutes. However, too much attention – washing, styling, drying and colouring – combined with the effects of a poor diet, pollution, air-conditioning and central heating, can strip your hair of its vitality, and leave it looking dull and lifeless. A daily haircare routine and prompt treatment when problems do arise are of vital importance in maintaining the natural beauty of healthy hair.

The haircare and styling section provides a complete guide to making the most of your hair. There are hints and tips for establishing good haircare habits, and tricks and treatments to get your hair in tip-top shape – from aromatic shampoos, herbal tonics and intensive conditioning treatments to colouring, bleaching and tinting – as well as a range of inspirational styling ideas for every season and occasion.

exercise and healthy eating

It is particularly important that you make regular exercise and healthy eating a key part of your beauty routine.

Walking, swimming, cycling, working out, yoga and Pilates are all great ways to stay fit, increase your stamina and keep your body toned and supple. Exercise boosts circulation,

allowing the body to absorb nutrients and eliminate toxins and waste more efficiently. The exercise and healthy eating section provides a complete guide to health and fitness, from finding the right sports to relaxation and stress-reducing techniques. Find out how to make the best of your body shape and improve your posture, and get tips and techniques for tackling specific trouble spots. There are simple step-by-step sequences for general fitness to fit into your daily routine, as well as an introduction to the benefits of Pilates.

A healthy diet involves eating foods that provide all the nourishment your body requires for growth, tissue repair, energy to carry out vital internal processes and to make sure you are fit and active. The healthy eating chapter has a clear, comprehensive breakdown of foods and nutritional values to help you achieve a balance in your daily diet. There is advice on the best foods to eat to improve your skin, hair and nails, and hints on how to change your eating habits

so that the food you eat peps you up instead of pulling you down. From advice on eating to lose weight, to detoxing to cleanse and refresh your whole system, you'll find all you need to know about healthy eating.

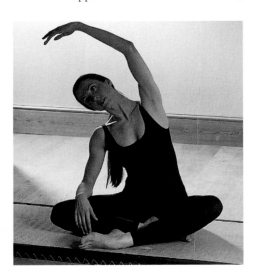

△ Pilates combines stretches and strengthening exercises. Side stretches like these are good for relieving the body of unwanted tension and liberating the spine and joints.

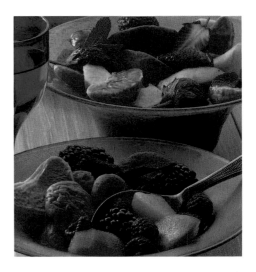

△ Eating a varied selection of fresh fruit every day will keep your body healthy. Fresh fruit provides the body with valuable fibre, vitamins and minerals.

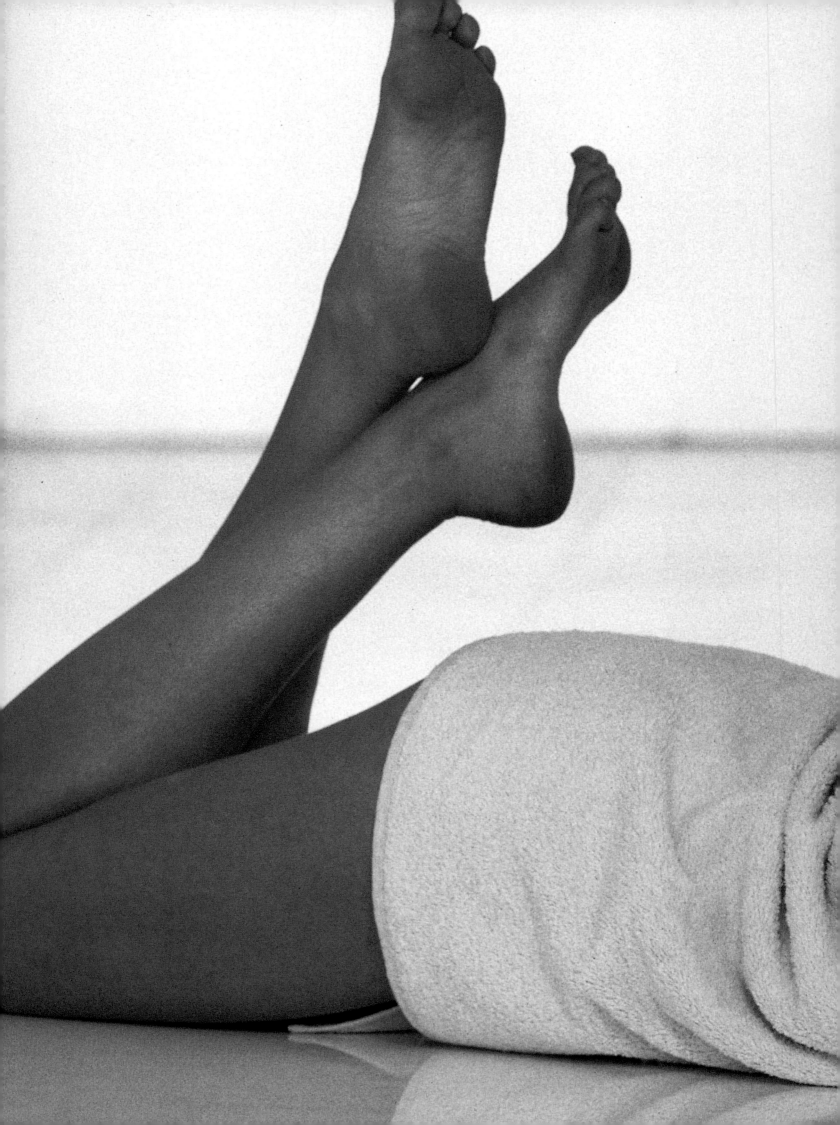

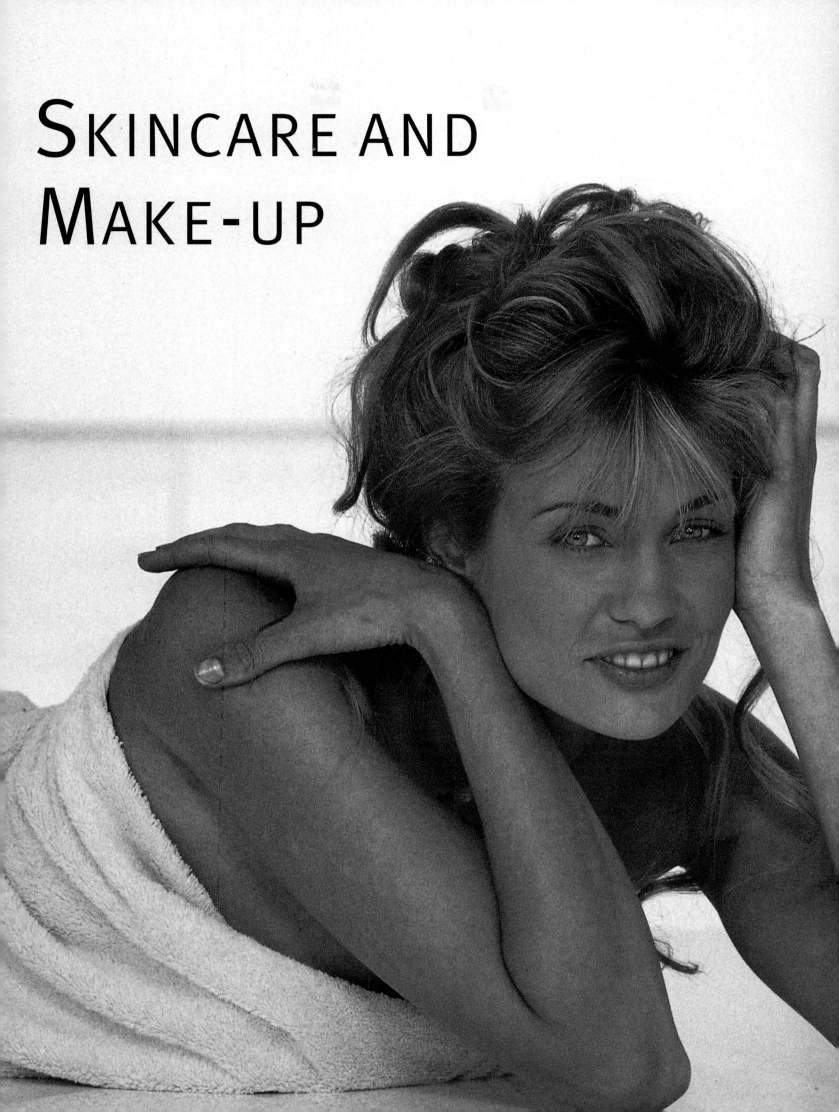

Skincare and Make-up

What is skin?

Skin is your body's largest organ, covering and protecting every single surface of your body. The secret of beautiful, healthy skin is to understand how your skin functions because this will help you to treat it correctly, keeping it strong and supple. Your skin is made up of two main layers, called the epidermis and the dermis.

the epidermis

This is the top layer of skin and the one you can actually see. It protects your body from invasion and infection and helps to seal in moisture. It's built up of several layers of living cells which are then topped by sheets of dead cells. It's constantly growing, with new cells being produced at its base. They quickly die, and are pushed up to the surface by the arrival of new ones. These dead cells eventually flake away, which means that every new layer of skin is another chance to have a soft, glowing complexion.

The lower levels of living cells are fed by the blood supply from underneath, whereas the upper dead cells only require a supply of water to make sure that they are kept plump and smooth.

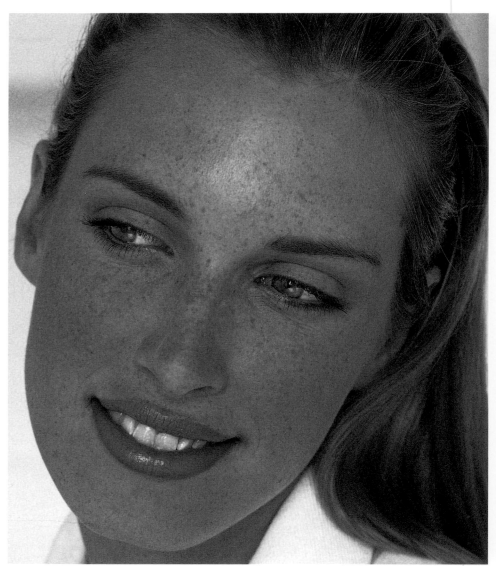

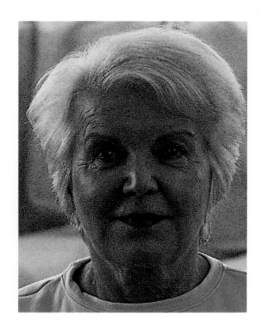

△ Every woman can have beautiful skin regardless of age, race or colouring.

The epidermis is responsible for your colouring, because it holds the skin's pigment. Its thickness varies from area to area. For instance, it's much thicker on the soles of your feet than on your eyelids.

the dermis

The layer that lies underneath the epidermis is called the dermis, and it is composed entirely of living cells. It consists of bundles of tough fibres, which give your skin its elasticity, firmness and strength. There are also blood vessels, which feed vital nutrients to these areas.

The epidermis is usually able to repair and restore itself to make itself as good as

△ **Understanding your skin the way a beauty therapist would allows you to give it the care it deserves and to appreciate why certain factors are good for it – and others are not.**

new, but the dermis will be permanently damaged by injury. The dermis also contains the following specialized organs:

Sebaceous glands: These are tiny organs that usually open into hair follicles on the surface of your skin. They produce an oily secretion, called sebum, which is your skin's natural lubricant. The sebaceous glands are concentrated on the scalp and face, around the nose, cheeks, chin and forehead (the T-zone), which are usually the most oily areas.

▷ The condition of your skin is an overall sign of your health. It reveals stress, a poor diet and a lack of sleep. Taking care of your health will benefit your skin.

Sweat glands: These are located all over your body. There are millions of them and their main function is to control and regulate your body temperature. When sweat evaporates on the skin's surface, the temperature of your skin drops.

Hairs: Growing out of the hair follicles, these can help to keep your body warm by trapping air underneath them. There are no hairs on the soles of your feet or the palms of your hands.

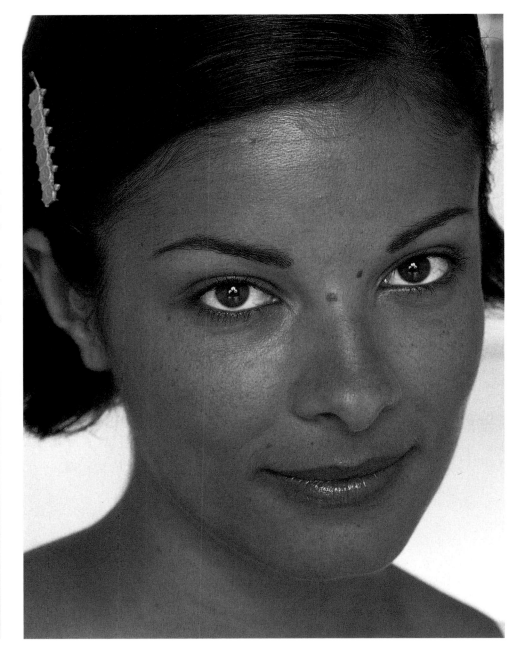

THE MAIN FUNCTIONS OF YOUR SKIN

• It acts as a thermostat, retaining heat or cooling you down with sweat.

• It offers protection from potentially harmful things.

• It acts as a waste disposal system. Certain waste is expelled from your body 24 hours a day through your skin.

• It provides a sense of touch, which enables you to interact and communicate with other people and function in your environment.

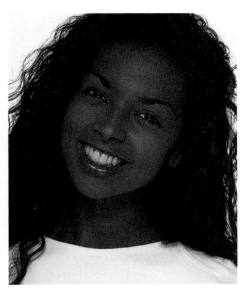

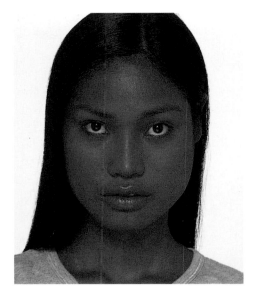

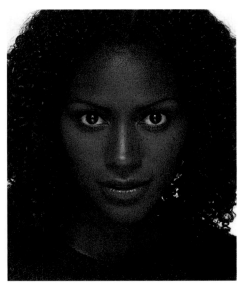

△ Skin is a barometer of your emotions. It becomes red when you're embarrassed and quickly shows the signs of stress.

△ Your skin can cleanse, heal and even renew itself. How effectively it does these things is partly governed by you.

△ Your skin is a sensor of pain, touch and temperature, offering protection and a means of eliminating waste.

What is your skin type?

There's no point spending a fortune on expensive skincare products if you buy the wrong ones for your skin type and make a collection of assorted once-used bottles. The key to developing a skincare regime that works for you is to analyse your skin-type first.

skincare quiz

To develop a better understanding of your skin and what will suit it best, start by answering the questions here. Then add up your score and check the list at the end to discover which of the skin types you fit into.

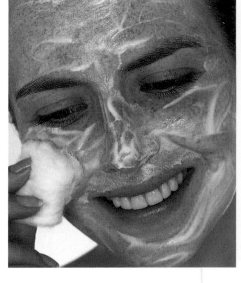

2 How does your skin feel if you cleanse it with cream cleanser?

A Relatively comfortable.

B Smooth and comfortable.

C Sometimes comfortable, sometimes itchy.

D Quite oily.

E Oily in some areas and smooth in others.

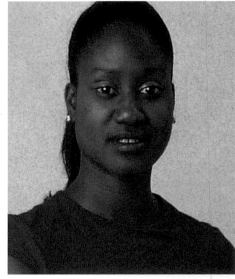

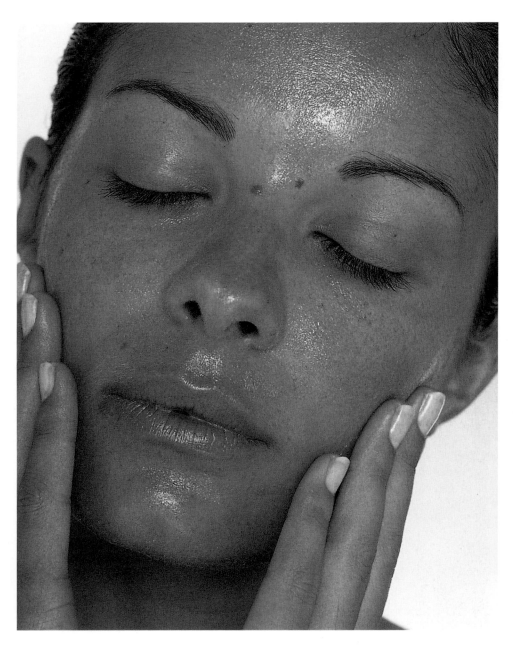

3 How does your skin usually look by the middle of the day?

A Flaky patches appearing.

B Fresh and clean.

C Flaky patches and some redness.

D Shiny.

E Shiny in the T-zone.

1 How does your skin feel if you cleanse it with facial wash and water?

A Tight, as though it's too small for your face.

B Smooth and comfortable.

C Dry and itchy in places.

D Fine – quite comfortable.

E Dry in some areas and smooth in others.

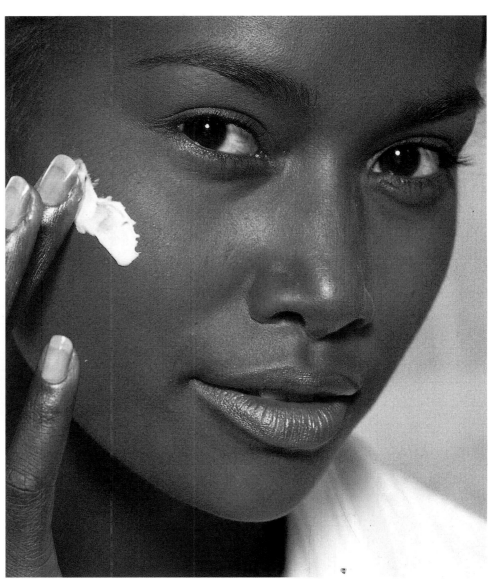

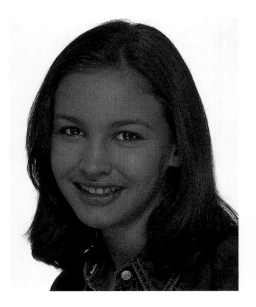

4 How often do you break out in spots?

A Hardly ever.

B Occasionally, perhaps before or during your period.

C Occasionally.

D Often.

E Often – in the T-zone.

6 How does your skin react when you have applied a rich night cream?

A It feels very comfortable.

B Comfortable.

C Sometimes feels comfortable, other times feels irritated.

D Makes your skin feel very oily.

E Oily in the T-zone, comfortable on the cheeks.

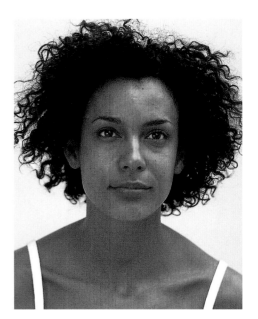

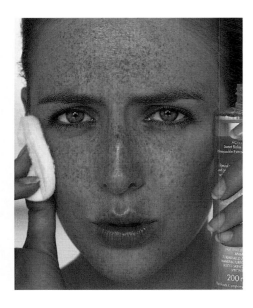

5 How does your skin react when you use facial toner?

A It stings.

B No problems.

C Stings and itches.

D Feels fresher.

E Feels fresher in some areas but stings in others.

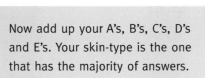

Now add up your A's, B's, C's, D's and E's. Your skin-type is the one that has the majority of answers.

Mostly A's: Your skin is DRY.

Mostly B's: Your skin is NORMAL.

Mostly C's: Your skin is SENSITIVE.

Mostly D's: Your skin is OILY.

Mostly E's: Your skin is COMBINATION.

△ **You know best how your skin reacts to different things so check your skin type before you buy lots of skincare products. Even if you've been told what your skin type is at some stage, it is a good idea to run through this quiz now as your skin will change over a period of time.**

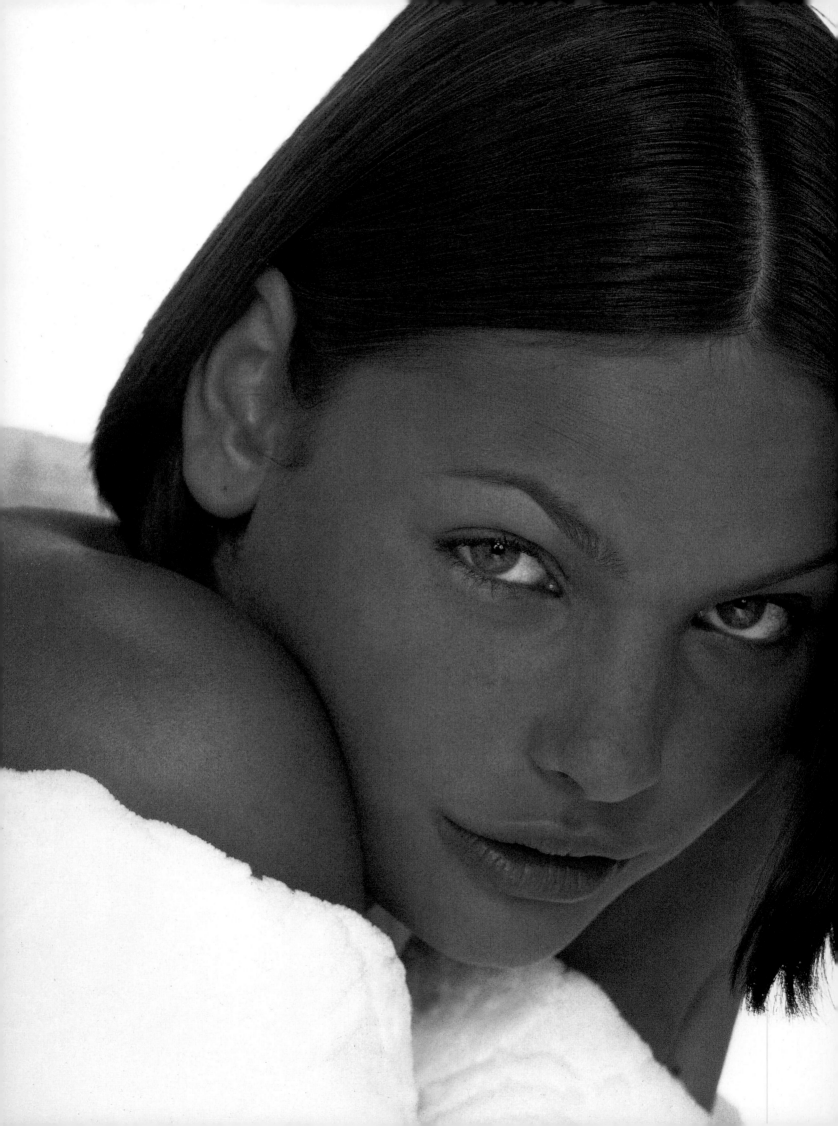

Caring for your skin

Clear, soft and supple skin is one of the greatest beauty assets, and there is plenty you can do every day to ensure that your skin always looks as good as possible. You'll soon realize the benefits of regularly spending time on your skin, and the results will last a lifetime.

Top 10 skin products

Before you can devise the best regime for yourself and give your skin some special care, you need to understand what the main skincare products are designed to do.

the key treatments

From the old soap and water cleansing routine, today's skincare has evolved into a modern range of products.

facial washes

These liquids are designed to be lathered with water to dissolve grime, dirt and stale make-up from the skin's surface.

cleansing bars

Ordinary soap is too drying for most skins. Now you can foam up with these special bars, which will cleanse your skin without stripping it of moisture. They're refreshing for oilier skin-types, and help keep pores clear and prevent pimples and blackheads.

cream cleansers

A wonderful way to cleanse drier complexions, they generally have a light, fluid consistency that spreads more easily on to the skin. They contain oils to dissolve surface dirt and make-up, and can be quickly removed with cotton wool (cotton).

toners and astringents

Refreshing and cooling your skin, they quickly evaporate after being applied with cotton wool. They can also remove excess oil from the surface layers of your skin. The word "astringent" means it has a higher alcohol content, and is suitable only for oily skins. The words "tonic" and "toner" mean that they're useful for normal or combination skins, as they are gentler. Those with dry and sensitive skins should avoid these products, as they can be too drying. Generally, if the product stings your face, move on to a gentler foundation or weaken it by adding a few drops of distilled water (available from a pharmacist).

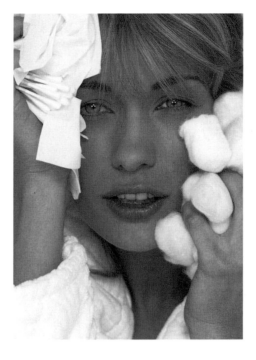

moisturizers

The key function of a moisturizer is to form a barrier film on the skin's surface to prevent moisture loss. This makes the skin feel softer and smoother. Generally, the drier your skin the thicker the moisturizer you should choose. All skin types need a moisturizer, and one of the most valuable ingredients to look for is a UV filter. This ensures your moisturizer will give your skin year-round protection from the burning rays of the sun.

eye make-up removers

Ordinary cleansers aren't usually sufficient to remove stubborn eye make-up, which is why these special products are so useful.

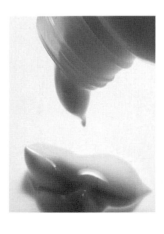

◁ **Put some zing into your skincare regime with a refreshing toner or astringent.**

If you wear waterproof mascara you will probably need to check that the cleanser you use is designed to remove it.

special treatments

In addition to a basic wardrobe of skincare products, you can add a few extras.

face masks

These intensive treatments deep-cleanse your skin or boost its moisture levels.

facial scrubs and exfoliators

These creams or gels contain hundreds of tiny abrasive particles. When massaged into damp skin, the particles dislodge dead surface skin cells, revealing the younger, fresher cells underneath.

eye creams

The delicate skin around your eyes is usually the first to show the signs of ageing. These gels and creams contain ingredients to plump out fine lines. They can also reduce puffiness and under-eye shadows.

night creams

These intensive creams are designed to pamper your skin while you sleep. They can have a thicker consistency because you won't need to apply make-up over the top.

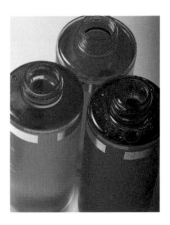

◁◁ **Creamy cleansers should be a top priority for drier complexions, as they cleanse and nourish at the same time.**

◁ **Before you tailor-make a skincare regime for yourself, you need to know the key benefits of each product.**

A fresh approach to oily skin

This skin type usually has open pores and an oily surface, with a tendency towards pimples, blackheads and a sallow appearance. This is due to the over-production of the oily substance called sebum by the oil glands in the lower layers of the skin. Unfortunately, this skin-type is the one most prone to acne. The good news is that this oiliness will make your skin stay younger-looking for longer – so there are some benefits!

ACNE ALERT

This is a distressing condition that usually appears in our lives at a time when we're already feeling insecure – adolescence. A condition that often runs in families, it is thought to be triggered by a hormonal change which causes your skin to produce more sebum. It can be aggravated by stress and poor diet, and careful skincare helps keep acne under control. Avoid picking at pimples, as this can lead to scarring. Try over-the-counter blemish treatments, as today's formulations contain ingredients that are successful at treating this problem. Products containing tea tree oil can also be effective. If these aren't successful, consult your doctor who may provide treatment, or can refer you to a dermatologist.

special care for oily skin

It's very important not to treat oily skin too rigorously, although you may well feel that you want to take drastic action when you are faced with a fresh outbreak of pimples. Remember that over-enthusiastic cleansing treatments can actually encourage the oil glands to produce even more sebum, and they will also leave the surface layers of your skin dry and dehydrated.

The best approach for oily skin is to use a range of products that gently cleanse away oils from the surface and unblock pores, without drying out and damaging the skin. The visible part of your skin actually requires water, not oil, in order to stay soft, healthy and supple.

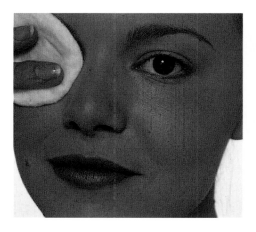

△ **1** Even though your skin is prone to oiliness, the skin around your eyes is delicate, so don't drag it when removing eye make-up. Soak a cotton wool (cotton) pad with a non-oily remover and hold over your eyes for a few seconds to dissolve the make-up, then lightly wipe it away from the eyelids and lashes.

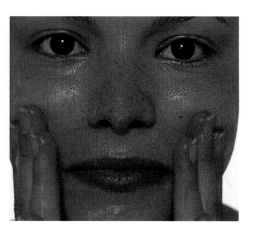

△ **2** Lather up with a gentle foaming facial wash. This is a better choice than ordinary soap, as it won't strip away moisture from your skin, but will remove grime, dirt and oil. Massage gently over damp skin with your fingertips, then rinse away the soapy suds with lots of warm water.

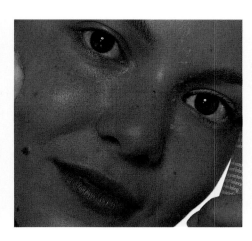

△ **3** Soak a cotton wool ball with astringent lotion, and sweep it over your skin to refresh it. This shouldn't irritate your skin – if it does, change to a gentler one. Continue until the cotton wool comes up clean.

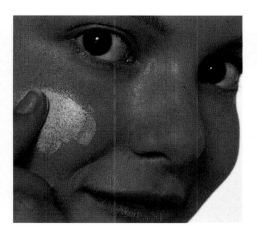

△ **4** Even oily skins need moisturizer, because it helps seal water into the top layers to keep the skin soft and supple. Don't load the skin down with a heavy formulation. Instead, choose a light, watery fluid.

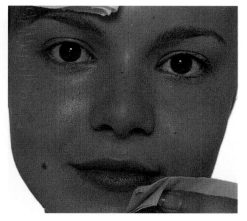

△ **5** Allow the moisturizer to sink in for a few minutes, then press a clean tissue over your face to absorb the excess, and to prevent a shiny complexion.

Nourishing care for dry skin

If your skin tends to feel tight, as if it is one size too small, it's a fair bet you've got a dry complexion. This is caused by too little sebum in the lower levels of skin, and too little moisture in the upper levels. At its best, it can feel tight and itchy after washing. At its worst it can be flaky, with little patches of dandruff in your eyebrows, and a tendency to premature ageing with the emergence of fine lines and wrinkles. It requires a regular routine of soothing care to keep it looking its best.

special care for dry skin

The condition of dry skin can be aggravated by over-use of soap, detergents and toners. It can also be adversely affected by exposure to hot sun, cold winds and central heating. For these reasons it is advisable to opt for a gentle, nourishing approach that concentrates on boosting the skin's moisture levels. This will plump out fine lines and keep the skin soft and supple.

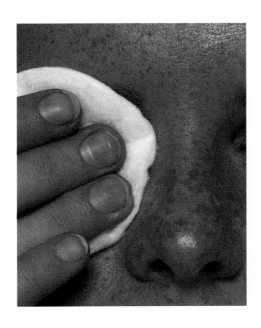

△ **1** Pour a little oil-based eye make-up remover on to a cotton wool (cotton) pad and sweep it over the eye area. This oily product will also help soothe away dryness in the delicate eye area, but a little goes a long way. If you overload the skin here with an oily product it can cause puffiness and irritation.

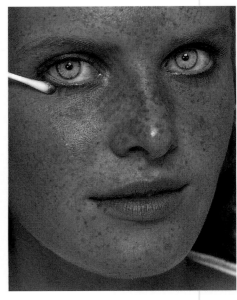

△ **2** If there are any stubborn flecks of mascara left behind, tackle them with a cotton bud (swab) dipped in the eye make-up remover. Take great care that the remover does not get in your eyes, but you will need to work as closely as you can to the eyelashes to remove all signs of make-up.

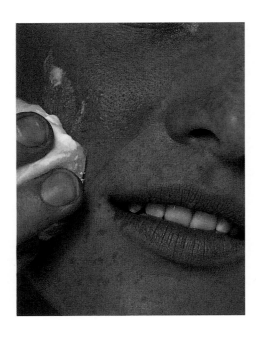

△ **3** Choose a creamy cleanser as it's vital that your skin is really clean. Leave the cleanser on for a few moments, before sweeping it away with a cotton wool pad. Use gentle upward movements to prevent stretching the skin and encouraging lines.

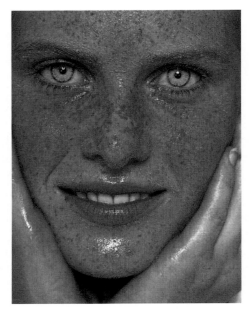

△ **4** Many women with dry skin complain that they miss the feeling of water on their skin. However, you can splash your face with cool water to remove excess cleanser and to refresh your skin. This also helps boost the circulation.

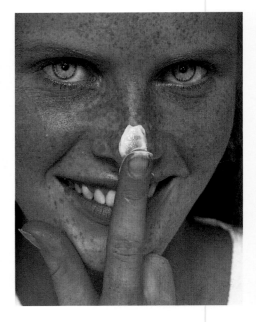

△ **5** Finally, apply a nourishing cream to seal in moisture. Opt for a thick cream, not a runny lotion, as this contains more oil than water, and helps seal in moisture. Give the moisturizer a few minutes to sink in before applying make-up.

Balanced care for combination skin

Combination skin needs careful attention because it has a blend of oily and dry patches. The centre panel or T-zone, across the forehead and down the nose and chin, tends to be oily, and needs to be treated like oily skin. However, the other areas are prone to dryness and flakiness from lack of moisture, and need to be treated like dry skin.

Having said this, some combination skins don't follow the T-zone pattern and can have patches of dry and oily skin in other arrangements. If you're unsure of your skin's oily and dry areas, press a tissue to your face an hour after washing it. Any greasy patches on the tissue signify oily areas.

special care for combination skin

Skin that has a combination of dry and oily patches requires a dual approach to skincare. Treating your entire complexion like oily skin will leave the dry areas even drier and tighter than before. In the same way, treating it only like dry skin can provoke excess oiliness and even an outbreak of blemishes. This means that you need to deal with the different areas of skin individually, with products to suit. This isn't as complicated and difficult as it sounds, and the result will be a softer, smoother and clearer complexion than before!

A dual approach to skincare will double the benefits for combination skin, and it needn't be terribly time-consuming.

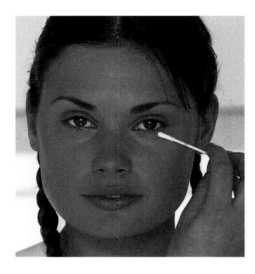

△ **1** Choose an oil-based eye make-up remover to clear away every trace of eye make-up from this delicate area which is prone to dryness. Use a cotton bud (swab) to remove any stubborn traces. Splash with cool water afterwards to rinse away any excess oil.

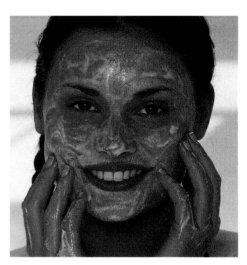

△ **2** Use a foaming facial wash in the morning. This ensures oily areas are clean, and clears pores to prevent blackheads. Massage a little on to damp skin, especially oily areas. Leave for a few seconds to dissolve the dirt, then splash clean with cool water.

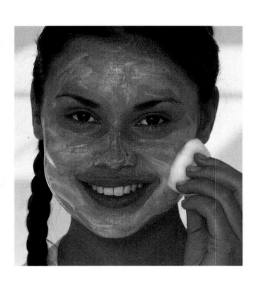

△ **3** In the evening, switch to a cream cleanser, to keep dry areas of skin clean and soothed. This will balance excess oiliness or dryness in your complexion. Massage well into your skin, concentrating on the drier areas, then gently remove with cotton wool (cotton) pads.

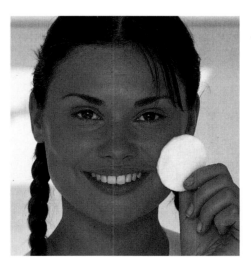

△ **4** To freshen your skin, you need two different strengths of toner to deal with the differing skin types. Choose a stronger astringent for oily areas, and a mild skin freshener for drier ones. This isn't as costly as you think, because you will use only a little of each. Sweep over your skin with cotton wool pads.

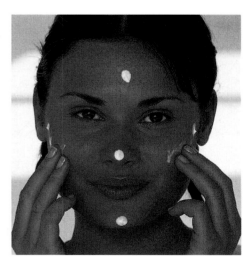

△ **5** Smooth moisturizer on to your entire face, concentrating on the drier areas. Then blot off any excess from the oily areas with a tissue. This will give all your skin the nourishment it needs.

Maintaining normal skin

This is the perfect, balanced skin-type. It has a healthy glow, with a fine texture and no open pores. It rarely develops spots or shiny areas. The truth is that it is actually quite rare to find a perfectly normal skin, especially because all skins tend to become slightly drier as you get older.

special care for normal skin

Your main concern is to maintain normal skin, to keep it functioning well, and as a result of this let it continue the good job it's already doing! It naturally has a good balance of oil and moisture levels. Your routine should include gently cleansing your skin to ensure surface grime and stale make-up are removed, and to prevent a build-up of sebum. Then you should boost moisture levels with moisturizer, to protect and pamper your skin.

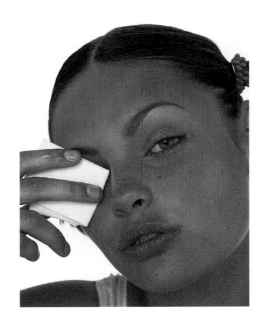

△ **1** Always remove eye make-up carefully. Going to bed with your mascara still on can lead to sore, puffy eyes. Applying new make-up on top of old, stale make-up is unhygienic, too! Choose your cleanser according to whether you're wearing ordinary or waterproof mascara.

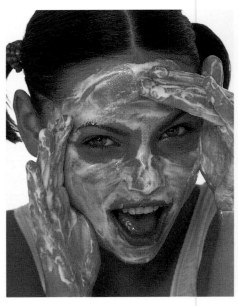

△ **2** Splash your face with water, then massage in a gentle facial wash and work it up to a lather for about 30 seconds. It is a good idea to massage your skin lightly, because this will boost the supply of blood to the surface of your skin – which means a rosier complexion.

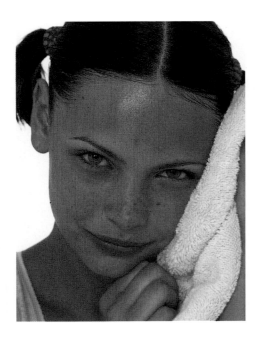

△ **3** Rinse with clear water until every soapy trace has been removed from your face. Then pat your face with a soft towel to absorb residual water from the surface of your skin. Don't rub at your skin, especially around the eyes, as this can encourage wrinkling.

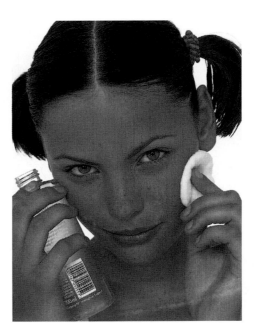

△ **4** Cool your skin with a freshening toner. Again, avoid the delicate eye area as this can become more prone to dryness.

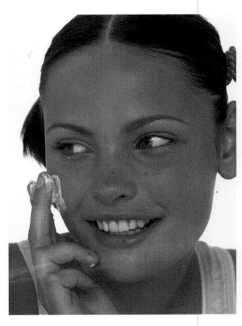

△ **5** Smooth your skin with moisturizing lotion. Dot on to your face, then massage in with your fingertips using light upward strokes. This leaves a protective film on the skin, so make-up can be easily applied and the moisture content is balanced.

Soothing care for sensitive skin

Sensitive skin is usually quite fine in texture, with a tendency to be rosier than usual. Easily irritated by products and external factors, it's also prone to redness and allergy, and may have fine broken veins across the cheeks and nose. There are varying levels of sensitivity. If you feel you can't use any products on your skin without irritating it, cleanse with whole milk and moisturize with a solution of glycerin and rosewater. These should soothe it.

special care for sensitive skin

Your skin needs extra-gentle products to keep it supple and healthy. Choose from a wide range of hypo-allergenic products that are specially formulated to protect sensitive skin. These products are free of common irritants, such as fragrance, that can cause dryness, itchiness or even an allergic reaction.

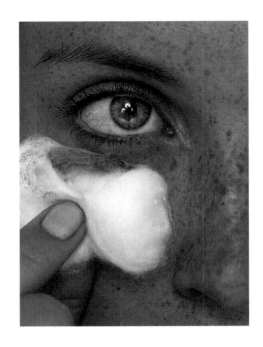

△ **1** Make sure the make-up you use is hypo-allergenic, too, and remove it thoroughly. First use a soothing eye make-up remover. Apply with a cotton wool (cotton) ball, then remove every last trace with a clean cotton bud (swab).

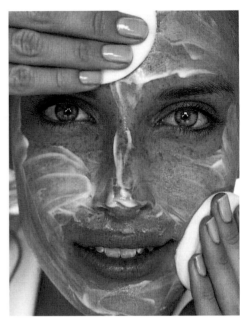

△ **2** It is advisable not to use facial washes and soaps, as these are likely to strip your skin of oil and moisture which can increase its sensitivity even more. So, instead, choose a light, hypo-allergenic cleansing lotion.

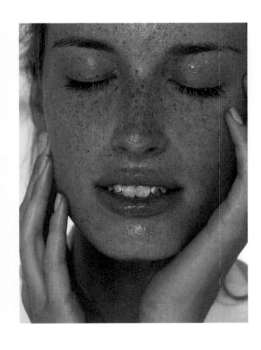

△ **3** Even mild skin fresheners can break down the natural protection your delicate skin needs against the elements. So freshen it by splashing with warm water instead. This also removes the final traces of cleanser and eye make-up remover from your skin.

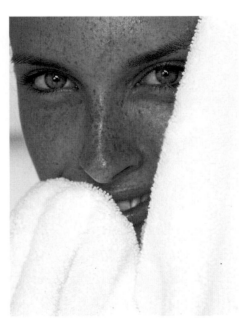

△ **4** To dry your skin, lightly pat your face with a soft towel, taking care not to rub the skin because this could irritate it.

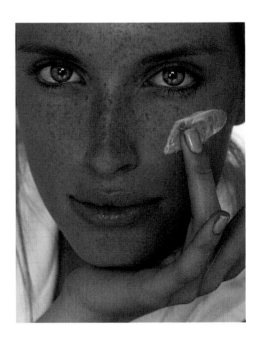

△ **5** It is vital to keep your skin moisturized to keep it strong and supple and provide a barrier against irritants that can lead to sensitivity. Dryness can make sensitive skin more uncomfortable, so it is a good idea to choose an unscented moisturizer.

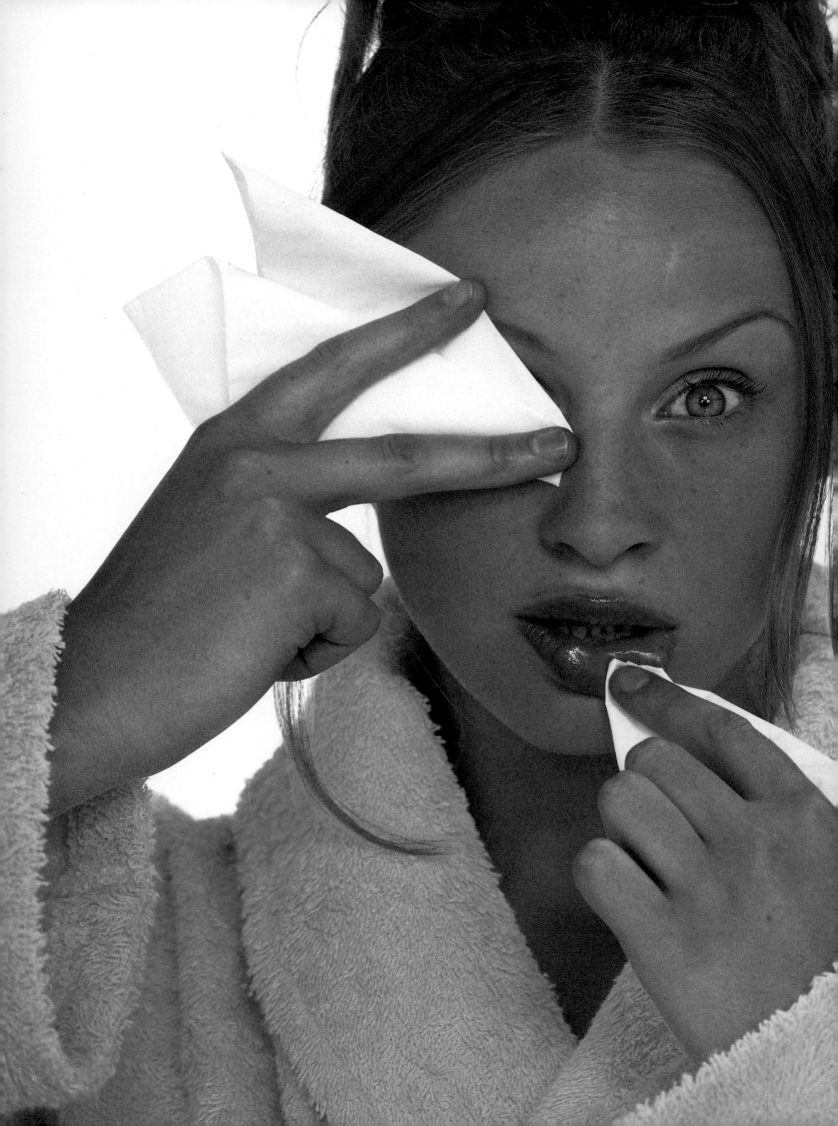

Special treatments

However well you care for your skin on a daily basis, from time to time a special treatment can make it feel even better. This chapter is packed with fabulous facials, healing masks, invigorating scrubs and soothing massages, as well as hints and tips on tackling particular problems.

Miraculous masks

If there's one skincare item that can work miracles, it's a face mask. But, like any other skincare product, you should choose carefully to pick the right one for you.

mask it!

Choose from the wonderful selection of face masks on the market to find one that is perfect for your skin.

moisturizing masks

These are ideal for dry complexions because they boost the moisture levels of your skin. This means they can help banish dry patches, flakiness and even fine lines. They work quickly like an intensive moisturizer, and are usually left on the skin for 5–10 minutes before being removed with a tissue. The slight residue left on your skin will continue to work until you next cleanse your skin. They are a soothing treat, particularly after too much sun, or when your skin feels "tight".

clay and mud masks

Ideal for oily skins, they absorb excess grease and impurities. They're an ideal way to "shrink" open pores, reduce shine and clear troublesome blemishes. They dry on your skin over a period of 5–15 minutes, then you simply wash them away with warm water, rinsing dead skin cells, dirt and grime away at the same time. They're a fantastic pick-me-up for skin.

exfoliating masks

Masks with a light exfoliating action can keep your skin in tip-top condition. Even normal skins sometimes suffer from the build-up of dead skin cells, which can create a dull look and lead to future problems such as blackheads. Masks that cleanse and exfoliate are the perfect solution. They smooth on like a clay mask, and are left to dry. When you rinse them away, their tiny abrasive particles slough away the skin's surface debris.

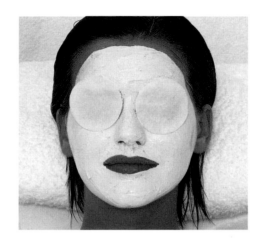

peel-off masks

Ideal for all skin types, the gel is smoothed on, left to dry and peeled off. The light formulation refreshes oily areas, clears clogged pores and nourishes drier skins.

gel masks

These are suitable for sensitive skins, as well as oily complexions, as they have a wonderfully soothing and cooling effect.

◁ **Clay and mud masks dry on your skin over a period of 5–15 minutes.**

Simply apply the gel, lie back, then wipe off excess after 5–10 minutes. Ideal after too much sun, or if your skin feels irritated.

face mask tips

Your skin can change with the seasons. Skin that becomes oily in the hot summer months can become drier in winter and in central heating. So take your skin's quirks into account when choosing your mask.
• Cleanse your face before applying your chosen mask. Afterwards, rinse with warm water, than apply moisturizer.
• Most masks should be left on the skin for between 3 and 10 minutes. For the best results, read the instructions carefully.
• If you have combination skin, use two masks – one suitable for oily skin and one for dry skin. Just apply each one to the area that needs it.

NATURAL NOURISHERS
Making masks from natural ingredients is easy to do and can be very effective.

avocado mash
Avocados make excellent face masks for dry skin. They boast 14 minerals as well as the antioxidant vitamins E and A. To prepare a face mask, mash up an avocado, add a touch of sweet almond oil and smooth the mixture over your face; keep it on for as long as possible to nourish and soften your skin.

gentle oatmeal mask
A good face mask for oily skin, this recipe is sufficient for one treatment and must be applied as soon as it is mixed.

ingredients
• 15ml/1 tbsp runny honey
• 1 egg yolk
• up to 60ml/4 tbsp fine oatmeal

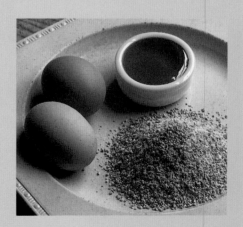

Mix honey and egg yolk together in a small bowl, then slowly stir in enough oatmeal to make a soft paste. Smooth the mask on to the skin of the face and neck and leave for 15 minutes. Rinse off with lukewarm water and pat your skin dry.

Facial scrubs

Brighten up your complexion in an instant with this skincare treat – if you don't include a facial scrub in your weekly skincare regime, then you've been missing out! Technically known as exfoliation, it's a simple method that whisks away dead cells from the surface of your skin, revealing the plumper, younger ones underneath. It also encourages your skin to speed up cell production, which means that the cells that reach the surface are younger and better-looking. The result is a brighter, smoother complexion – no matter what your age or skin type.

action tactics

Use an exfoliater on dry or normal skin once or twice a week. Oily or combination skins can be exfoliated every other day. As a rule, avoid this treatment on sensitive skin, or if you have bad acne. However, you can gently exfoliate pimple-prone skin once a week to help keep pores clear and prevent break-outs.

getting to the nitty-gritty

Apply a blob of facial scrub cream to damp skin, massage gently, then rinse away with lots of cool water. Opt for an exfoliater that contains gentler, rounded beads, rather than scratchy ones such as crushed kernels.

You could also try a mini exfoliating pad, lathering up with soap or facial wash.

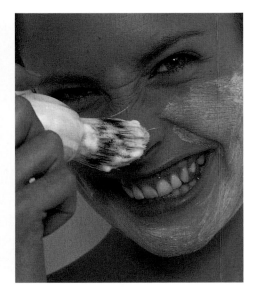

△ **Instead of using a facial scrub, gently massage your skin with a soft flannel, facial brush or old, clean shaving brush and facial wash.**

applying a facial scrub
Using a facial scrub is a quick and invigorating way to cleanse and smooth your skin.

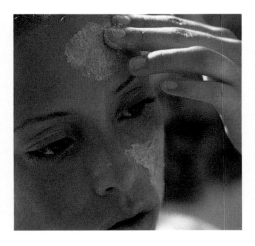

△ **1** With a light touch, gently rub the facial scrub into damp skin, using a circular motion and taking care to avoid the delicate area of skin around the eyes.

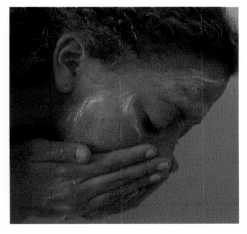

△ **2** Rinse the facial scrub off thoroughly and slowly with splashes of warm water and then gently pat your face dry with a soft towel.

GENTLE FACE SCRUB

This is a luxurious blend of almonds, oatmeal, milk and rose petals. The rose petals should be bought from a herbalist or, if you want to use petals from your garden, be sure that they have not been sprayed with chemicals. The rose petals can be powdered in a pestle and mortar or in an electric coffee grinder. When mixed with almond oil, the scrub will cleanse the face and leave it silky soft.

ingredients

Makes enough for 10 treatments.
- 45ml/3 tbsp ground almonds (without skin)
- 45ml/3 tbsp medium oatmeal
- 45ml/3 tbsp powdered milk
- 30ml/2 tbsp powdered rose petals
- almond oil
- mixing bowl
- spoon
- lidded glass jar

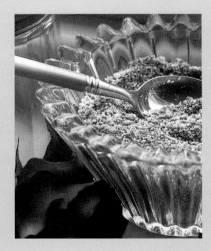

Put all the ingredients in a bowl and combine thoroughly. Then store the mixture in a sealed glass jar. When you are ready to use the facial scrub, take a handful of the mixture and blend it to make a soft paste with a little almond oil. Apply and remove as shown (left).

Fabulous face pampering

For deep-down cleansing and a definite improvement in skin tone, try an at-home facial. If you apply this treatment just once a month you will notice an improvement in your complexion. Simply follow these step-by-step instructions for a fabulous facial to recreate the benefits of the beauty salon in the comfort and privacy of your own home.

SKIN TONIC RECIPE

This flower skin tonic is suitable for normal skin, and can be applied to soothe and freshen the skin.

ingredients
• 75ml/5 tbsp orangeflower water
• 25ml/1½ tbsp rosewater

Pour the ingredients into a glass bottle and shake to mix. Apply to skin with a cotton wool (cotton) pad.

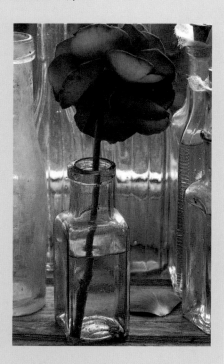

△ **If you make your own rosewater any fragrant roses are suitable for this recipe, as long as they have not been sprayed with pesticide. Pink or red ones are best.**

freshening facial

Facial skin is delicate and needs regular cleansing to keep the pores dirt-free so the skin can breathe.

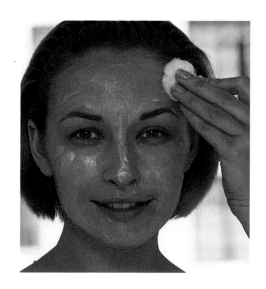

△ **1** Smooth your skin with cleansing cream. Leave on for 1–2 minutes to give it time to dissolve grime, oil and stale make-up. Then gently smooth away with a cotton wool (cotton) ball.

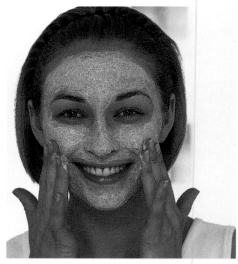

△ **2** Dampen your skin with warm water. Then gently massage with a blob of facial scrub, taking care to avoid the delicate eye area. This will loosen dead surface skin cells, and leave your skin softer and smoother. It will also prepare your complexion for the beneficial treatments to come. Rinse away with splashes of warm water.

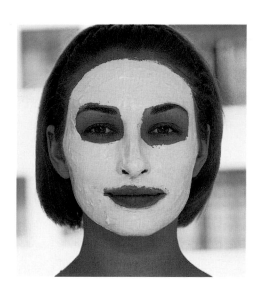

△ **4** Smooth on a face mask. Choose a clay-based one if you have oily skin, or a moisturizing one if you have dry or normal skin. Leave the mask on your skin for 5 minutes, or for as long as specified by the instructions on the product.

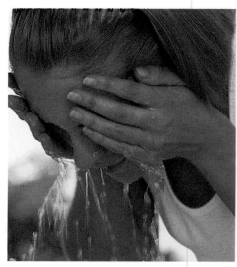

△ **5** Rinse away the face mask with warm water. Once all the mask is removed, finish off with a few splashes of cool water to close your pores and freshen your skin, then pat dry with a towel.

face massage

**Dot your skin with moisturizer and smooth in. Following your facial, continue the pampering by taking
the opportunity to massage your skin, as this encourages a brighter complexion and can help to
reduce puffiness.**

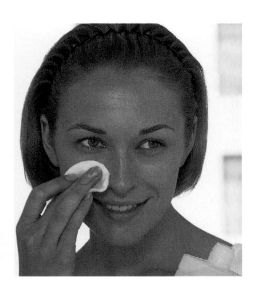

△ **3** Fill a bowl or washbasin with boiling water. Lean
over it, capturing the steam with a towel placed over
your head. Allow the steam to warm and soften your
skin for 5 minutes. If you have blackheads, try to
remove them gently with tissue-covered fingers after
this treatment. If you suffer from sensitive skin, or are
prone to broken veins, you should avoid this step.

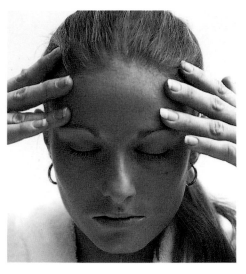

△ **1** Starting in the centre of your forehead, make
small circular motions with your fingertips and work
slowly out towards the temples. Repeat 3 times.

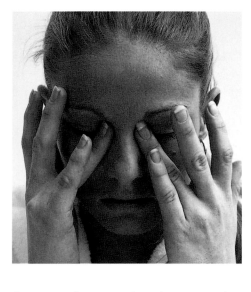

△ **2** Use your fingers to apply gentle pressure to the
area where the eye socket meets your nose. Repeat
at least 3 times.

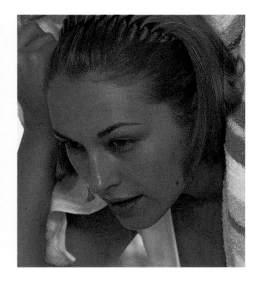

△ **6** Soak a cotton wool pad with a skin toner lotion
or a homemade tonic, and smooth over oily areas,
such as the nose, chin and forehead.

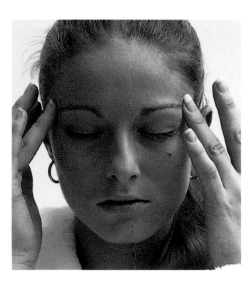

△ **3** Move your fingers outwards along the brow
bone from the top of your nose. Repeat 5 times. The
skin around the eyes is the most delicate on the face
and the first to show signs of stress, so it is important
that you treat this area very gently.

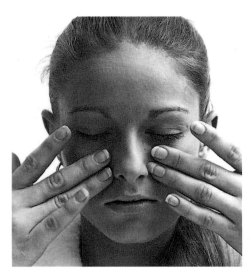

△ **4** Starting either side of your nose, move your
fingers outwards using circular motions along the
cheekbone to the jaw. Pay particular attention to
the jaw area. Repeat 5 times. Finally, gently smooth
your undereye area with a soothing eye cream to
reduce fine lines and wrinkles, and make the skin
ultra-soft.

Care for eyes

The fine, delicate skin around your eyes is the first to show the signs of ageing. However, don't be tempted to deal with the problem by slapping on heavy oils and moisturizers because they are usually too heavy for the skin in the eye area. They can also block tear ducts, causing puffiness. The delicate skin around your eyes needs particularly special care because it is significantly thinner than the skin on the rest of your face, and this means that it is less able to hold in moisture. There are also fewer oil glands in this area, making it particularly susceptible to dryness, and also meaning that there is no fatty layer underneath to act as a shock absorber. Consequently this area of skin quickly loses its suppleness and elasticity.

choosing an eye treatment

There is a huge range of products to choose from, and it is important to find the right one for you. Gel-based ones are suitable for young or oily skins, and are refreshing to use. However, most women find light eye creams and balms more effective.

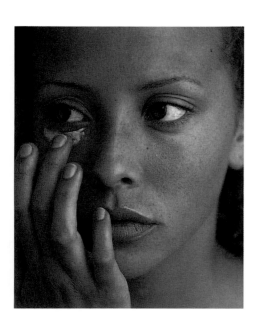

△ **The skin around the eyes is soft and delicate so it is important to apply moisturizer to this area very gently.**

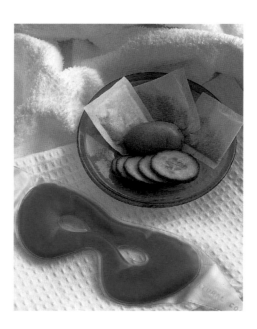

△ **There is a range of remedies for eyes, from special pads to home-made therapies. Experiment to find out which works best for you.**

Use a tiny amount of the eye treatment, as it's better to apply it regularly in small quantities than apply lots occasionally. Apply with your middle finger, as this is the weakest one and won't stretch the delicate skin. This will help keep your skin more supple and prevent premature wrinkling in this area.

preventing puffy eyes

This is one of the most common beauty problems. These ideas can help:
• Gently tap your skin with your ring finger when you're applying eye cream to encourage the excess fluid to drain away.
• Store creams in the refrigerator, as the coldness will also help reduce puffiness.
• Place thin strips of potato underneath your eyes to reduce swelling. The starch in the potato seems to tighten the skin.
• Fill a small bowl with iced water or ice-cold milk. Soak two cotton wool (cotton) pads and lie down with the pads over your eyes. Replace the pads as soon as they become warm. Continue for 15 minutes. This treatment reduces puffiness and brightens the whites of your eyes.

cooling cucumber

This is a super-quick and simple treatment. Place a slice of cucumber over each eye, then just lie back and relax for 15 minutes. Cucumber will gently tone and soothe the skin around the eyes.

herbal eyepads

A compress over your eyes will refresh them, reduce puffiness and relieve itchiness.

fennel decoction

Make a decoction by boiling 10ml/2 tsp fennel seeds in 300ml/$\frac{1}{2}$ pint/$1\frac{1}{4}$ cups purified water for 30 minutes. Strain and cool, then use to soak cotton wool pads.

teabag treatments

Use a teabag to make tea then apply to the eyes when cool. Chamomile is good for tired eyes. The tannin in Indian tea is an astringent and will firm the skin.

rosewater

Soak cotton wool pads in an infusion of rose petals and purified water.

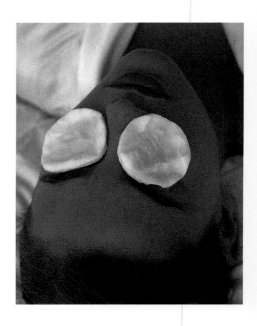

△ **Whichever eye treatment you decide to use, it is vital that you take time to lie down and relax for at least 10 minutes.**

Goodnight creams

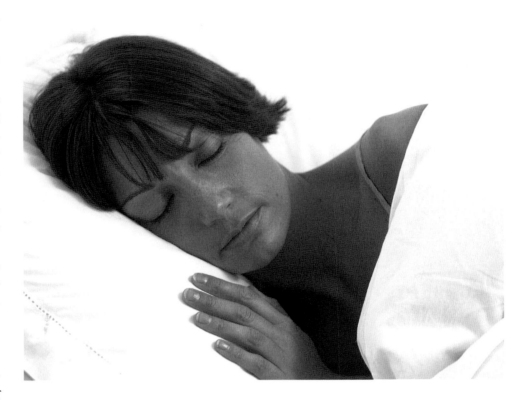

Going to bed with night cream on your face can benefit your skin while you are sleeping. The main difference between night creams and ordinary daily moisturizers is that most night creams have special added ingredients such as vitamins and anti-ageing components. They can also be thicker and more intensive than creams you apply during the day because you won't need to apply make-up on top of them.

Your skin's cell renewal is more active during the night, and night creams are designed to make the most of these hours. Using a night cream gives your skin the chance to repair the daily wear and tear caused by pollution, make-up and ultra-violet light.

who needs night creams?

While very young skins do not generally require the extra nourishing properties of night creams, most women will benefit from using one regularly. Dry and very dry skins will respond particularly well to this treatment. Remember that you don't have to choose very rich formulations, as there are lighter alternatives that contain the same special ingredients. Choose the formulation carefully on the basis of how dry your skin is – it is important that your skin shouldn't feel overloaded.

△ **Applying night cream before you go to bed means waking up to a softer, smoother complexion. If you apply cream to slightly damp skin this can really boost its performance, as it seals in extra moisture.**

▽ **Dab a little night cream in your palm, then gently rub your hands together. The heat will liquefy the cream so that it is more easily absorbed as you massage it into your skin.**

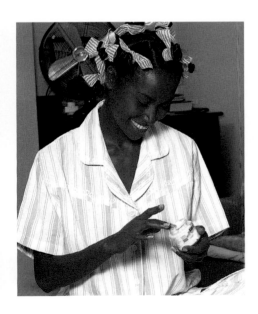

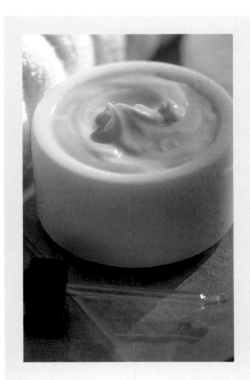

NOURISHING NIGHT CREAM

As we get older, our skin becomes drier and more in need of regular care. Jasmine and rose oils help to rehydrate the skin, while frankincense helps to reduce wrinkles and restore tone to slack muscles.

ingredients

• 50g/2oz jar of unperfumed base cream with a close-fitting lid
• 3 drops of rose essential oil
• 2 drops of frankincense essential oil
• 1 drop of jasmine essential oil

Add the oils to the cream, and mix well together. Apply a little of the cream just before going to bed.

Special skin treatments

As well as basic moisturizers, there is a vast range of special treatments, serums and gels that have been carefully formulated to treat specific problems.

key treatments

Special skin treatments come in all shapes and sizes, and in various formulations:

serums and gels

These have an ultraviolet formulation, a non-greasy texture and a high concentration of active ingredients. They're not usually designed to be used on their own, except on oily skins. They're generally applied under a moisturizer to enhance its benefits and boost the anti-ageing process.

skin firmers

You can lift your skin instantly with creams that are designed to tighten, firm and smooth. They work by forming an ultra-fine film on the skin, which tightens your complexion and reduces the appearance of fine lines. The effects last for a few hours, and make-up can easily be applied on top. These products are a wonderful treat for a special night out or when you're feeling particularly tired.

skin energizers

These creams contain special ingredients designed to accelerate the natural production and repair of skin cells. As well as producing a fresher, younger-looking skin, they are also thought to help combat the signs of ageing.

ampule treatments

These concentrated active ingredients are contained in sealed glass phials or ampules, to ensure that they're fresh. Typical extracts include herbs, wheatgerm, vitamins and collagen – used for their intensive and fast-acting results. Vitamin E is another great skin saver. Break open a capsule and smooth the oil on to your face for a fast skin treat.

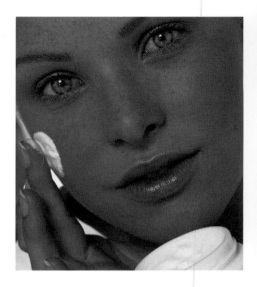

△ Choose a cream that contains specialized ingredients to improve your skin.

liposomes creams

These are tiny spheres in the cream which carry special ingredients into the skin. Their shells break down as they're absorbed into your skin, releasing the active ingredients.

AHA KNOW-HOW

Alpha-hydroxy acids, also commonly known as fruit acids, are found in natural products. These include citric acid from citrus fruit, lactic acid from sour milk, tartaric acid from wine, and malic acid from apples and other fruits. Incorporated in small amounts, AHAs are often a key ingredient in specialized skincare products.

They work by breaking down the protein bonds that hold together the dead cells on the surface of your skin. They then lift them away to reveal brighter, plumper cells underneath. This gentle process cleans and clears blocked pores, improves your skintone and softens the look of fine lines. Basically, they're the ideal solution to most minor skincare problems. You should see results within a couple of weeks, although many women report an improvement after only a few days.

Without even realizing it, women have used AHAs for centuries and have reaped the benefits for their skins. For example, Cleopatra is said to

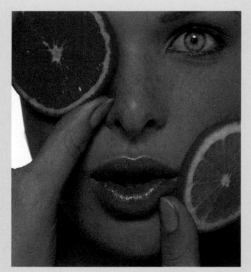

◁ AHAs (also known as fruit acids) are an effective way to replace the zing in your skin.

have bathed in sour asses' milk, and ladies of the French court applied wine to their faces to keep their skin smooth and blemish-free – both these ancient beauty aids contain AHAs.

AHA products are best used under your ordinary everyday moisturizer as a treatment cream. You should avoid applying them to the delicate eye and lip areas. If you have sensitive skin, you may find they're not suitable for you, but some women do experience a slight tingling sensation as the product gets to work. The great news is that AHA products are now becoming more affordable, and not just the preserve of more expensive skincare companies. Many mid-market companies are including the benefits of AHAs in their products, so everyone can give their skin the treatment it deserves. You can also find AHA products for the hands and body, so you can reap the benefits from top to toe.

10 ways to beat wrinkles

Fine lines and wrinkles aren't inevitable. In fact, skin experts believe that most skin damage can be prevented with some special care. Here are the 10 main points to bear in mind, no matter what your age.

1 sun protection
The single biggest cause of skin ageing is sunlight. You should use a sunscreen every day because the aging effects of the sun are as prevalent in the cold winter months as in the hot summer ones. This will help prevent your skin from aging prematurely, and will guard against burning.

2 stop smoking
Cigarette smoke speeds up the ageing process as it strips your skin of oxygen and slows down the regeneration of new cells. It can give the skin a grey, sluggish look, and cause fine lines around the mouth because heavy smokers are constantly pursing their lips to draw on a cigarette.

3 deep cleanse
Many older women don't cleanse their skin as thoroughly as they should, believing this can lead to dryness and lines. However, it's essential to ensure your skin is clear of dead skin cells, dirt and make-up to give it a youthful, fresh glow.

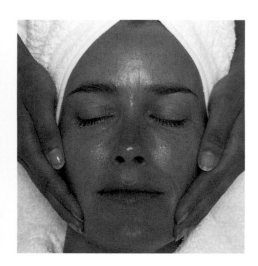

△ **Relax and enjoy a beneficial facial!**

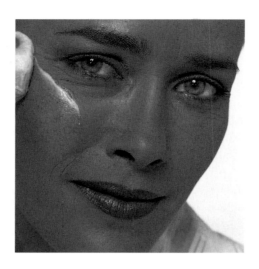

△ **Whatever you are applying to your skin, always use gentle strokes and an upward motion.**

Don't use harsh products – a creamy cleanser removed with cotton wool (cotton) is effective for most women. If your skin is very dry, massage with an oily cleanser. Leave on your skin for a few minutes, then rinse away the excess with warm water.

4 deep moisturize
As well as using a daily moisturizer, you can also boost your skin's water levels weekly. Either use a nourishing face mask, or apply a thick layer of your usual moisturizer or night cream. Whichever you choose, leave on the skin for 5–10 minutes, then remove the excess with tissues. Apply to damp skin for greater effect.

5 boost the circulation
Buy a gentle facial scrub or exfoliater, and use once a week to keep the surface of your skin soft and smooth. This increases the blood-flow to the top layers of skin, and encourages cell renewal. You can get the same effect by lathering a facial wash on your skin using a clean shaving brush.

6 disguise lines
Existing lines can be minimized to the naked eye by opting for the latest light-reflecting foundations, concealers and powders. These contain luminescent particles to bounce light away from your skin, making lines less noticeable and giving your skin a wonderful luminosity.

7 pamper regularly
As well as daily skincare, remember to treat your skin from time to time with special treatments such as facials, serums and anti-ageing creams.

8 be weather vain
Extremes of cold and hot weather can strip your skin of essential moisture, leaving it dry and more prone to damage. Central heating can have the same effect. For this reason, ensure you moisturize regularly, changing your products according to the seasons.

For instance, in the winter you may need a more oily product, which will keep the cold out and won't freeze on the skin's surface. In hot weather, lighter formulations are more comfortable on the skin, and you can boost their activity by using a few drops of special treatment serum underneath.

9 be gentle
Be careful not to drag at your skin when applying skincare products or make-up. The skin around your eyes is particularly likely to show signs of ageing. A heavy touch can cause the skin to stretch. So, always use a light touch, and take your strokes upwards, rather than drag the skin down. Also, avoid any products that make your skin itch, sting or feel sensitive. If any product causes this sort of reaction, stop using it at once and switch to a gentler formulation.

10 clever make-up
Skincare benefits aren't limited to skincare products. In fact, many make-up products now contain UV filters and skin-nourishing ingredients to treat your skin as well as superficially improve its appearance. So investigate the latest products – it's well worth making use of them.

Eating for beautiful skin

While lotions and potions can improve your skin from the outside, a healthy diet works from the inside out. A nutritious, balanced diet isn't only a delicious way to eat – it can work wonders for your skin.

you are what you eat

A diet for a healthy body is the same one as for a healthy, clear complexion. That is, one that contains lots of fresh fruit and vegetables, is high in fibre, low in fat and low in added sugar and salt. This should provide your body and skin with all the vitamins and minerals they need to function at their very best.

healthy skin checklist

These are the essentials your body needs to keep your skin in tip-top condition.

• The most essential element is water. Although there's water in the foods you eat, you should drink at least two litres (quarts) of water a day to keep your body healthy and your skin clear.

• Cellulose carbohydrates, better known as fibre foods, have another less direct effect on the skin. Their action in keeping you

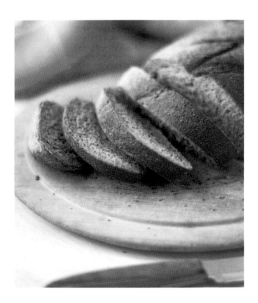

△ **Wholegrain cereals, such as bread, are an excellent source of B vitamins and also provide the fibre that your body needs to stay healthy.**

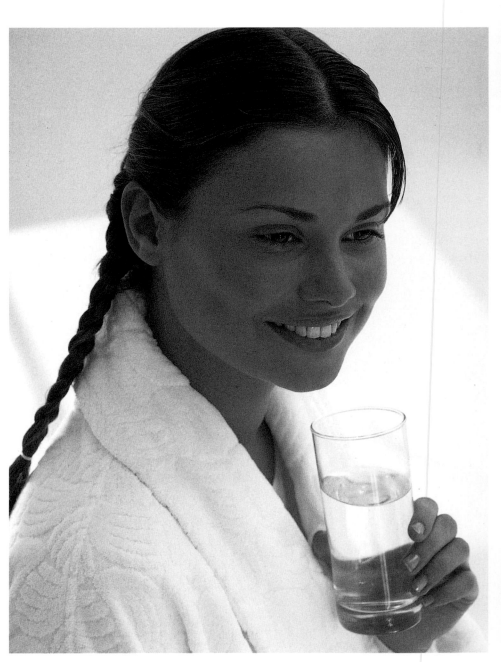

regular can help to give you a brighter, clearer complexion.

• Vitamin A is essential for growth and repair of certain skin tissues. Lack of it causes dryness, itching and loss of skin elasticity. It's found in foods such as carrots, spinach, broccoli and apricots.

• Vitamin C is needed for collagen production, to help keep your skin firm. It's found in foods such as strawberries, citrus fruits, cabbage, tomatoes and watercress.

• Vitamin E is an antioxidant vitamin that

△ **Drinking plenty of water during the day helps rehydrate and purify your body.**

neutralizes free radicals – highly reactive molecules that can cause ageing. It occurs in foods such as almonds, hazelnuts and wheat germ.

• Zinc works with vitamin A in the making of collagen and elastin, the fibres that give your skin its strength, elasticity and firmness. It occurs in shellfish, wholegrains, milk, cheese and yoghurt.

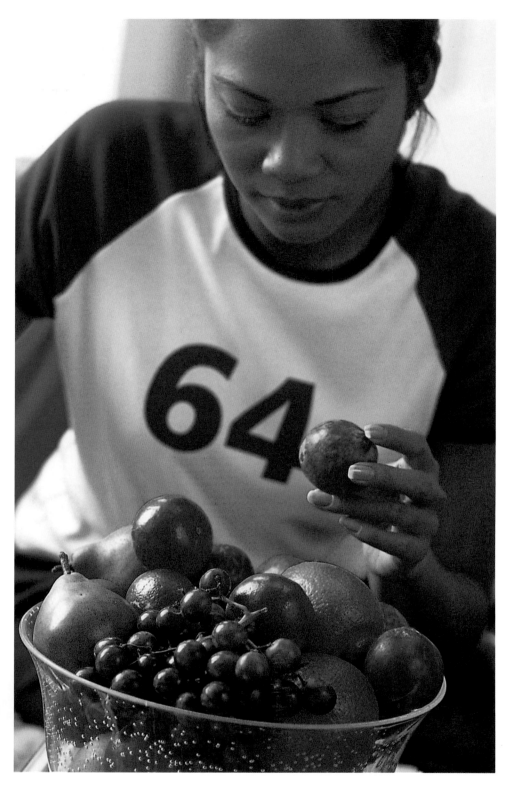

diet Q & A

A healthy diet and a beautiful complexion go hand in hand. Check you know the facts.

yo-yo dieting

Q *"Is it true that if you are constantly losing and then gaining weight it can have a bad effect on your skin?"*

A Yes. Eating too much and becoming overweight thickens the layer of fat under your skin and consequently stretches it. Crash dieting can then result in your skin collapsing, leading to the appearance of lines and wrinkles. What's more, a crash diet will deprive your skin and body of the essential nutrients they need to stay healthy and look good. If you need to lose weight, do it slowly, sensibly and steadily, to give your skin time to acclimatize. Consult your doctor before starting any weight-loss programme.

daily diet

Q *"What would be a good typical day's diet for a clearer complexion?"*

A One that follows the rules already outlined. For example, here's a typical day you could follow:

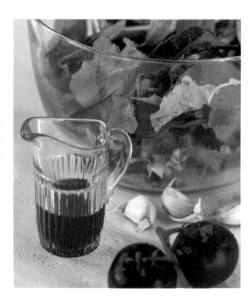

△ Fresh raw vegetables and salads provide your body and your skin with valuable nutrients. Aim to eat five portions of fruit and vegetables a day.

Breakfast: Glass of unsweetened fruit juice; bowl of unsweetened muesli (granola), with a chopped banana and semi-skimmed (low-fat) milk; two slices of wholewheat toast with a scraping of low-fat spread.
Lunch: Baked potato filled with low-fat cottage cheese and plenty of fresh, raw salad; one low-fat yogurt, any flavour.
Evening meal: Grilled fish or chicken with boiled brown rice and plenty of steamed vegetables. Fresh fruit salad, topped with natural yogurt and nuts.

on the spot

Q *"I love eating chocolate but have heard that it cause pimples. Is this true?"*

A There isn't any scientific evidence that links eating chocolate to having break-outs of spots, but as a healthy low-fat, high-fibre diet is known to be good for the skin, keep snacks such as chocolate to a minimum and eat them only as an occasional treat. If you find yourself craving sweet snacks, try eating a low-fat yoghurt or a delicious bowl of strawberries.

Your top 20 skincare questions answered

Here are quick and simple remedies, and sound advice, for a range of common skincare problems.

1 night watch

Q *"My dry skin needs night cream, but I seem to lose most of it on my pillow."*

A Try placing the cream in a teaspoon, and heating it gently over a low heat on the cooker until just warm, before applying. It sounds strange, but it really works!

2 polished perfection

Q *"I spend a fortune on skincare, but resent paying for exfoliators. Are there alternatives?"*

A Yes. After washing your skin, gently massage with a soft facecloth or natural sponge to ease away the dead surface skin cells. If you have dry skin, massage cream cleanser on to damp skin, then rub over the top with your flannel. Rinse afterwards, then apply moisturizer in the normal way. It is essential to wash the facecloth after every couple of uses, and to hang it up to dry in between to prevent the build-up of bacteria.

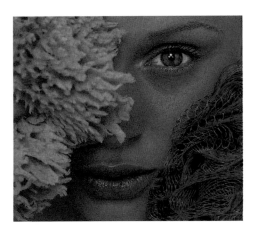

△ **The soft touch of a natural sponge is a cheap and effective alternative to a facial scrub.**

3 lip tricks

Q *"How can I stop my lips getting so chapped and flaky in winter?"*

A This three-step action plan will help:
• Massage dry lips with petroleum jelly. Leave for a couple of minutes to soften the skin, then gently rub your lips with a warm, damp facecloth. As the petroleum jelly is removed, the flakes of skin will come with it!
• Smooth your lips morning and night with a lip balm.
• Switch to a moisturizing lipstick to prevent lips from drying out during the daytime.

4 red nose day

Q *"How can I cover my red winter nose?"*

A Try smoothing a little green foundation or concealer over the red area before applying foundation and powder. The green works by cancelling out the redness.

5 winter sun

Q *"Is it true that you should still wear a sunscreen in winter?"*

A Yes. Exposure to sunlight is thought to be the main cause of wrinkling, and the ultraviolet A rays that are responsible for this process are around all year, so choose a moisturizer that contains sunscreens.

6 lighten up

Q *"My skin feels as though it needs a richer cream in the winter months, but I find most of them too heavy"*

A A heavier moisturizer doesn't necessarily mean it's more effective, so choose one that feels right for you. Help seal moisture into your skin by spritzing your face with water before applying it. Also, choose a nourishing foundation or tinted moisturizer to ensure your skin stays smooth and soft all day long.

7 water factor

Q *"I like the feeling of water on my face, but I find soap too drying. Should I switch to a cream cleanser instead?"*

A For dry skin, it's generally better to use a creamy cleanser – applied with your fingertips and removed with cotton wool (cotton) or soft tissues. This prevents too much moisture from being lost from the skin's surface. Normal and oily skins should

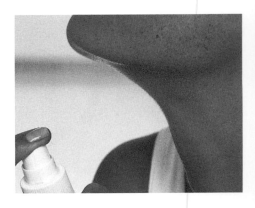

△ **Boost the moisture in your skin with a refreshing spritz.**

be fine with water but a facial wash or wash-off cleanser is formulated to be non-drying, while still cleaning your skin.

8 age spots

Q *"I've noticed 'liver spots' on the back of my hands. How are they caused – and how can I get rid of them?"*

A Many people find these light-to-dark-brown patches on the back of their hands as they grow older. They can also appear on the forehead and temples. They're caused by an uneven production of the melanin tanning pigment in the skin. This can be caused by excess sun exposure, or merely highlighted by it.

You can use a cream containing hydroquinone, which penetrates the skin tissue to 'dissolve' the melanin. In six to eight weeks, your skin should be back to normal. However, you must use a safe level of hydroquinone – the recommended amount in a cream is two per cent. Using a sunscreen on a daily basis can prevent these patches from appearing again.

9 sensitive issue

Q *"Why does my skin feel more sensitive in winter than in summer?"*

A Eighty per cent of women claim to have sensitive skin – which tingles, itches and is prone to dryness. It can be aggravated by harsh winter winds and cold, because this breaks down the natural protective oily layer. Moisturizing regularly with a hypo-allergenic cream formulated for sensitive skin should help.

10 pregnant pause

Q *"I'm pregnant and have patches of darker colour on my face, particularly under my eyes and around my mouth. What is this?"*

A This is called chloasma, or "the mask of pregnancy". It's triggered by a change in hormones, and is made more obvious by sunbathing. Cover up in the sun and use sunblock to stop patches becoming denser. It usually fades within a few months of having your baby. Chloasma can also be triggered by birth-control pills, but disappears once you stop taking them.

11 on the spot

Q *"I suffer from oily skin, but find blemish creams too drying. What can you suggest?"*

A Choose an antibacterial cream to kill off the cause of your blemishes while soothing the skin around them.

12 treatment sprays

Q *"I find body lotions too hot and sticky to wear after bathing. What else can I try?"*

A There are body treatment sprays, combining moisturizer, toner and fragrance. Your skin will be lightly moisturized and smell fantastic.

13 the throat vote

Q *"The skin on my neck looks grey and dull. Are there any special treats to use?"*

A Necks show the signs of ageing, mainly because they lack sebaceous glands. Using a creamy cleanser can help. Massage in, leave

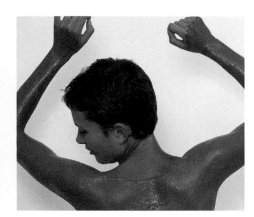

△ **Back to basics with a clay mask for the body.**

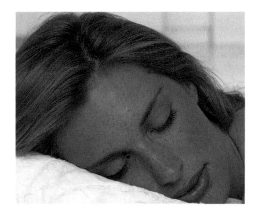

△ **Don't forget your beauty sleep.**

to dissolve dirt, and remove with cotton wool (cotton) pads. Dull grey skin benefits from regular exfoliation – scrub briskly with a facecloth or soft shaving brush. Boost softness by smoothing on moisturizer.

14 beautiful back

Q *"What can I do for pimples on my back?"*

A Backs are hard to reach, so they're prone to break-outs. Keep your back blemish-free by exfoliating daily with a loofah or back brush to remove dead skin. For stubborn pimples, try a clay mask to draw out deep-seated impurities.

15 mole watch

Q *"I understand you need to keep an eye on moles on your skin to monitor the risk of skin cancer. What should I look for?"*

A Moles are clumps of clustered pigment cells, usually darker than freckles. All changes in existing moles should be checked by your doctor. Any that cause concern will be removed and sent off for analysis. You should also check moles yourself once a month. Try the following A.B.C.D. code: check for A (asymmetry); B (border irregularity); C (colour change); D (change in diameter).

16 shadow sense

Q *"What's best for shadows under my eyes?"*

A Dark shadows can have a variety of causes, including fatigue, anaemia, lack of fresh air and poor digestion. They can also be hereditary. If in doubt, consult your doctor. Take steps to cut out causes such as getting a good night's sleep and keeping to a low-fat, high-fibre diet. Try bathing the eyes with pads soaked in ice-cold water for 15 minutes, to lessen the shadow effect temporarily. Or cover by dotting on concealer.

17 brown baby

Q *"Is there any way to prolong my tan?"*

A Your skin is dried by sunbathing, and so sheds old cells more quickly. Prolong colour by applying lots of body lotion. Use while your skin is damp to make it extra effective. Apply a little fake tan every few days to keep your colour topped up. Better still, protect your skin by using fake tan all the time.

18 sticky situation

Q *"I exercise a lot, and find body odour a problem. How can I prevent it?"*

A Sweating is your body's natural cooling device. Sweat itself has no odour, but smells when it comes into contact with bacteria on the skin. So, opt for an antiperspirant deodorant. Antiperspirants prevent sweating, while deodorant helps prevent odour. Also wear fresh, natural fibres next to your skin.

19 massage magic

Q *"Can I give myself a facial massage?"*

A A massage is the ideal way to give your complexion a workout. Pour a few drops of vegetable oil into the palms of your hands and smooth it on to your face and neck. Then follow these steps:

• Use finger pads to stroke upwards from the base of your neck to your chin.

• Continue with long strokes up one side of your face, then the other. Then go around your nose and up towards your forehead.

• When you get to your forehead, stroke it across from left to right using one hand. Finish off by gently drawing a circle around each eye using one finger.

20 stretch marks

Q *"Can I get rid of the stretch marks on my stomach, breasts and thighs?"*

A Stretch marks are a sign of your skin's inability to cope with the rapid expansion of flesh underneath. The collagen and elastin fibres underneath actually tear with the strain. They usually appear in times of rapid weight gain, such as puberty and pregnancy. They look quite red at first, although with time, they fade away to a pale silvery shade. There's nothing you can do once you've got them, except wait until they start to fade. However, moisturizing well can help guard against them. Apply body lotion after a bath or shower, and give it time to sink in.

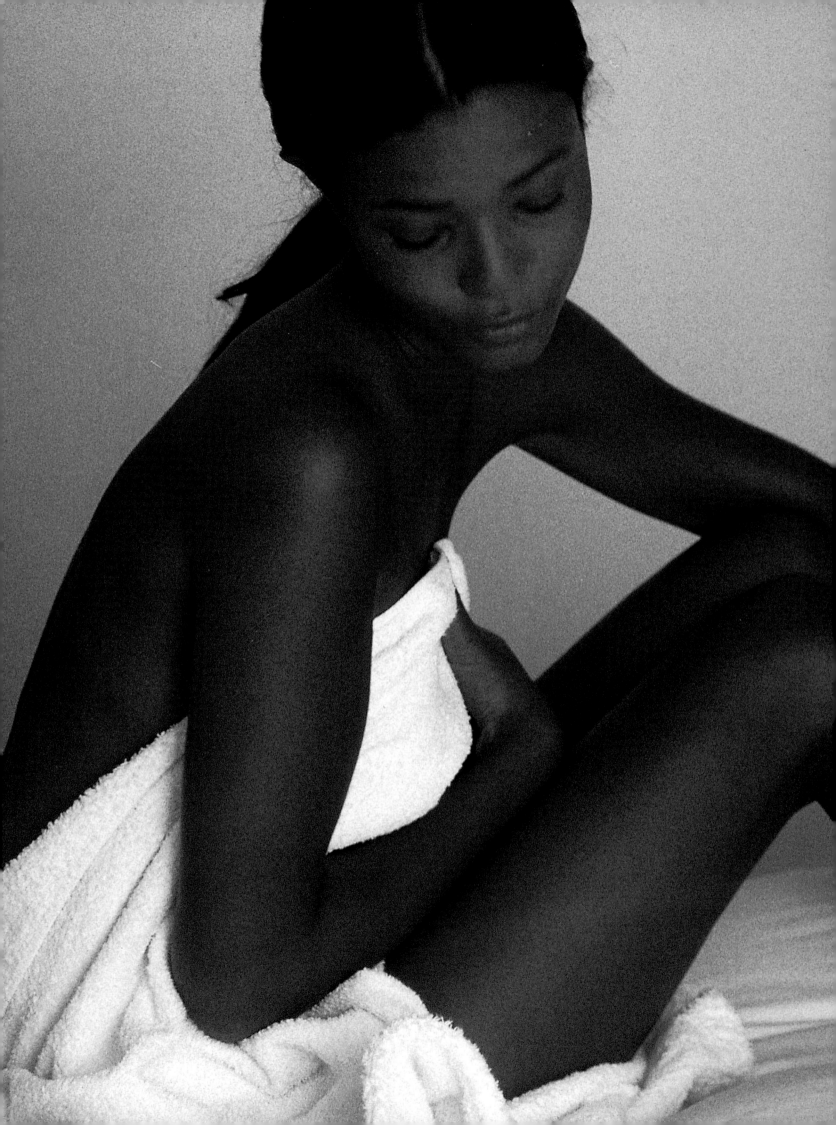

Complete bodycare

The secret to a beautifully maintained body is to lavish the same care on it as you do on your complexion and make-up. You need to take into account both general maintenance and any special needs it may have. Whatever beauty boosts your body needs, you'll find the help you need in this section of the book.

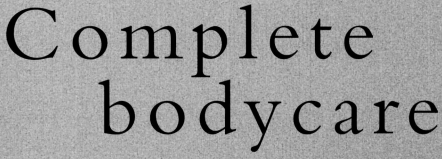

Caring for your body

One of the most effective ways to care for your body is to build bodycare treatments into your everyday bathroom routine. Hands and feet, elbows and necks can be forgotten and neglected because we are not in the habit of focusing our attention on them. Regular pampering may seem like an indulgence but in fact taking care of your whole body is vital to keeping it healthy. The power of touch to identify problem areas and notice changes, as you moisturize, scrub and massage, should not be underestimated.

throat
• Does skincare stop at your neck?
• Is the skin rough and grey?
• Do you indulge yourself with special treats to keep your skin in tip-top condition?

chest
• Do you give your breasts the care they need?
• Is your chest prone to break-outs?
• Do you protect this area of your skin from the harmful rays of the sun?

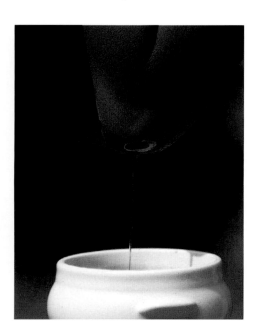

△ The skin on your elbows can miss out on moisturizing and become very dry. Evening primrose oil is especially nourishing for dry skin.

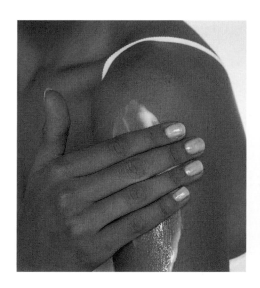

△ **Tops and especially the backs of arms need care too, so that they stay soft, smooth and firm.**

arms
• Are your elbows grey and dull in tone?
• Is the skin soft and supple, or rough and dry?
• Do darker hairs on your lower arms need bleaching?
• If you remove hair from your underarms, have you found the best method, the one that suits you for convenience and results?
• Have you found the solution to underarm freshness?

hands
• Do they suffer from too much housework?
• Do they need some moisturizing care?
• Are your nails neatly filed and shaped?
• Would a lick of polish or a French manicure give them a helping hand?

legs
• Are they free from stubbly hairs?
• Is the skin as smooth as it could be?
• Would they benefit from a light touch of fake tan?
• Are they prone to cellulite?
• Would bathtime treats improve the look of your skin?

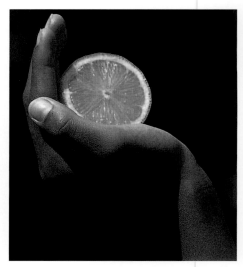

△ **The juice of a lemon is a good natural bleach for nails stained by dark nail polish.**

bikini line
• If you remove hair from this area, have you found the best method for you?

feet
• Are they free from hard skin, corns and calluses?
• Are your nails neatly trimmed?
• Do you smooth a foot cream on them regularly to ensure that the skin stays soft?

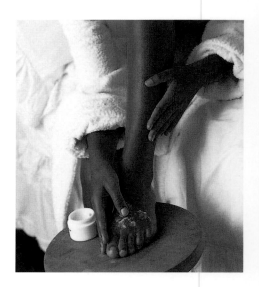

△ **As you massage your feet, take care to apply cream to the soles of your feet, as the skin on the heels can often become dry and cracked.**

Bathroom essentials

A pleasing, well-stocked bathroom can make all the difference at the start of a busy day and can be transformed into a sensual haven to help you unwind at the end of it.

The skin is the body's largest organ and forms a protective barrier against bacteria and other invaders. Although it continually sheds and renews itself, the skin has a lot to cope with and it deserves special attention. Scrubbing our skin removes dead skin cells and stimulates the blood supply, leaving skin tingling and toned. So keeping clean is vital for the overall health of the skin and body.

sponges and facecloths

These are useful for lathering soaps and gels on your skin, and dislodging dirt and grime from your body. Wash your facecloth regularly, and allow it to dry between uses. Natural sponges are a more expensive but long-lasting alternative. Squeeze out afterwards in warm clear water and allow to dry naturally.

pumice stone

These are made from very porous volcanic rock, and work best if you lather up with soap before rubbing at hardened areas of skin in a circular motion. Don't rub too fiercely or you'll make the skin sore. Little and often is best.

loofah or back brush

Try using a loofah as an exfoliator as its length makes it useful for scrubbing difficult-to-reach areas such as the back. Loofahs are actually the pod of an Egyptian plant and need a bit of care if they're going to last. Rinse and drain them thoroughly after use to prevent them going black and mouldy. Avoid rinsing them in vinegar and lemon juice as this can be too harsh for these once-living things.

Back brushes are also useful for areas of skin that are hard to reach, and are easier to care for: you simply rinse them in cool water after use and leave them to dry.

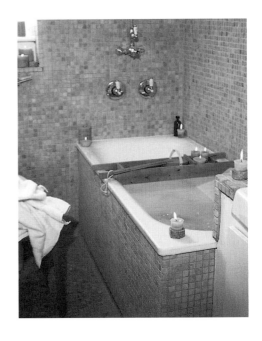

△ **A well-organized bathroom can be transformed into a haven to help you unwind.**

soaps and cleansing bars

These are a cheap and effective way of cleansing your body. If you find them too drying, choose ones that contain moisturizing ingredients to minimize these effects. Most people can use ordinary soaps and cleansers without any problem. However, if you have particularly dry or sensitive skin, it is advisable to opt for the pH-balanced variety.

BATHROOM BASICS

From cleaning your teeth to preventing underarm odour, there are a few basics that are essential for a well-stocked bathroom:

• **Toothbrush:** It is vital to choose the right toothbrush. A nylon brush is best, as bristle tends to split and lose its shape quickly. Choose one with a small head so you can easily clean your back teeth. A soft or medium brush is best as harder brushes may damage the tooth enamel and gums. Change your toothbrush approximately every month.

• **Dental floss:** Use floss at least once a day to clean between the teeth where the toothbrush can't reach. Waxed floss is best as it's less likely to catch on fillings or uneven edges. To floss, wind a short length around the second finger of each hand. Slide it gently down between two of the teeth, taking care to press it against the side of the tooth. Then gently slide it upwards out of the teeth, removing any food particles with it. Repeat between all of the teeth.

• **Antiperspirant deodorant:** Deodorants do not prevent perspiration – they only stop the bacteria from decomposing the sweat. If you perspire heavily, it is advisable to use an antiperspirant or even better an antiperspirant deodorant. The antiperspirant element prevents the production of sweat. Remember, though, not to use it on inflamed or broken skin or immediately after shaving.

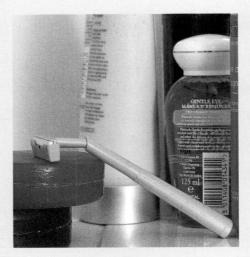

◁ **Stock your bathroom with bodycare products and bathtime treats for top-to-toe health and freshness.**

• **Talcum powder:** This white powder is made from finely ground magnesium silicate and is usually perfumed. It is considered to be rather old-fashioned, which is a shame because a good talcum powder makes you smell fresh and helps you slide into your clothes after bathing or swimming. However, there is no substitute for a thorough drying with a towel, especially between the toes, for keeping your skin healthy.

Fresh ideas for the bath and shower

As well as a chance to cleanse your body, bath- or shower-time is the perfect opportunity to pamper and polish your skin, and indulge in some refreshing and energizing beauty treats.

bathing beauty

The time of day and even the time of year will affect what you like using, so why not take the opportunity to try different products, adding any you particularly like to those you already know well.

shower gels and bubble baths

These are mild detergents that help cleanse your body while you soak in the water. There are hundreds of varieties to choose from, including those containing a host of additives, ranging from herbs to essential oils. If you find them too harsh for your skin, look for the ones that offer 2-in-1 benefits – these also contain moisturizers, to soothe your skin.

bath oils

These are a wonderful beauty boon for those with dry skins. They float on the top of the water, and your entire body becomes covered with a fine film when you step out

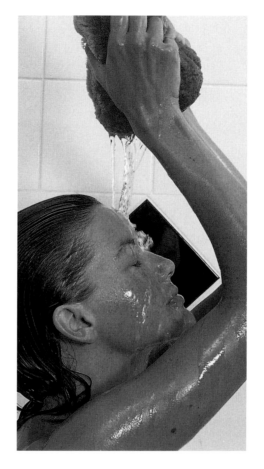

of the bath. Most cosmetic houses produce a bath oil, but if you're not worried about the fragrance, you can use a few drops of any vegetable oil, such as olive, corn or peanut.

◁ Just splashing water on your face will refresh and revive you. Take time to relax and enjoy your bath or shower.

bath salts

Made from sodium carbonate, these are particularly useful for softening hard water, and for preventing your skin from becoming too dry. Combined with warm water, they are a popular way to soothe away aches and pains.

bath-time treats

Once you've armed yourself with some bathroom treats and luxuries, try these water-baby bath treats to boost your body, beauty and mood.

sleepy "sitz" bath

The combination of hot and cold temperatures is an effective way of helping you get to sleep. Try a "sitz" bath, which helps you relax by drawing energy away from your head and stopping your mind from racing. Here's how to create your own "sitz" bath:
• Ensure the bathroom is warm, then run approximately 7.5–10cm (3–4in) of cold water into the bath.
• Wrap the top half of your body in a warm sweater or towel, then immerse your hips and bottom in the cold water for 30 seconds.
• Get out of the bath, pat yourself dry, then climb into bed and fall asleep.

learning to relax

Turn bathtime into an aromatherapy treat by adding relaxing essential oils such as chamomile and lavender to the water. Just add a few drops once you've run the bath, then lie back, inhale the vapours and relax completely. Salts and bubble baths that

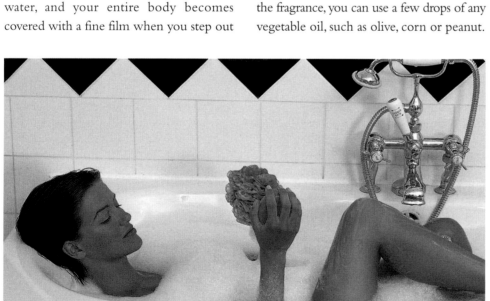

◁ Soaking in a warm bubble bath is a great opportunity to pamper and polish your skin, and has to be one of the most popular ways to relax.

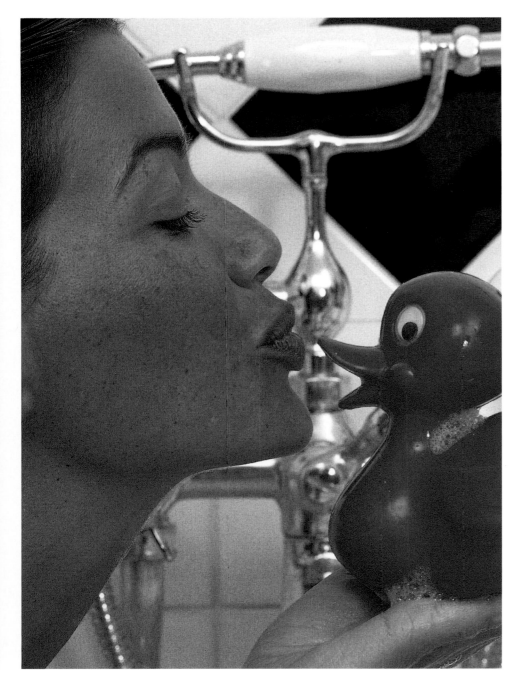

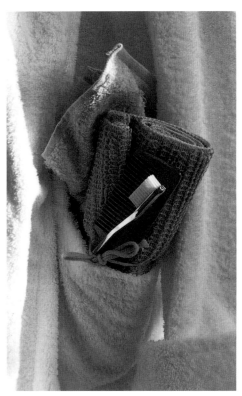

◁ There is nothing like a leisurely soak to melt away tension and to lift your spirits.

△ Make sure all the bath products you plan to use are close to hand, so you won't have to disturb your relaxing soak to fetch them.

contain sea minerals and kelp also have a relaxing effect, and purify your skin too. Bathing by candlelight and listening to calming music will make it even more of a treat. Put on soothing eye pads and relax for 10 minutes.

be a natural beauty

You don't have to splash out on expensive bath additives – try adding some simple, natural remedies:

• Soothe irritated skin by adding a cup of cider vinegar to the running water.

• A cup of powdered milk will soothe rough skin.

• Sprinkle a cupful of oatmeal or bran to the water to cleanse, whiten and soothe your skin.

sleek skin

Smooth your body with body oil before getting into the bath. After soaking for 10 minutes, rub your skin with a soft facecloth – you'll be amazed at how much dead skin you remove!

shower-time treats

Showers are a wonderful opportunity to cleanse your body quickly and cheaply, and to wake yourself up. Here are some of the other benefits.

circulation booster

Switch on the cold water before finishing your shower to help boost your circulation. It will also make you feel warmer once you get out of the shower! It also works well if

you concentrate the blasts of cold water on cellulite-prone areas, as this stimulates the sluggish circulation in these spots.

boosting benefits

If you pat yourself dry after a bath, it'll help you to unwind, whereas briskly rubbing your skin with a towel will help to invigorate you.

shower sensation

Add a few drops of essential oils to the floor of the shower itself. As they evaporate you will find that you're surrounded by a sensuous-smelling mist while you wash your body. Rosemary, peppermint and basil are classic refreshers, while grapefruit blended with geranium makes a stimulating mix.

Natural bathing treats

Enjoyed in the evening, a warm bath helps the body to relax and can pave the way for a good night's sleep. Although you may be tempted, especially in cold weather, to have a steaming hot bath, a short soak in body-temperature water is far more effective at helping you unwind. Bathing in water that is too hot can cause thread veins and may make you feel unwell. The skin is also better able to release impurities at body temperature and to absorb the healing properties of any herbs and minerals that are added to the bathwater.

essential oils

To make bathing a real indulgence you can create your own aromatic bath products. Lavender, chamomile, clary sage, neroli and rose all have a relaxing, soporific effect.

Add 5–10 drops of your chosen oil blend to your bath, then sink in and relax. Inhaling the wonderful aromas will soothe your mind, and the oils will also have a beneficial effect on your skin and body.

▽ **A good supply of clean, fluffy towels and beautiful candles can make taking a bath a glorious indulgence.**

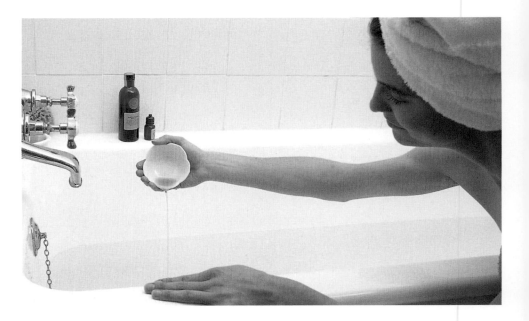

△ **Essential oils evaporate very quickly in hot water so the oils will be much more effective if you pour them into the bath water just before you climb in.**

orange and grapefruit bath oil

At the end of the day, a scented bath is a therapeutic treat. Choose the oils depending on whether you want to be relaxed or invigorated. An orange and grapefruit bath will gently refresh you. Add one teaspoon once you have run the bath, otherwise the oils will evaporate before you get in.

ingredients

- 45ml/3 tbsp sweet almond oil
- 5 drops grapefruit oil
- 5 drops orange oil

Pour the oils into a bottle and shake so that they are well combined before you add one teaspoon to the bathwater.

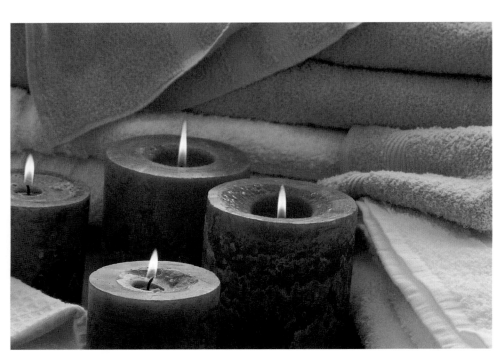

THERAPEUTIC BATH OIL BLENDS

Mix two or three essential oils in a base of sweet almond oil or jojoba oil. These quantities are for a 50ml/¼ cup bottle of base oil. Add 20 drops of the mixed oil to the bathwater.

Alternatively, you can mix the oils with milk or honey because this will help to disperse them in the water.

- **Anti-stress mix**: 10 drops each marjoram, lavender and sandalwood.
- **Invigorating mix**: 5 drops rosemary, 5 drops camphor, 20 drops peppermint.
- **Healing mix for colds and flu**: 10 drops each eucalyptus, thyme and lavender.
- **Soothing arthritis**: 30 drops eucalyptus.

▷ **Lavender is a versatile and widely used essential oil, well known for its fabulous scent and its soothing, relaxing and healing properties.**

lavender and olive oil soap

Use a good-quality pure olive oil soap to make this home-made soap. Enrich it with other oils and scent it with lavender to produce a gently rejuvenating cleanser.

ingredients

- 175g/6oz good-quality olive oil soap
- 25ml/1¹/₂ tbsp coconut oil
- 25ml/1¹/₂ tbsp almond oil
- 30ml/2 tbsp ground almonds
- 10 drops lavender essential oil
- lavender buds for decorating

Grate the soap and place in a double boiler. Leave the soap to soften over a low heat. When soft, add all the other ingredients and mix evenly. Press the mixture into oiled moulds and leave to set overnight. Unmould, and decorate by pressing the top of each block of soap into a shallow tray of lavender buds.

goodnight bath salts

Chamomile is a widely recognized sedative; for these bath salts it has been combined with sweet marjoram, which is an effective treatment for insomnia.

ingredients

- 450g/1lb/2¹/₄ cups coarse sea salt
- 10 drops chamomile essential oil
- 10 drops sweet marjoram essential oil
- 1–3 drops green food colouring (optional)

Combine all the ingredients and pour into a glass storage jar with a close-fitting lid. Put the lid on firmly. Just before bedtime, light a scented candle, add a handful of the salts to your bath, immerse yourself in the warm water and relax.

herbal bath mix

All the ingredients for this mix are easily available to buy, or they can be grown in a herb garden or window box. They are associated with purification and cleansing.

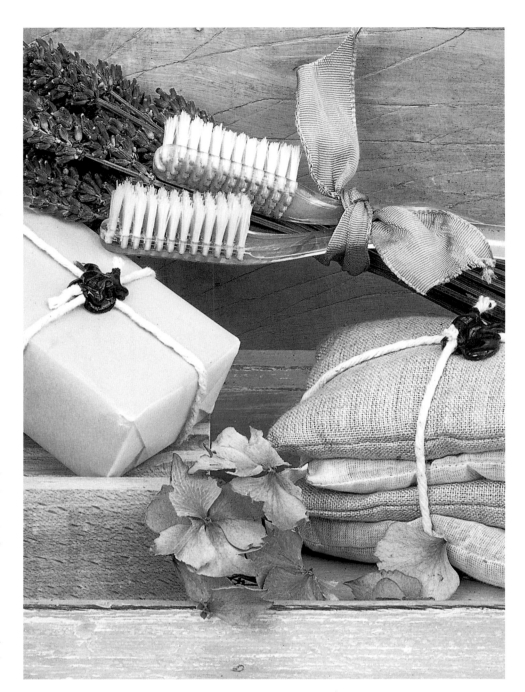

ingredients

- 7 basil leaves
- 3 bay leaves
- 3 sprigs oregano
- 1 sprig tarragon
- small square of cotton muslin
- 10ml/2 tsp organic oats
- pinch rock or sea salt
- thread to tie up muslin

Use fresh herbs for this recipe if possible. Pile the herbs in the centre of the muslin square, then sprinkle the oats on top. Top with the rock or sea salt, pick up the corners of the muslin and tie with thread. Hang the sachet from the bath tap so that as the water runs over the bag it is infused with the essence of the mixture.

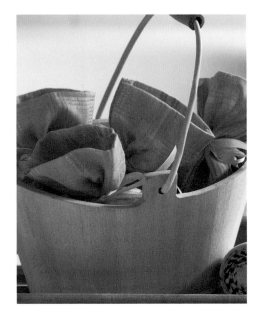

△ **Fragrant bath bags will lightly scent the bath.**

Be a smoothie

Most women aspire to smooth, healthy skin free of dry patches, superfluous hair, and blemishes. And the chances are, even if your skin isn't prone to spottiness or flaky patches, it will suffer from dullness and poor condition from time to time. This is where body scrubs and exfoliators come into their own. They work by shifting dead cells from the skin surface, revealing the younger, fresher ones underneath. This process also stimulates the circulation of blood in the skin tissues, giving it a rosy glow.

Hair on a woman's body is completely natural, but fashion and cultural practices mean that it is usually removed. There are a number of ways of removing hair for smooth, soft skin and it is simply a matter of finding the method that suits you best.

exfoliation methods

There are lots of different ways you can exfoliate your body – so there's one to suit every budget and preference.

• Your first option is to buy an exfoliating scrub, which is a cream- or gel-based product containing tiny abrasive particles.

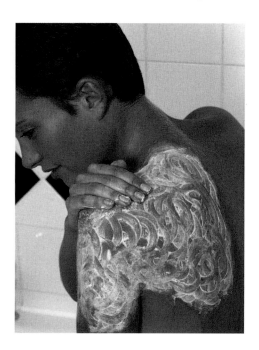

△ **A body scrub is a quick and easy way to keep your skin sleek and smooth.**

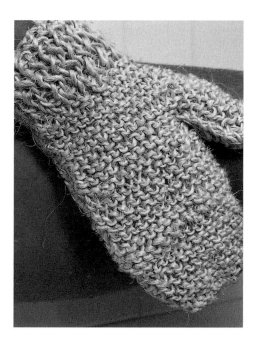

△ **Keep a sisal mitt to hand for super-soft skin.**

Look for the type with rounded particles which won't irritate delicate skin. Simply massage the scrub into damp skin, then rinse away with lots of warm water.

• Bath mitts, loofahs and sisal mitts are a cinch to use, and cost-effective too. They can be quite harsh on the skin if you press too hard, so go easily at first. Rinse them well after use, and allow them to dry naturally. Simply sweep over your body when you're in the shower or bath.

• Your ordinary facecloth or bath sponge can also double up as an exfoliator. Lather up with plenty of soap or shower gel, and massage over damp skin before rinsing away with clear water.

• Copy what health spas do, and keep a large tub of natural sea salt by the shower. Scoop up a handful when you get in, and massage over your skin. Rinse away thoroughly afterwards.

• You can also make your own body scrub at home by mixing sea salt with body oil or olive oil. Allow the mixture to soak into your skin for a few minutes to allow the edges of the salt crystals to dissolve before massaging in, then rinsing away.

• Body brushes are also useful. The best way to use them is on dry skin before you get in the bath or shower, as this is particularly good for loosening dead skin cells. You can also use them in the water, lathering them up with soap or gel.

perfecting your exfoliation technique

Whichever method you use, the best thing to do is concentrate on problem areas such as upper arms, thighs, bottom, heels and elbows. Also sweep over the rest of your body. However, go gently on delicate areas of skin, such as the inner arms, stomach and inner thighs. Work in large strokes, in the direction of your heart.

Oilier skin types will benefit from exfoliation 2–3 times a week, while once a week is sufficient for others. Never exfoliate broken, inflamed or acne-prone skins.

After exfoliating, always apply body lotion to seal moisture into the fresh new skin you've exposed.

BEAUTY TIP

For speedy super-soft skin, you should massage your body with oil before climbing into the bath or shower. Then proceed as usual with your preferred exfoliating method.

hair removal

These are the main removal methods for superfluous hair. Each method has advantages and disadvantages, and these have been outlined here:

shaving

Using a razorblade, shaving works by cutting the hair at the skin surface. Shaving is most effective for legs and underarms.

Pros: Cheap, quick and painless.

Cons: Regrowth (stubble) appears very quickly, usually within a couple of days.

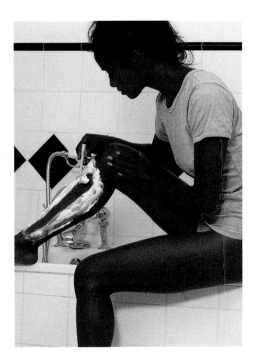

◁ For many women, shaving is the no-fuss option for silky smooth legs.

SHAVING TIPS
• Use with a moisturizing shave foam or gel for a close shave. Moisturize afterwards to soothe your skin.
• A closer shave means you will have to shave your legs less frequently.
• Let the shaving cream get to work and soften the hair for a few moments before using your razor.

tweezing
This rather time-consuming method involves plucking out hairs one at a time so it is most effective for small areas such as eyebrows, or for removing the odd stray hair missed by waxing.

Pros: Good control for shaping.

Cons: Can be painful and may make skin slightly reddened for a while afterwards. You also need to remember to check the area regularly in a mirror to see that you don't need to re-tweeze.

TWEEZER TIP
Before you begin, hold a warm facecloth over the area of skin you are going to work on. This will dampen and soften the skin, and open the pores, making tweezing easier. Or you could try pressing an ice cube over the area to numb the skin first if you find it really painful.

waxing
This method uproots the hair from below the skin's surface. Either wax is smoothed on to the skin and removed with strips, or pre-prepared wax strips are used. This is a form of hair removal that can be safely used on any part of the body.

Pros: The results last for 2–6 weeks.

Cons: This method can be extremely painful and there is also the risk of sore, red and blotchy legs and of ingrowing hairs. Also, hair has to be left to grow until it is long enough to wax effectively, so you have to put up with regrowth to give the hairs time to grow back sufficiently. If the hair is too short, it won't come out, or it will be removed patchily.

WAXING TIPS
• After waxing the bikini area, apply an antibacterial cream to prevent infection or a rash.
• Wear loose clothing after waxing.
• Never wax a sore area.

depilatory creams
These creams contain chemicals that weaken the hair at the skin's surface, so hair can be wiped away. Simply apply, leave for 5–10 minutes, then rinse away. (Check the packaging for exact instructions.) You can use a depilatory cream anywhere, especially as some companies produce different formulations for specific areas. Do a patch test 24 hours before use to make sure it won't cause irritation or an allergy.

Pros: It is cheap, and the results last a bit longer than a razor – up to a week.

Cons: Can be messy, and takes time. The smell of some products can be off-putting although formulations have improved.

bleaching
This is not technically hair removal, but it's a good way to make hair less noticeable. A hydrogen peroxide solution is used to lighten the hair. Bleaching is best for arms, upper lip and face.

Pros: Results last between 2 and 6 weeks, and there's no regrowth.

Cons: Not suitable for coarse hair.

BLEACHING TIP
It is a good idea to carry out a patch test on your skin first to ensure you don't react to the product's bleaching agents.

sugaring
This works in a similar way to waxing, but uses a paste made from sugar, lemon and water. It's well known in the Middle East, and is growing in popularity elsewhere.

Pros: Has the same benefits as waxing and can be used anywhere on the body.

Cons: Can be fairly painful and there is a risk of ingrowing hairs.

electrolysis
A needlelike probe conducts an electric current into the hair follicle, inactivating it. This method is best for small areas such as breasts and face. Go to a qualified practitioner (and ask to see proof of their qualifications).

Pros: A permanent solution.

Cons: Expensive, and more painful for some people than others, depending upon the pain threshold. You may find that you are more sensitive to the pain just before or during your period.

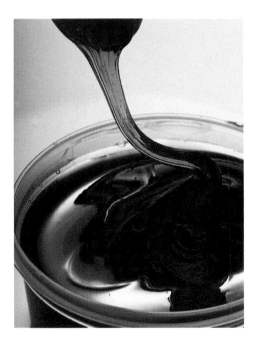

△ Sugaring – the sweeter way to removing superfluous hair.

Simple steps to softer skin

Slick on a body moisturizer to create a wonderfully silky body. Add a moisturizing body treat to your daily beauty regime, and you'll soon reap the benefits.

moisturizing matters

Just as you choose a moisturizer for your face with care, you should opt for the best formulation that is suited to the skin type on your body.

• Gels are the lightest formulation and are perfect for very hot days or oilier skin types. They contain many nourishing ingredients even though they're very easy to wear.

• Lotions and oils are good for most skin types, and easy to apply, as they're not sticky. Creams give better results for those with dry skins, especially on very dry areas.

make the most of body moisturizer

• Apply using firm strokes to boost your circulation as you massage in the product. Apply the moisturizer straight on to clean, damp skin – after a bath or shower is the ideal time. This helps seal extra moisture into the upper layers of your skin, making it softer than ever.

• Soften cracked feet by rubbing them with rich body lotion, pulling on a pair of cotton socks and heading for bed. They'll be beautifully soft by the next morning!

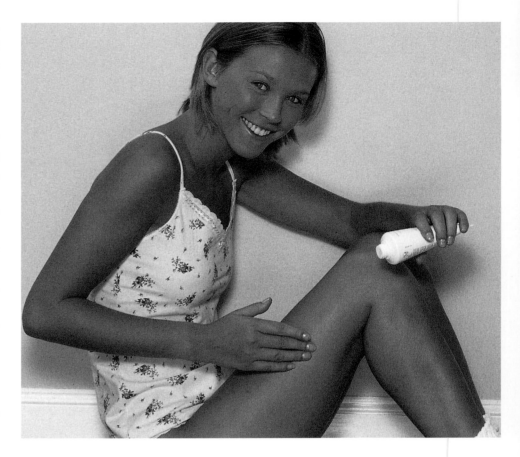

△ Take the time before dressing to moisturize your skin. Why not apply body lotion and then allow your skin to absorb it while you clean your teeth or dry your hair?

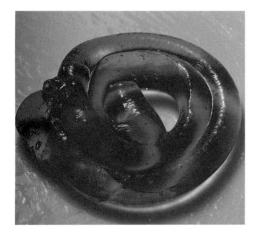

△ Opt for the light touch with a moisturizing gel.

• Concentrate on rubbing moisturizer into particularly dry areas such as heels, knees and elbows. The calves are also very prone to dryness because there aren't many oil glands present there.

• If you don't have time to apply moisturizer after your bath, simply add a few drops of body oil to the water. When you step out of the bath, your skin will be coated with a fine film of nourishing oil. Always remember to rinse the bath well afterwards to prevent you from slipping the next time you climb into the bath.

• Your breasts don't have any supportive muscle from the nipple to the collarbone and skin is very fine here. Firming creams won't work miracles, but can help maintain the elasticity and suppleness of this delicate area. Regular application of body lotion can have similar effects.

SMELLING SENSATIONAL

Opt for a scented body lotion as a treat. They can often be longer-lasting than the fragrances themselves. Alternatively, use them as part of "fragrance layering". This simply means taking advantage of the various scent formulations available. Start with a scented bath oil and soap, move on to the matching body lotion and powder, and leave the house wearing the fragrance itself sprayed on to pulse points.

However, be careful you don't clash fragrances. Choose unscented products if you're also wearing perfume, unless you're going to be wearing a matching scented body lotion. You don't want cheaper products to compete with your more expensive perfume.

▷ For super-soft skin apply moisturizer immediately after showering or bathing. Cream is better absorbed by warm, damp skin and this will help to seal in extra moisture.

home-made lotions

For pure pampering pleasure nothing beats a tailor-made beauty preparation, and you can choose the ingredients specially to suit your own skincare needs. Mixing oils or adding your favourite essential oil to a ready-made unscented cream is easy to do and very rewarding.

geranium body lotion

This is a spicy, fragrant lotion. Geranium oil is derived from a relative of the scented geranium leaf and the fragrance is pleasantly sharp and aromatic.

ingredients

• 175ml/6 fl oz unscented body lotion

• 15 drops geranium essential oil

Add the geranium oil to the body lotion, mix them well and pour into a bottle with a tight lid.

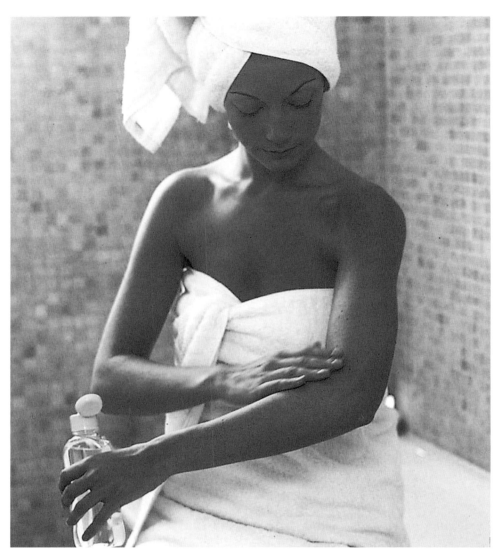

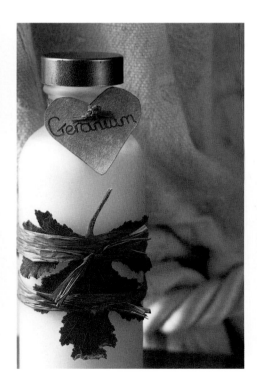

△ It is a good idea to label and date home-made lotion. It should keep for a month or so if it is stored in a sealed bottle in a cool place, but will not keep indefinitely.

coconut and orangeflower body lotion

This creamy preparation is soothing and nourishing for dry skin. Wheatgerm oil is rich in vitamin E, an antioxidant that protects skin cells against premature aging.

ingredients

• 50g/2oz coconut oil

• 60ml/4 tbsp sunflower oil

• 10ml/2 tsp wheatgerm oil

• 10 drops orangeflower essence or 5 drops neroli essential oil

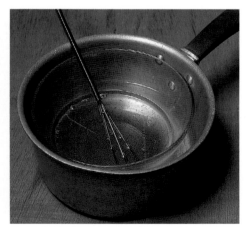

△ 1 Melt the coconut oil in a heatproof bowl over gently simmering water. Stir in the sunflower and wheatgerm oils. Leave to cool, then add the fragrance and pour into a jar.

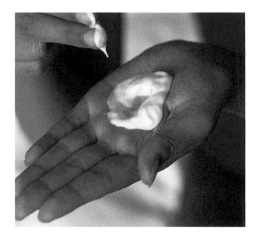

△ 2 The lotion will solidify after several hours. For the best results warm the cream on your hands briefly before applying to dry areas of skin.

Simple aromatherapy recipes

Many more of us are waking up to the benefits of aromatherapy and natural beauty products these days, and for very good reasons. Natural therapies are wonderful to use, easily available and can give immediate results.

Aromatherapy uses essential oils, which are the distilled essences of herbs, plants, flowers and trees. These oils smell wonderful and are a pleasure to use. It's this smell that usually attracts people to them for treating a variety of physical and mental conditions, from skin infections to stress.

aromatherapy massage

Mix 3–4 drops of essential oil into 10ml/ 2 tsp of a neutral carrier oil such as sweet almond oil, and use to massage your body – or ask someone else to massage you.

tips for using essential oils
• Essential oils are natural products but their effects can be powerful, so they must be used with care.
• If you don't want to buy individual essential oils, buy them ready-blended, or treat yourself to bath and body products that contain them.
• Some oils are thought to carry some risk during pregnancy. For this reason, consult a qualified aromatherapist for advice if you are pregnant and want to use essential oils.
• Don't try to treat medical conditions with them – always consult your doctor.
• Essential oils can be expensive, but a little goes a long way.
• Do not apply essential oils to the skin undiluted as they're far too concentrated in this form, and can result in inflammation. The only exception is lavender, which can be used directly on the skin for insect bites and stings. Otherwise, essential oils should be mixed with a carrier oil.
• Don't take essential oils internally. Essential oils are approximately 50 to 100 times more powerful than the plant from which they were extracted.

• Don't apply oils to areas of broken, inflamed or recently scarred skin.
• Whichever method of aromatherapy you use, shut the door to the room to prevent the aroma from escaping!
• For immediate results add about 4 drops of your chosen oil to a bowl of hot water, lean over it and cover your head with a towel. Inhale deeply for about 5 minutes.
• Place a few drops of your favourite oil on a tissue, so you can inhale it whenever you like. Eucalyptus is great for blocked sinuses or if you have a cold. Alternatively, sprinkle a few drops of chamomile or lavender on your pillow to help you sleep.
• If you have sensitive skin it is a good idea to carry out a patch test before you use an oil. Apply diluted oil to a small patch of skin and leave it for a few hours to make sure you do not have an adverse reaction to it.

hand and foot creams

These creams are made by adding suitable essential oils to an unscented cream, which means that you can easily adapt the recipe

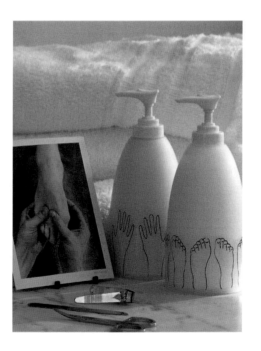

△ **Plastic pump-action bottles such as these make lotions easier to use so that you are much more likely to apply them regularly.**

to suit you. Look out for a lanolin-rich cream or one that includes cocoa butter, as both hands and feet benefit from something with a richer formulation. Although most creams and lotions are best stored in glass or ceramic containers, in this case it is practical to keep the lotion in a pump-action plastic bottle, which makes it much easier to use, and more likely that you will apply it regularly.

tea tree foot cream

Well-cared-for feet look and feel so much better. Tea tree is one of the best essential oils to add to a foot cream. It has healing, antiseptic properties and an effective fungicidal action.

ingredients
• 120ml/4fl oz unscented cream
• 15 drops tea tree essential oil
• bowl and spoon for mixing
• pump-action plastic bottle
• funnel

Blend the essential oils thoroughly into the unscented cream and pour into the plastic bottle through a funnel.

healing hand cream

The oils in this cream are good for the hands: the chamomile soothes, the geranium helps heal cuts and grazes and the lemon softens the skin.

ingredients
• 120ml/4fl oz unscented hand cream
• 10 drops chamomile essential oil
• 5 drops geranium essential oil
• 5 drops lemon essential oil
• bowl and spoon for mixing
• pump-action plastic bottle
• funnel

Blend the essential oils thoroughly into the unscented hand cream and pour into the plastic bottle through a funnel.

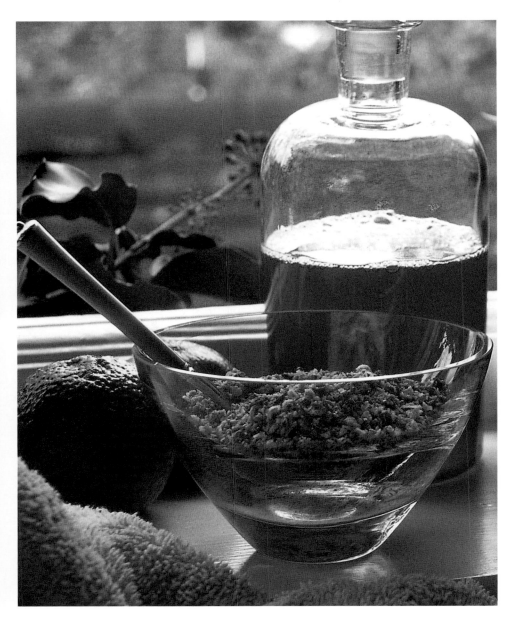

◁ The combination of aromatic orange peel and refreshing grapefruit oil in this body scrub gives it a stimulating, clean scent.

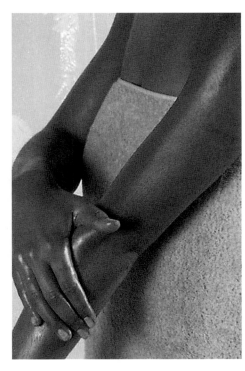

△ For a soothing and moisturizing massage on a problem area, mix 15ml/1 tbsp almond oil with a suitable essential oil and massage gently. Breathe deeply as you massage to maximize the therapeutic effect.

citrus body scrub

Orange peel is mixed with the slightly gritty texture of ground sunflower seeds, oatmeal and sea salt in this reviving scrub, helping to remove dead skin cells and stimulate the blood supply to the skin, leaving it feeling tingling and toned.

ingredients

- 45ml/3 tbsp freshly ground sunflower seeds
- 45ml/3 tbsp medium oatmeal
- 45ml/3 tbsp flaked sea salt
- 45ml/3 tbsp finely grated orange peel
- 3 drops grapefruit essential oil
- almond oil

Mix together all the ingredients except the almond oil and store in a sealed glass jar. Using just a little at a time, mix with some almond oil to make a thick paste, then rub over damp skin.

APPLYING A BODY SCRUB
For smoother, softer skin, mix the scrub with water or oil to make a paste.

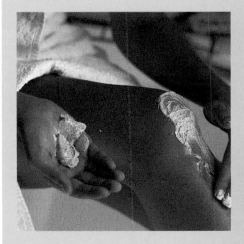

△ **1** Work the scrub into damp skin using a firm pressure and paying particular attention to areas of dry skin such as the elbows, knees and ankles.

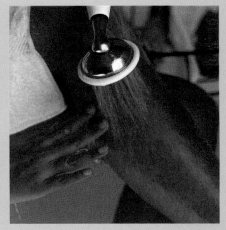

△ **2** Use a dry flannel to remove most of the scrub and then gently rinse the rest away with warm water.

Fabulous foot pampering

Setting aside time for a regular treatment will help you to care for your feet and keep them healthy all year round. A pamper session once a month will greatly improve their appearance, and will also soften the skin and help boost the circulation. You can also do it to pep up your feet at the start of the summer or before going on holiday.

You'll need at least an hour to do the treatment properly – or you can really indulge yourself and take two hours for the session. Use this as a time to relax – you will find that focusing on your feet is a great way to forget about day-to-day worries.

foot pamper routine

This routine uses the luxury foot scrub (opposite). If you don't have time to make this, buy one that includes essential oils so that you can benefit from their soothing properties. You also need foaming bath or foot gel, a large foot bowl, one large towel and two smaller ones, two plastic bags that are large enough to slip your feet into, a pumice stone and pedicure tools.

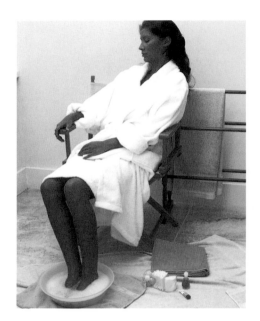

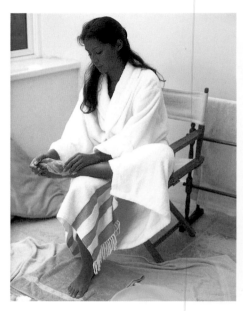

△ **1** Half fill a large bowl with warm water. Place the bowl on a large towel on the floor. Add a little foaming gel, and perhaps a couple of drops of essential oil which have been diluted first in a carrier oil. Swish the water around with your hand to create plenty of bubbles and to release the aroma of the essential oil. Put both feet into the water, then sit back and relax as you soak them for a good five minutes. Remove your feet from the bowl and rub on the floor towel to remove most of the water.

△ **2** Put a towel on your right knee and rest the left foot on top. Massage the foot scrub all over the sole, paying extra attention to any rough skin, and rub into cuticles. Place your foot in a plastic bag and secure.

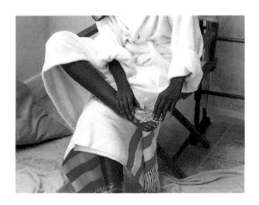

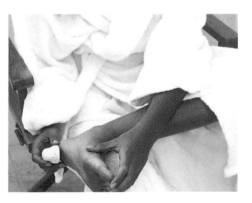

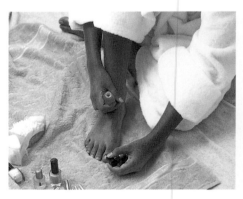

△ **3** Repeat on the right foot. Wait ten minutes, then remove the bag from the left foot, sliding it firmly down the foot to remove the foot scrub. Do the same for the right foot. Dip both feet into the water. This will have cooled down, so it will stimulate the circulation.

△ **4** Remove your feet from the bowl. Place your left foot on the right knee. Take the pumice stone and rub over the sole. Use firm pressure on the heel and ball, and light pressure on the arch. Now rub the pumice all over the top of the foot, using light pressure. This helps to improve the skin texture and bring nutrient-rich blood to the surface, which will help improve the appearance. Repeat on the left foot.

△ **5** Trim the nails straight across, then smooth the edges with an emery board. Use a cotton bud (swab) to apply cuticle remover, wait a few minutes, then gently push the cuticle back with a hoof stick. Soak the feet again, then carefully clean under the nail. Dry the feet, then apply base coat, polish and top coat, using cotton wool (cotton) to separate the toes and allowing each layer to dry before applying the next.

luxury foot scrub

The following recipe is an excellent cleanser and softener for the feet. It can be used whenever you feel they need a boost. For the best results, though, set aside enough time for a long pamper session.

ingredients

• 5ml/1 tsp each almond oil, jojoba oil and glycerine – to nourish and soften the skin

• 5ml/1 tsp each Fullers earth and rock salt – to soften and cleanse

• 10ml/2 tsp foaming foot or bath wash – to cleanse the skin and soften the cuticles

• 3 drops essential oil – for aromatic feel-good factor. Choose whichever oil you like best, or use a blend: mandarin and geranium, or lavender and lemon are relaxing, cleansing combinations

In a small clean bottle, mix the foaming wash, essential oil and glycerine. Shake and set aside while you prepare the other ingredients. Put the Fullers earth and rock salt into a medium-sized dish and mix together. Mix in the almond and jojoba oils. Add the glycerine mixture to the bowl, and mix all the ingredients together with a metal spoon. You should now have a runny paste.

lemon verbena and lavender foot bath

ingredients

• 15g/¹⁄₂oz dried lemon verbena

• 30ml/2 tbsp dried lavender

• 5 drops lavender essential oil

• 30ml/2 tbsp cider vinegar

Put the lemon verbena and lavender into a basin and pour in enough hot water to cover the feet. When it has cooled add the lavender oil and cider vinegar. Sit down and immerse your feet in the bath for 15 minutes. Dry your feet thoroughly afterwards.

CARING FOR YOUR FEET

A pedicure will help to keep your feet attractive and healthy. You will need a few special items, but because they will last a long time they are definitely a worthwhile investment.

• **Nail-polish remover**: It's a good idea to choose a conditioning one.

• **Cotton wool (cotton)**: Ideal for removing nail polish and also useful for separating toes while you paint them.

• **Nail brush or orange stick** (tip covered with cotton wool): Useful for cleaning under the nail.

• **Hoof stick or cotton buds (swabs)**: Vital for pushing back the cuticles.

• **Toenail clippers**: These are often easier to use than scissors.

• **Emery board**: Toenails are harder than fingernails so you'll need a strong one.

• **Cuticle remover**: Invaluable for softening and loosening the cuticle.

• **Nail polish and a clear top coat**: Great for sealing polish and preventing chipping.

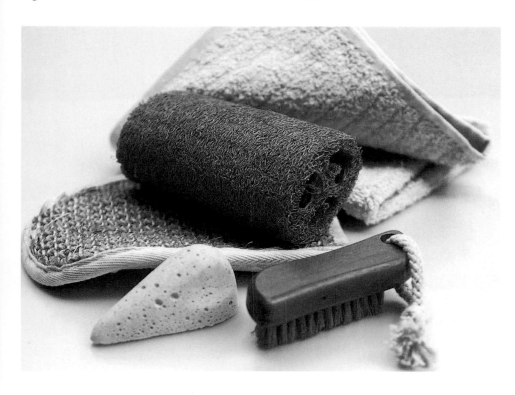

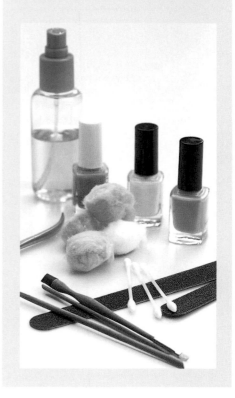

△ **After soaking your feet in a footbath for ten minutes, use a loofah or nail brush to scrub and deep-cleanse, then use a pumice on the dead skin all over the soles of the feet. Pat them dry, then give your feet a quick massage using a blend of neroli and lemon essential oils well diluted in almond oil.**

Beating cellulite

It's not just plumper, older women who suffer from "orange-peel skin" on their thighs, hips, bottom and even tummy – many slim, young women suffer too. Sadly, there is no miracle cure for cellulite, but there are some practical things you can do to see great results.

facts on cellulite

Experts disagree about what causes cellulite. It seems likely that it's an accumulation of fat, fluid and toxins trapped in the hardened network of elastin and collagen fibres in the deeper levels of your skin. This causes the dimpled effect and feel of cellulite areas. These areas also tend to feel cold to the touch because the flow of blood is constricted and the lymphatic system, which is responsible for eliminating toxins, can't work properly. This can worsen the problem and make the cellulite feel puffy and spongy.

testing for cellulite

Try squeezing the skin of your upper thigh between your thumb and index finger. If the flesh feels lumpy and looks bumpy, you have cellulite. Further clues may be that these areas look whiter and feel colder than elsewhere on your legs.

common causes

Cellulite can be caused and/or aggravated by the following:
• A poor diet is full of toxins and puts the body under great strain to get rid of vast quantities of waste. Also, an unhealthy low-fibre, high-fat diet means that the body's digestive system can't work effectively to expel toxins from the body.
• Stress and lack of exercise make your body sluggish and can slow down blood circulation and the lymphatic system.
• Hereditary factors – if your mother has cellulite, it's a fair bet you will have, too.
• Hormones, such as the contraceptive pill or hormone replacement therapy, may contribute.

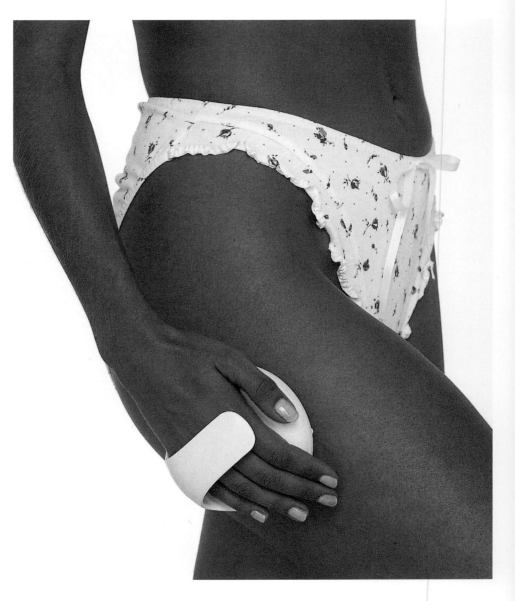

tackling cellulite

There are dozens of products around designed to deal with cellulite, but it is debatable how effective they really are. To actually tackle the problem effectively you should attempt to follow a three-pronged approach, combining:
• Circulation-boosting tactics
• Diet
• Exercise

boost your circulation

Here are several ways to boost your circulation and your lymphatic system. Whichever one you choose, aim to follow it for at least 5 minutes a day.

△ Pep up your circulation and lymphatic system to help beat that cellulite.

• Use a soft body brush on damp or dry skin. Brush the skin in long sweeping movements over the affected area, and make sure you are working in the direction of the heart.
• Use a massage glove or rough sisal mitt in the same way as above.
• Use a cellulite cream. These usually contain natural ingredients such as horse chestnut, ivy and caffeine to boost your circulation. However, you can make them doubly effective by massaging them thoroughly into the skin with your

step up your exercise

Exercise will boost your sluggish circulation and lymphatic system, and encourage your body to get rid of the toxins causing your cellulite. Do a regular aerobic workout, exercising for 20–40 minutes, 3–5 times a week, and choose from these: brisk walking, swimming, cycling, tennis, badminton, aerobic classes or running. (It is always wise to consult your doctor before embarking on a new form of exercise.)

tone it up!

You can also try these exercises to increase circulation, firm up your legs and give them a better shape. Carried out daily, they will help you win the cellulite battle.

fingertips. Some cellulite creams even come with their own plastic or rubber hand-held mitts to help boost the circulation.

anti-cellulite diet

To cleanse your body you need to follow a healthy low-fat, high-fibre diet – one that contains plenty of fresh fruit and vegetables. The great news is, if you have any excess weight to lose it will naturally fall away by following these rules.

• Eat at least five servings of fresh fruit and vegetables every day.

• Cut down on the amount of fat you eat. For instance, grill rather than fry foods, and cut off visible fat from meat. For many foods you buy, look out for a low-fat alternative. Water cleanses your system and flushes toxins from body cells, so drink at least 2 litres (quarts) of pure water every day.

• Change from caffeine-laden tea and coffee to herbal teas and decaffeinated coffee. Sip pure fruit juices rather than fizzy drinks.

• Steer clear of alcohol as much as possible as it adversely affects your liver – your body's main de-toxifier.

• Drink a glass of hot water containing the juice of a fresh lemon when you get up in the morning – it's a wonderful way to detoxify your body.

• Avoid eating sugary snacks between meals – eat a piece of fruit, raw vegetables or rice cakes instead.

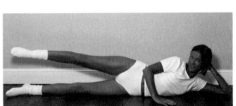

△ **Inner thigh toner:** Lie on your side on the floor, supporting your head with your arm. With your top leg resting on the floor in front, raise the lower leg off the floor as far as you can without straining, then gently lower it again. Repeat 10 times, then turn over and work the other leg.

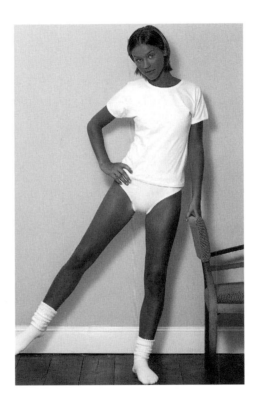

△ **Hip toner:** Stand sideways with your hand resting on a chair. Your knees should be slightly bent and your shoulders relaxed. Slowly raise your right leg out to the side, keeping your body and raised foot facing forward. Carefully and slowly lower your leg, and then repeat this movement 10 times. Turn round and repeat with the other leg.

△ **Outer thigh toner**: Lie on your side, supporting your head with your hand. Bend your lower leg behind you and tilt your hips slightly forward. Place your other hand on the floor in front of you for balance. Slowly lift your upper leg, then bring it down to touch the lower one, and repeat this action 6 times. Repeat on the other side.

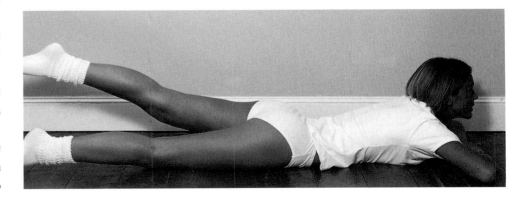

△ **Bottom toner:** Lie on your front with your hands on top of one another, resting your chin on them if you wish. Raise one leg about 13cm/5in off the floor and hold for a count of 10. Bring your leg back to the floor, and repeat 15–20 times with each leg.

Holiday skincare

There's nothing that lifts your spirits like spending time in the sunshine and a certain amount of exposure to the sun is actually good for our bodies. However, it is important that you take special care of your skin against the dangers of suntanning. The secret is to give your skin the protection it needs, while you gradually develop a light attractive colour.

the right product

There is a wide range of sun creams, lotions and blocks available, and it is vital to use the right one because burning ages your skin and increases your chances of skin cancer. Play safe by following our two-step plan:

step 1: know your SPFs

SPF stands for Sun Protection Factor. The higher the number of the SPF, the more protection the product will give you from the burning ultraviolet B (UVB) rays. For instance, an SPF 2 will let you stay out in the sun for twice as long as you usually could before burning, whereas an SPF 8 will let you stay out eight times as long.

step 2: go by skin type

To choose an SPF, you need to know how vulnerable your skin is to the sun's UVB rays. Dermatologists divide skins into six types, each needing a different level of protection, so you can ensure your skin is always well protected, wherever you travel.

Skin-type 1: Always burns, never tans. Fair-skinned, usually with freckles. Red or blonde hair. Typical Irish or Anglo-Saxon skin type.
UK/North Europe: Use total sunblock, or keep out of the sun.
USA/Tropics/Africa: Use total sunblock.
Mediterranean: Use total sunblock.
Skin-type 2: Burns easily and tans with difficulty. Fair hair and pale skin. Typical North European skin type.
UK/North Europe: Start with SPF 20 and use sunblock on delicate areas. Progress gradually to SPF 15.
USA/Tropics/Africa: Start with sunblock and progress gradually to SPF 20.
Mediterranean: Start with SPF 20, use sunblock on delicate areas, and progress gradually to SPF 15.

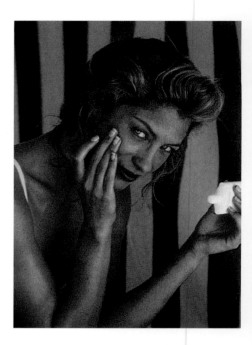

△ **If your skin is going to be exposed to the sun, make sure you apply plenty of sunscreen to protect it.**

Skin-type 3: Sometimes burns but tans well. Light brown hair and medium skin tone. Again, a typical North European skin type.
UK/North Europe: Start with SPF 10 and progress to SPF 8.
USA/Tropics/Africa: Start with SPF 20, moving to SPF 15, then SPF 10.
Mediterranean: Start with SPF 15, moving to SPF 10.
Skin-type 4: Occasionally burns but tans easily. Usually with brown hair and eyes, and olive skin. This is the typical Mediterranean skin type.
UK/North Europe: Start with SPF 8, moving to SPF 6.
USA/Tropics/Africa: Start with SPF 15, moving to SPF 8.
Mediterranean: Start with SPF 10, moving to SPF 6.
Skin-type 5: Hardly ever burns and tans very easily. Dark eyes, dark hair and olive skin. A

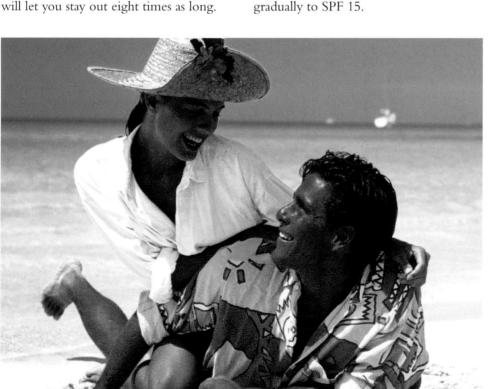

◁ **If you are out in the sun during the hottest part of the day, make sure you cover up with a shirt and a hat.**

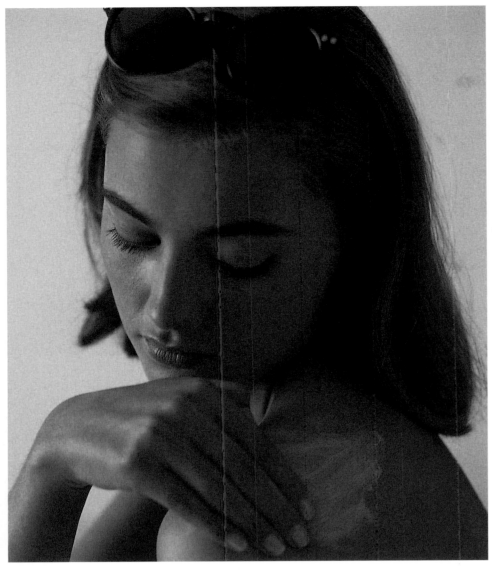

Always apply plenty of moisturizing after-sun lotion or a soothing oil preparation after a day in the sun.

55

complete bodycare

wash-off tanners

A quick way to create an instant tan on your face and body. Simply smooth on the cream, then wash it away at the end of the day.

self-tanners

If you haven't tried these formulations for years because you remember the awful smell, colour and streaky results, then you'll be pleasantly surprised at the improvements that have been made. In fact, choose carefully and you'll create an acceptable alternative to the real thing. These products contain an active ingredient called dihydroxyacetone (DHA), which is absorbed by surface skin cells and turns brown in the presence of oxygen, creating the "tan". This process usually takes 3–4 hours, and the effects last until these skin cells are naturally shed – which can be from a few days right up to a week.

self-tanning tips

• Use a body scrub first to rub away the dead flaky skin that can create a patchy finish.
• Massage plenty of body lotion into the area to be treated. This will combat any remaining dry areas, and give a smooth surface on which to apply the tanning lotion.
• If there's a shade choice, go with the lighter one, because you can always apply more to get a darker colour.
• Use a small amount of the product at a time – you can apply a second layer later.
• Work the product firmly into the skin until it feels completely dry. Any excess left on the surface is likely to go patchy.
• If you've applied self-tan to your body, wipe areas that don't normally tan with damp cotton wool (cotton) – armpits, nipples, soles of feet and fingers. On the face, work the cotton wool around eyebrows, hairline and jawline.
• While there are self-tanning products that offer some protection from the sun until you wash your skin, it's best to use them in conjunction with the best sunscreen for your skin type.

typical Middle Eastern or Asian skin type.
UK/North Europe: Use SPF 6 throughout.
USA/Tropics/Africa: Start with SPF 8 and move to SPF 6.
Mediterranean: Start with SPF 8 and move to SPF 6.
Skin-type 6: Almost never burns. Has dark hair, eyes and skin. Typical African or Afro-Caribbean skin type.
UK/North Europe: No sunscreen needed.
USA/Tropics/Africa: Start with SPF 8, moving to SPF 6.
Mediterranean: Use SPF 6 throughout.

safe tan plan

• Apply suntan lotion before you go into the sun, and before you dress, to ensure that you don't miss any areas.
• Gradually build up the time you spend in the sun. Never be tempted to stay in the sun so long that your skin burns – it's a sign of skin damage.
• Stay out of the sun between 12 noon and 3 o'clock when the sun is at its hottest. Move into the shade or cover up with a t-shirt and broad-brimmed hat.
• If you're playing a lot of sport or swimming, choose a special sports formula or waterproof formulation.
• Lips need a good lip screen to protect them from burning and chapping.
• If you have sensitive skin, there are hypo-allergenic products around, so ask your pharmacist.

fake tan plan

The safest tan of all is one that comes out of a bottle! There are three main ways to fake a tan.

bronzing powders

These are designed to be used on your face, and they act in the same way as a blusher. Make sure that the one you use is not too pearlized, or you'll shimmer a little too much in the sunshine.

Skincare glossary

If you are confused about the various claims and ingredients in your skincare products, check out what they mean here in our guide to the most commonly found skincare terms on bottles and jars.

Allergy-screened: This means that the individual ingredients in the product have gone through exacting tests to ensure that they're safe to use and that there's just the minimum risk of causing allergy.

Aloe vera: The juice from the leaves of this succulent plant is often used in skincare ingredients because of its soothing, protecting and moisturizing qualities.

Antioxidants: These work by mopping up and absorbing 'free radicals' from your skin. These highly reactive molecules can damage your skin and cause premature aging. Good antioxidants are the ACE vitamins, that is vitamins A, C and E.

Benzoyl peroxide: This is an ingredient commonly used in over-the-counter spot and acne treatments because it gently peels surface skin and unclogs blocked follicles, which can cause spots.

Cocoa butter: This comes from the seeds of the cacao tree in tropical climates. Cocoa butter is an excellent moisturizer, especially for dry skin on the body.

Collagen: Collagen is an elastic substance in the underlying tissues of your skin that provides support and springiness. Old collagen fibres are less elastic than young collagen, which is one of the main reasons why skin can become less springy as it ages. Collagen is a popular ingredient in skincare treatments, although it's doubtful if a molecule this size can penetrate the skin.

Dermatologically tested: This means the product has been patch-tested on a panel of human volunteers to monitor it for any tendency to cause irritation. This means it's usually suitable for sensitive skins.

Elastin: These are fibres in the underlying layer of your skin, rather like collagen, which help give it strength and elasticity.

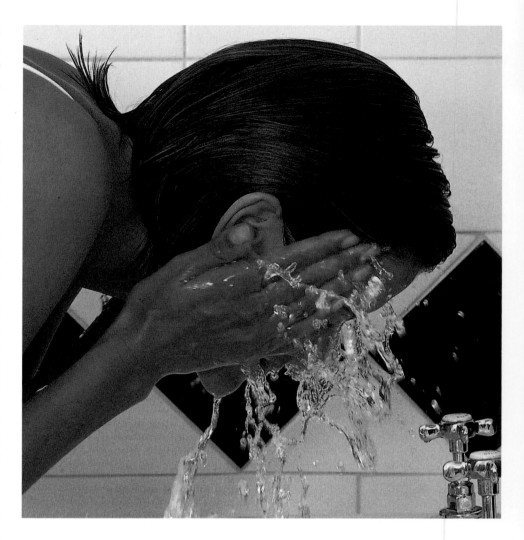

△ A pH-balanced facial wash will help prevent your skin from feeling tight.

Exfoliation: Exfoliating means whisking away the top surface layers of dead cells from your skin. This has the effect of making it look brighter and feeling smoother. To exfoliate, you massage a gritty exfoliating scrub over damp skin, then rinse it away with warm water.

Fruit acids: Also known as AHAs or alpha-hydroxy acids. They're commonly found in natural products such as fruit, sour milk and wine. AHAs are included in many face creams because they work by breaking down the protein bonds that hold together the dead cells on the skin's surface, to reveal newer, fresher skin underneath.

Humectants: These ingredients are often found in moisturizers, as they work by attracting moisture to themselves, and so keep the surface layers of your skin well hydrated.

Hypo-allergenic: These products are usually fragrance-free and contain the minimum of colouring agents and no known irritants or sensitizers. This is not a total guarantee that no one will have an allergic reaction to them. Some people are even allergic to water.

Jojoba oil: Jojoba is a liquid wax obtained from the seeds of a Mexican shrub. It was used for centuries by American Indians. It's a gentle, non-irritant oil that makes an excellent moisturizer as it is easily absorbed into the skin and helps improve the condition of the hair and scalp.

Lanolin-free: This means a product doesn't contain the ingredient lanolin – the fat stripped from sheep's wool. At one time it

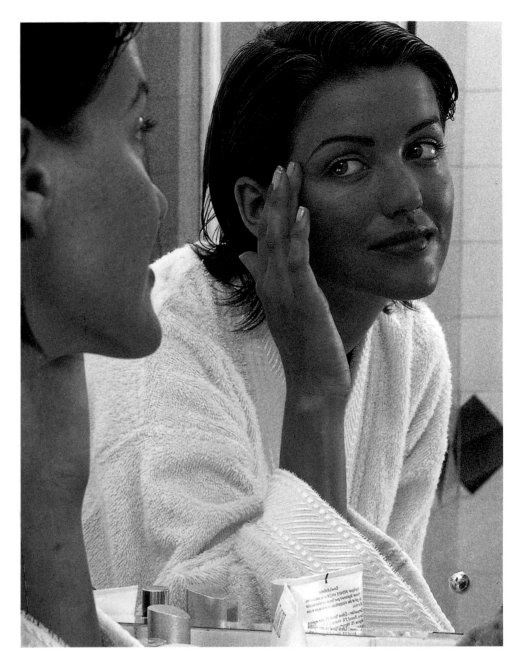

was thought that lanolin was a common skin allergen, although evidence does now seem to show that lanolin is even suitable for sensitive skins.

Liposomes: These are tiny fluid-filled spheres made of the same material that forms cell membranes. Their very small size is said to let them penetrate into the skin's living cells, where they act as delivery parcels and release their active ingredients.

Milia: Another word for whiteheads – small pimples on the skin. Oil produced from the sebaceous glands gathers to form a white plug, which is trapped under the skin. You can try to remove these by gentle squeezing with tissue-covered fingers or treat them with an antibacterial cream.

Non-comedogenic: A comedo is a blackhead, so this means the product has been screened to eliminate ingredients that can clog the follicles and encourage blackheads and spots. It's particularly useful for oily skins.

Oil of evening primrose: The oil taken from the seeds of the evening primrose plant is very useful for helping your skin retain its moisture. It's a wonderful moisturizer, particularly for dry or very dry skins, as it hydrates, protects and soothes. It also improves the skin's overall softness and suppleness. Many sufferers of eczema find it useful.

pH-balanced: The pH scale measures the acidity or alkalinity of a solution, with 7 meaning that it is neutral. Any number below that is acidic, and numbers above are alkaline. Healthy skin has a slightly acidic reading, so pH-balanced skincare products are slightly acidic to maintain this natural optimum level.

Retin A: Also known as Retinoic Acid, this is a derivative of vitamin A that has been used for years to treat acne. Now it's available on prescription, to be used under medical supervision, to help reverse the visible signs of ageing on the skin.

SPF: This stands for Sun Protection Factor. It will tell you how long the sun cream or moisturizer will protect you from the sun's

burning ultraviolet B rays. The higher the number, the more protection it will give.

T-zone: This is the area across the forehead and down the centre of the face where the oil glands and sweat glands of the face are most concentrated.

Ultraviolet (UV) rays: Ultraviolet light damages your skin. UVB rays will burn your skin if you sunbathe for too long. UVA rays are strong all year round and cause ageing and wrinkling of the skin. Guard against this with a broad-spectrum sun cream, which contains both UVA and UVB filters.

Vitamin E: This is often used in moisturizers because it can help combat dryness and the signs of ageing. It's also useful for helping to heal scars and burns.

Water-soluble: When they contain oils to dissolve grime and make-up from your

skin, cleansers are described as water-soluble, with the bonus that they can be quickly and easily rinsed away.

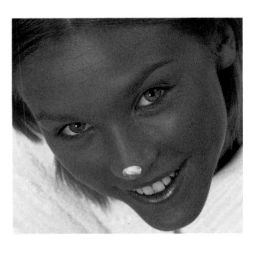

△ Discover the healing properties of vitamin E on your skin.

Make-up magic

The key to making-up successfully is to understand how to enhance your features using the best cosmetic formulations and colours. Buy the best products, brush up your techniques and experiment to find the perfect look.

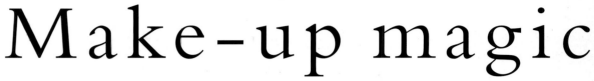

Make-up basics

Being considered beautiful today no longer means conforming to one accepted ideal. The contemporary approach to beauty places the emphasis firmly on the individual and her own particular needs, aspirations and lifestyle. For although every woman is concerned to some extent about how she looks, everyone is very different. For instance, the make-up needs of a blue-eyed blonde are not the same as those of a dark-eyed woman with an Oriental skin-tone.

The great news is that make-up can be used to enhance everyone's features. Applied with a sensitive touch it should create a subtle emphasis, rather than a mask disguising the features.

Many women are wary of cosmetics because they are not sure which colours suit them or which make-up methods and textures are the most flattering. Good make-up hinges on experience: you learn what suits you by trial and error. Nobody wants to waste money on a lipstick that turns out to be the wrong colour when you try it at home; but it's easy to get stuck in a rut – so be brave and experiment a little.

product know-how

No two women are alike. When we're buying a pair of jeans, we don't just pick the same size, colour and pair as our sister, because we have different requirements. Make-up is the same. We need to choose carefully from the vast array of products and formulations around to create a look that's made-to-measure for our own complexions and features. Simply buying the most expensive product on the shelves is no guarantee of success, as it may not be the most suitable for your colouring or skin type.

These pages will take you through the myriad bottles, compacts and colours, and show you how to find the ones that work best for you, and how to apply them.

tailor-made make-up

The perfect make-up for you will be effortless once you choose the correct shades for your skin tone and hair colour. It'll also work wonderfully, because you'll still look like you, only better! Checking your hair colour is easy – whether it's natural or comes out of a bottle. Deciding whether your skin is "warm" or "cool" seems slightly more difficult – however, there is an easy way to check. Simply look in a mirror and hold a piece of gold and a piece of silver in front of your face. These can just as easily be pieces of foil or costume jewellery as the real thing. The right metal will bring a healthy glow to your skin, whereas the wrong will make it look grey. If gold suits your skin, then it's "warm" toned. If silver suits it, it's "cool" toned. A further clue is how well you tan in the sun – cool skin tones tend to colour less easily.

inspirational ideas

Sometimes make-up should be used just for the sheer fun of it. Try out a different look for a special occasion, bringing out the

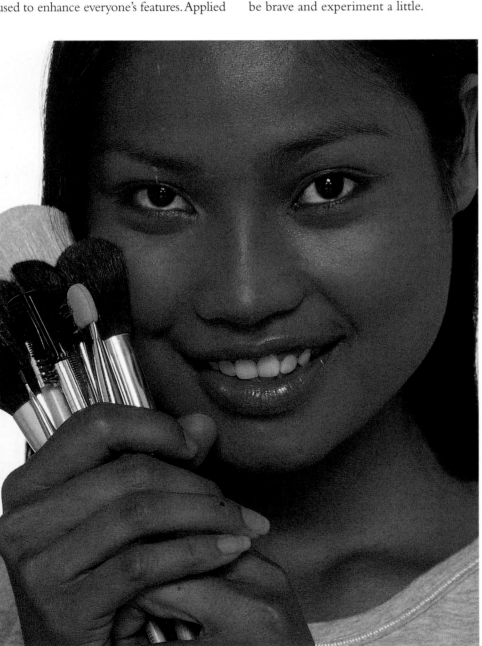

◁ **Every woman can use make-up to emphasize her best features.**

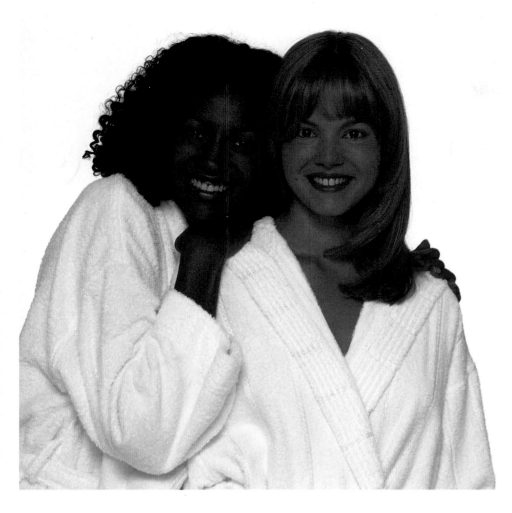

◁ We're all different. What works for one woman may not work for another. Understanding this helps you to bring out the best in yourself.

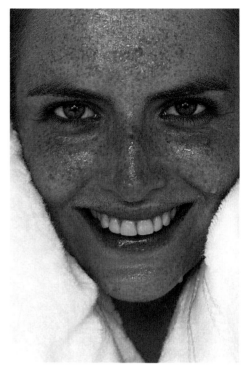

△ Take a close look at your face while you are washing or getting ready for bed. Which features would you like to enhance? Which would you like to play down?

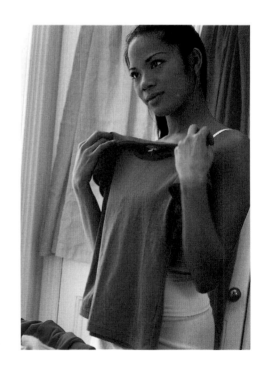

△ We already have a pretty good idea of colours that suit us, and it is important to work out what make-up colours and styles work best for you.

make-up artist in you. Whether you want to create an impact in the office or turn heads at a party, there are lots of ideas to help you put on the perfect face.

how to reassess your image

Take a careful look at your make-up bag or drawer. How old are the cosmetics? Six months, a year or more? Now study your face when you are wearing your usual make-up, and ask yourself what your make-up does for you: does it widen or narrow your eyes or mouth, enhance the shape of your face, make you look younger or older? If it does not produce the effect you require and your cosmetics are more than a year old, it is time for a complete change. Bear these points in mind:

Your age: Make-up that suited you when you were 25 is not going to look right 10 years down the line. Changes in skin tone and texture, as well as in hair colour, require different make-up shades and textures: the right make-up can take years off your face.

Your face shape and skin tone: Make-up can improve face shape by illusion; it can also improve skin tone and texture.

Your eye colour and size: Deftly applied make-up can make small eyes look bigger, blue eyes look bluer and round eyes look longer; can your current make-up do this for you?

Your hair colour: Make-up should complement hair; if your hair is jet black and your skin is pale, deep red lipstick and black eye make-up (mascara and kohl) look stunning. If you are blonde, earthy tones look best (the bright colours can be a bit brassy). If you have brown or black hair, you will have almost limitless colour freedom.

Your lifestyle: Make make-up easy; there is no point choosing make-up that requires a great deal of time to apply properly if you have a very busy lifestyle.

brush up your techniques

Don't just read about them but actually put new ideas into practice! Brush up on tips and tricks to help you maximize your looks, and deal with your own particular beauty needs. Perhaps you need a new look on a budget, speedy ideas or some expert help. The main thing is to spend a little time on making the most of yourself.

Foundation that fits

Many women avoid foundation because they're scared of an unnatural, mask-like effect. In fact, finding the right product for your skin is simpler than you might think. There are two keys to success: the first is to pick the right formulation, and the second is to choose the perfect shade for your skin.

find your formulation

Long gone are the days when you could only buy heavy pancake foundation. Now you can choose from many formulations, so you can get the best coverage for your particular skin type. Here are the products on offer, and who they're best for.

tinted moisturizers

These are a cross between a moisturizer and a foundation, as they'll soothe your skin while giving a little coverage. They're ideal for young or clear skins. They're also great in the summer, when you want a sheer effect or to even out a fading tan. Unlike other foundations, you can blend tinted moisturizers on with your fingertips.

liquid foundations

These are the most popular and versatile of all foundation types, because they smooth

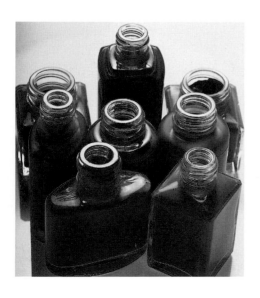

△ It is well worth spending time to find the right foundation colour for you.

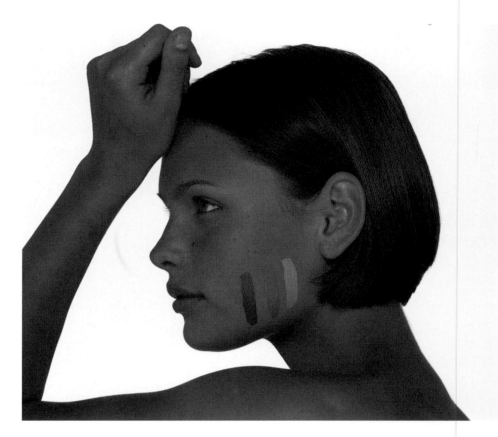

△ Before buying, check different foundation colours on your jawline for the perfect match.

on easily and offer natural-looking coverage. They suit all but the driest skins. If you have oily skin or suffer from occasional spot break-outs, look for an oil-free liquid foundation, to cover the affected areas without aggravating them.

cream foundations

These are thick, rich and moisturizing, making them ideal for dry or mature skins. As they have a fairly heavy texture, make sure you blend them well into your skin with a damp cosmetic sponge.

mousse foundations

Again these are quite moisturizing and ideal for drier skins. The best way is to dab a little of the product on to the back of your hand, then dot on to your skin with a sponge.

compact foundations

These are all-in-one formulations, which already contain powder. They come in a compact, usually with their own sponge for

application. However, they actually give a lighter finish than you'd expect. They're great on all but dry skin types.

stick foundations

These are the original foundation. They have a heavy texture, and so are best confined for use on badly blemished or scarred skin. Dot a little foundation directly on to the affected area, then blend gently with a damp sponge.

shade selection

Once you've chosen the ideal formulation for you, you're ready to choose the perfect matching shade to your skin. At last cosmetic companies have woken up to the fact that not everyone has an "American tan" complexion! Now, there is a good selection of foundation shades from a pink-toned English rose to a yellow-hued, olive

▷ Blend, blend, blend for a professional finish. And don't forget to give all angles of your face a final check in the mirror to make sure you haven't got any unnatural lines where your foundation finishes.

▽ Liquid foundations are popular because they provide natural-looking coverage.

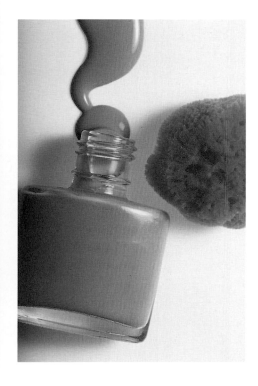

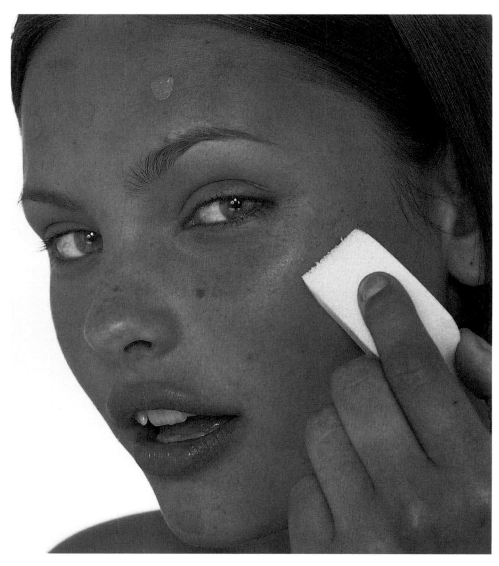

skin, as well as from the palest skin to the darkest one. There are some tried-and-tested methods for choosing the perfect one for your skin tone:

• Ensure you're in natural daylight when trying out foundation colours, so you can see exactly how your skin will look once you leave the shop or counter.

• Select a couple of shades to try that look as though they'll match your skin.

• Don't try foundation on your hand or on your wrist – they're a different colour to your face.

• Stroke a little colour on to your jawline to ensure you get a tone that will blend with your neck as well as your face. The shade that seems to "disappear" into your skin is the right one for you.

application know-how

Apply foundation to freshly moisturized skin to ensure you have a perfect base on which to work.

• Use a cosmetic sponge to apply most types

of foundation – using your fingertips can result in an uneven, greasy finish.

• Apply foundation in dots, then blend each one with your sponge.

• Dampen the sponge first of all, then squeeze out the excess moisture – this will prevent the sponge from soaking up too much costly foundation.

• Check for tell-tale "tidemarks" on your jawline, nose, forehead and chin.

high performance foundation

Companies these days have made great improvements to their foundations. Here are some benefits to look out for:

• Many companies have added sunscreens to their foundations, so they'll protect you from the ageing effects of the sun while you wear them. Look out for the words UV Protection and Sun Protection Factor (SPF) numbers on the tube or bottle.

• Look for the new "light-diffusing" foundations, which are great for older skins. They contain hundreds of tiny light-

reflective particles that bounce light away from your skin – making fine lines, wrinkles and blemishes less noticeable.

correct colour

You can wear a colour corrective foundation under your normal foundation to alter your skin-tone. They can seem quite strange at first glance but are, in fact, highly effective at toning down a high colour or boosting the colour of your complexion. Use them sparingly at first until you feel confident that you have achieved an effective, but subtle, result.

• Green foundation cools down rosiness and is great for those who blush easily.

• Lavender foundation will brighten up a sallow complexion, and is great for when you're feeling tired.

• Apricot foundation will give a subtle glow to dull skin, and is a great beauty booster in the winter.

• White foundation gives a wonderful glow to all complexions, and is perfect for a special night out.

Clever concealer

Concealers are a fast and effective way to disguise blemishes, shadows, scars and red veins, so your skin looks perfect.

find your formulation

Concealers are concentrated foundation with a high pigment content, giving complete coverage to problem areas. Make-up artists argue as to whether concealer should be applied before or after foundation. Applying it after foundation is often best, as it's applied to specific areas which would be disturbed when the foundation was applied. If you're after a light effect, apply concealer to clean skin, then apply powder or all-in-one foundation/powder on top.

stick concealers

These are easy to apply as you can simply stroke them straight on to the skin. Some have quite a thick consistency, so it's worth trying samples before buying.

cream concealers

These usually come in a tube, with a sponge-tipped applicator. The coverage isn't as thick as the stick type, but the finished effect is natural.

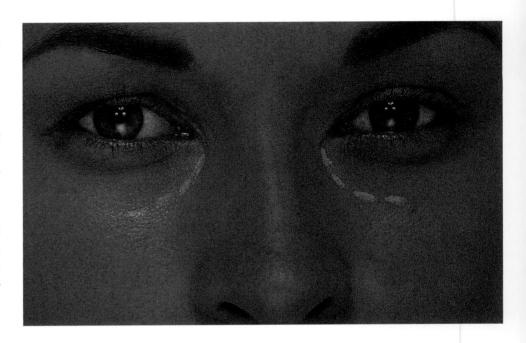

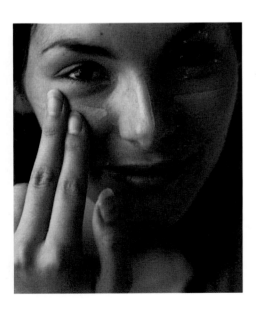

△ **Cream concealer is easier to apply smoothly on larger areas.**

liquid concealers

Again, these come in a tube. Just squeeze a tiny amount on to your finger and smooth over the affected area. Look for the cream-to-powder formulations, which slick on like a cream and dry to a velvety powder finish.

taking cover

Here's how to conceal all your beauty problems effectively.

spots and blemishes

The ideal solution is to use a medicated stick concealer as this contains ingredients to deal with the pimple or blemish as well as cover it. Only apply the concealer on the pimple or blemish, as it can be quite drying, and then smooth away the edges with a clean cotton bud (swab). Applying concealer all around the area will make the spot more noticeable.

> **CONCEALER TIP**
> When choosing a concealer look for the colour that is nearest your own skin tone rather than a lighter one. Covering a problem area with a paler shade will simply accentuate it.

△ **If you have noticeable shadows under your eyes, you can tone them down very effectively with a few dots of concealer.**

under-eye shadows

Opt for a creamy stick concealer or a liquid one, as dry formulations emphasize fine lines around your eyes. If you're blending with your fingertips, use your ring finger, as this is the weakest finger and less likely to drag at the delicate skin around your eyes.

scars

Scars, including old acne or chickenpox marks, can be effectively covered using a concealer but it can be a time-consuming process. Begin by building the indentation up to skin level by dotting on layers of concealer. This is best applied using a fine brush. Take your time and allow each layer to settle into the skin properly.

red veins

Stick or liquid concealer is ideal for tackling this problem. Apply a layer of concealer over the area with a fine eyeliner brush or clean cotton bud, then carefully feather and soften the edges to blend them in and make them less noticeable.

The power of powder

Face powder is the make-up artist's best friend, as it can make your skin look really wonderful and is very versatile in its uses.

why use powder

Here are four good reasons for putting on that powder!
• Powder gives a super-smooth sheen to your skin – with or without foundation.
• It "sets" your foundation, so it stays put and looks good for longer.
• Powder absorbs oils from your skin, and helps prevent shiny patches appearing.
• It helps conceal open pores.

choose your powder

You'll need two types of powder – a loose form at home, and a powder compact for your handbag.

loose powder

This gives the best and longest-lasting finish and is the choice of professional make-up artists and models. The best way to apply loose powder is to dust it lightly on to your skin using a large, soft powder brush. Then lightly brush over your face again to dust off the excess.

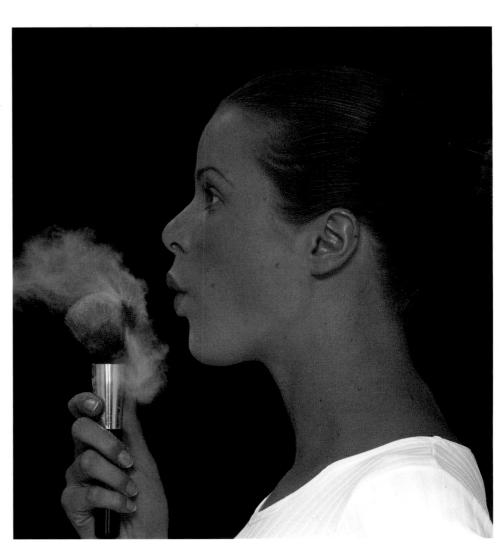

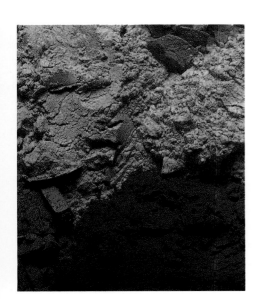

△ Take time to experiment so you choose the shade that best suits your colouring.

pressed powder

Compacts containing pressed powder are ideal for carrying in your make-up bag as they're very quick to use and lightweight. Most come with their own application sponges, but you'll find you get a better result if you apply them with a brush. Look for brushes with retractable heads to carry in your make-up bag.

If you do use the sponge, use a light touch and wash it regularly, or you'll transfer the oils in your skin on to the powder and get a build-up.

shade away

Don't make the mistake of thinking that one shade of powder suits all. Instead, choose one that closely matches your skin-

△ Careful application of the right powder as the final finishing and fixing touch should give your skin a soft, glowing and natural feel.

> **POWDER TIP**
> When dusting excess powder away from your skin, use your brush in light, downward strokes to help prevent the powder from getting caught in the fine hairs on your skin. Pay particular attention to the sides of the face and jawline which aren't so easy for you to see.

tone for a natural effect. Do this by dusting a little on your jawline, in the same way as you would with foundation.

Beautiful blusher

Give your complexion a bloom of colour with this indispensable beauty aid.

blush baby

Blusher is an instant way to give your looks a lift. It's old-fashioned to use blusher to sculpt your face, as it looks so unnatural. Instead, it should be applied in the way it was first intended to be used – to recreate a youthful flush.

powder blusher

This should be applied over the top of your foundation and face powder. To apply powder blusher, dust over the compact with a large soft brush. If you've taken too much on to your brush, tap the handle on the back of your hand to remove the excess. It's better to waste a little blusher than to apply too much! A good guide is to use half as much blusher and twice as much blending as you first think you need.

Start applying the colour on the fullest parts of your cheeks, directly below the centre of your eyes. Then smile and dust the blusher over your cheekbones and up towards your temples. Blend the colour well towards the hairline, so you avoid harsh edges. This will effectively place colour where you would naturally blush.

cream blusher

Breaking all the traditional beauty rules, cream blusher is applied with your fingertips. It's put on after foundation and before face powder. It drops out of fashion from time to time, but it's never long before it makes a comeback. This is for good reason, as it can give a lovely fresh glow to every skin type.

To apply, dab a few dots of cream blusher over your cheeks, from the plump part up towards your cheekbone. Using your fingertips, blend well. Build up the effect gradually, adding more blusher to create just the look you want. Or, if you prefer, you can use a foundation wedge to blend in cream blusher.

colour choice

There is a kaleidoscope of blusher shades to choose from. However, as a rule, it's best to opt for a shade that tones well with your skin colouring, and co-ordinates with the rest of your make-up. You can opt for lighter or darker shades, depending on the season.

Blusher colour guide

COLOURING	CHOOSE
Blonde hair, cool skin	Baby pink
Blonde hair, warm skin	Tawny pink
Dark hair, cool skin	Cool rose
Dark hair, warm skin	Rosy brown
Red hair, cool skin	Soft peach
Red hair, warm skin	Warm peach
Dark hair, olive skin	Warm brown
Black hair, dark skin	Terracotta

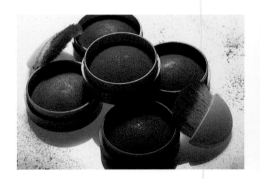

△ **Powder blusher is a quick and easy option.**

▽ **Be a blushing beauty with a light touch of powder blusher (left). Or go for more of a glow with cream blusher (right).**

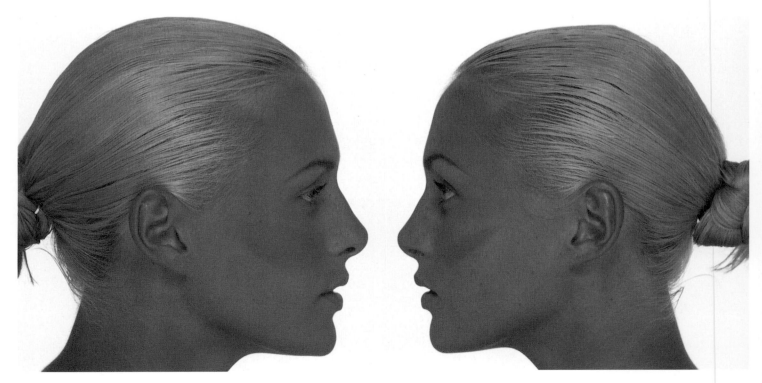

Brush up your make-up

Even the most expensive make-up in the world won't look particularly great if it's applied carelessly and using your fingertips.

basic tools

For a professional finish you need the right tools. This means investing in a set of good brushes and applicators.

make-up sponge

Have a wedge-shaped one, so you can use the finer edges to help blend in foundation round your nose and jawline, and the flatter edges for the cheeks, forehead and chin. However, if you prefer not to use a synthetic sponge try the small, natural ones instead. Remember to use it damp, not dry.

powder brush

Get used to using a powder brush each time you put make-up on. To prevent a caked or clogged finish to your face powder, use a large, soft brush to dust away any excess.

blusher brush

Use to add a pretty glow to your skin with a light dusting of powder blusher. A blusher brush is slightly smaller than a powder brush to make it easier to control.

eyeshadow brush

Smooth on any shade of eyeshadow with this brush.

eyeshadow sponge

A sponge applicator is great for applying a sweep of pale eyeshadow that doesn't need much blending, or for applying highlighter to your brow bones.

all-in-one eyelash brush/comb

Great for combing through your lashes between coats of mascara for a clump-free finish. Flip the comb over and use the brush side to sweep your eyebrows into shape, or soften pencilled-in brows.

lip brush

Create a perfect outline and then use it to fill in the shape with your lipstick.

eyebrow tweezers

It is essential to have a good pair of tweezers for regularly tidying up the eyebrows.

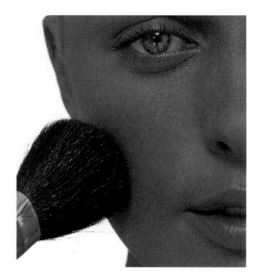

△ **Use a big soft brush to blend the colour on to your cheeks.**

eyelash curlers

Once used, they'll soon become a beauty essential! Curlier eyelashes make a huge difference to the way your lashes look and help open up the eyes.

▽ **Bring out the creative make-up artist in you with a good-quality set of brushes and a basic make-up tool kit.**

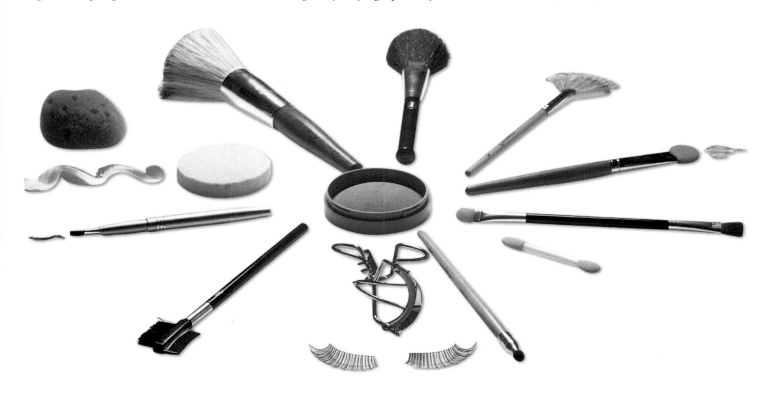

Eye-catching make-up

Eye make-up is the most popular type of cosmetic, and for good reason. Just the simplest touch of mascara can open up your eyes, while a splash of colour can transform them instantly. Whatever your eye shape and colour, you can take steps to ensure that they always look stunning.

mastering the basics

Many women hesitate to experiment with eye make-up, because it seems too time-consuming and complicated. The sheer quantity of products on the shelves and make-up counters can make it even more intimidating. However, you can create a huge variety of looks – from the simplest to the most extreme – by opening your eyes to the basic techniques.

eyebrow know-how

Many women tend to ignore their eyebrows completely. Or sometimes, which is usually even worse, they will overpluck them. When it comes to eye make-up, the eyebrows make a very important impression. They can provide a balanced look to your face so it's well worth making the effort to master the techniques and to get them looking right.

natural brows

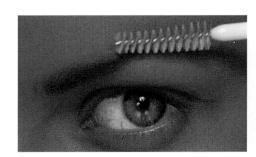

△ For perfectly groomed brows in an instant, try combing through them with a brush to flick away any powder or foundation. Comb the hairs upwards and outwards. This will also help give you a wide-eyed look. Then lightly slick them with clear gel to hold the shape in place.

lining up liner

Eyeliner can be applied to flatter all eye shapes and sizes. If you have never applied eyeliner before, try this straightforward technique. Sit down in front of a mirror in a good light. Take your eyeliner in your hand and rest your elbow on the table to keep your arm and hand steady. You might want to give yourself extra support by resting your little finger on your cheek. Eyeliner should be applied after eyeshadow and before mascara.

liquid liners

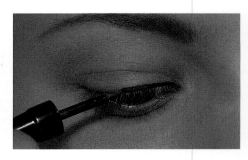

△ These have a fluid consistency, and usually come with a brush attached to the cap. To apply, look down into a mirror to prevent smudging. Stay like this for a few seconds after applying to give it time to dry.

pencil liners

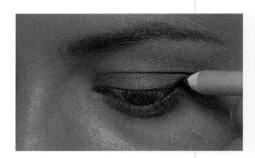

△ This is the easiest way, and one of the most effective, to add extra emphasis to your eyes. Using a pencil, carefully draw a soft line, keeping close to your upper lashes, then repeat under your lower lashes.

define your eyebrows with powder or pencil colour

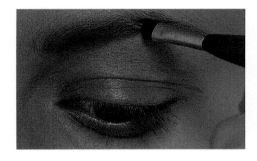

△ **1** To define your brows you can use eyebrow powder or pencil. Apply powder with an eyebrow brush, dusting it through your brows and taking care not to sweep it on to the surrounding skin. This gives a natural effect, and requires little blending.

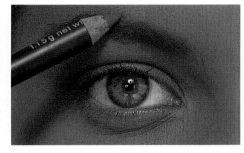

△ **2** Alternatively, use a well-sharpened pencil to draw on tiny strokes, taking care not to press too hard or the finished effect will be unnatural.

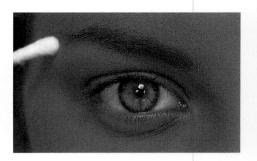

△ **3** Then soften the lines you've made with the eye pencil by lightly stroking a clean cotton bud (swab) through your brows.

false eyelashes

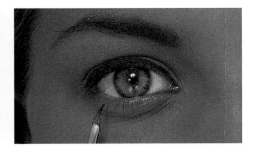

△ These luscious lashes are great for party looks but they can be tricky to apply. The strip lashes can look too obvious unless you apply them perfectly. It's a better idea to use the individual lashes on the outer corners of your eyes. Dot the roots with a little glue, then use a pair of tweezers to position them exactly.

magic mascara

Mascara creates a flattering fringe to your eyes – particularly if your lashes are fair. Most mascaras are applied with spiral wands that are quick and easy to use. Some contain fibres to add length and thickness. Opt for a waterproof variety to withstand tears, showers and swimming – but remember you'll need a special eye make-up remover as it clings more fiercely to your lashes.

EYEING UP EYESHADOWS

Choose neutral colours to enhance your looks subtly, or play with a kaleidoscope of different shades.

• **powder eyeshadows**: The most popular type, these come in pressed cakes of powder either with a small brush or a sponge applicator. You can build up their density from barely-there to dramatic. Apply using a damp brush or sponge if you want a deep colour for an evening look.

• **cream shadows**: These are oil-based and come in little pots or compacts. They're applied with either a brush or fingertips. They're a good choice for dry or older skins that need extra moisturizing.

• **stick shadows**: These are wax-based and smoothed on to eyelids from the stick. Ensure they have a creamy texture before you buy, so they won't drag at your skin.

• **liquid shadows**: Usually these come in a slim bottle with a sponge applicator. Look out for the cream-to-powder ones that smooth on as a liquid and then blend to a velvety powder finish.

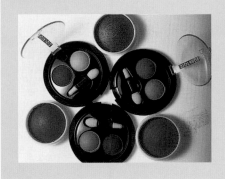

eyeshadow as eyeliner

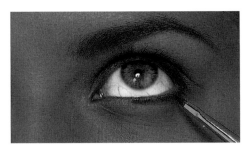

△ **1** Make-up artists often use eyeshadow to outline the eyes, and it's a trick worth stealing! It looks very effective because it gives a soft smoky effect. Use a small brush to apply shadow under your lower lashes and to make an impact over the top of the eyelid, taking care to keep the shadow close to the eyelashes.

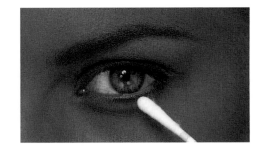

△ **2** To create an even softer effect, simply sweep over the eyeshadow liner with a cotton bud.

simple steps for creating perfect lashes

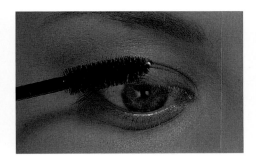

△ **1** Start by applying mascara to your upper lashes. Brush them downwards to start with, then brush them upwards from underneath. Use a tiny zig-zag movement to prevent mascara from clogging on your lashes.

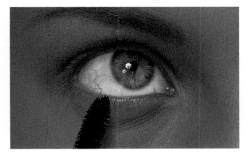

△ **2** Next, use the tip of the mascara wand to brush your lower lashes, using a gentle side-to-side technique. Take care to keep your hand steady while you are applying the mascara, and don't blink while the mascara is still wet.

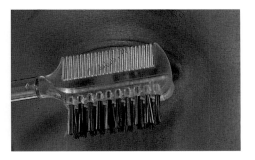

△ **3** Comb through your lashes with an eyelash comb to remove any excess, and to prevent your lashes from clumping. For a more defined effect, repeat the two previous steps twice more, allowing each layer of mascara to dry before applying the next.

Eye make-up masterclass

Now that you know where to start and have mastered the basic techniques, you can begin to experiment with more sophisticated eye make-up methods to create a variety of stunning looks.

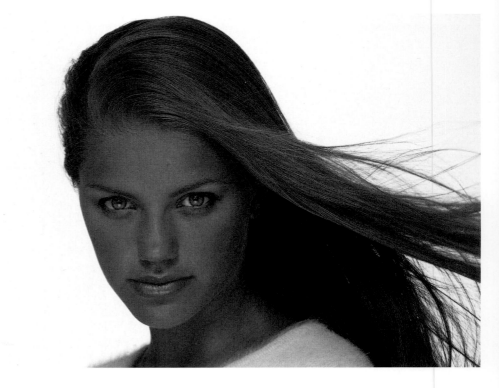

step-by-step to beautiful eyes

Here's a look you can try, using a wide range of techniques to create the ultimate in glamorous eye make-up.

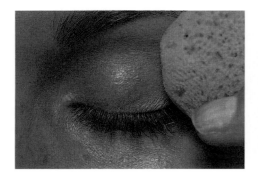

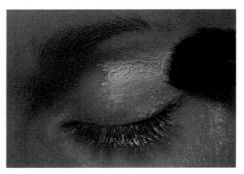

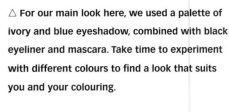

△ **For our main look here, we used a palette of ivory and blue eyeshadow, combined with black eyeliner and mascara. Take time to experiment with different colours to find a look that suits you and your colouring.**

△ **1** Smooth over your eyelids with foundation to create an even base on which to work, and to give your eye make-up something to cling to.

△ **2** Sweep over your eyelids with a brush loaded with translucent face powder.

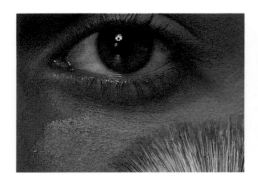

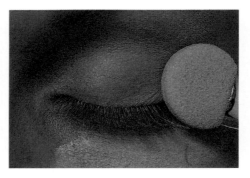

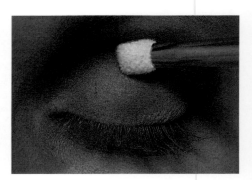

△ **3** Dust a little translucent powder under your eyes to catch any flecks of fallen eyeshadow. Use a very soft brush for this.

△ **4** Use a sponge applicator to sweep a neutral ivory shade over your eyelids. Work it right up towards your eyebrows for a balanced overall effect.

△ **5** Smudge a brown eyeshadow into the socket line of your eyes, using a sponge applicator. A slightly shimmery powder is easier to blend on.

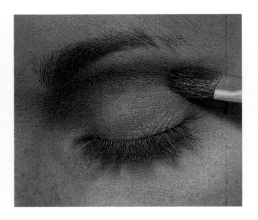

△ **6** Use a brush to sweep over the top of the brown shadow as this will remove any harsh edges.

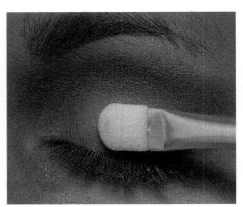

△ **7** To create a perfectly blended finish, sweep some more ivory shadow over the edges of the brown eyeshadow using a sponge applicator.

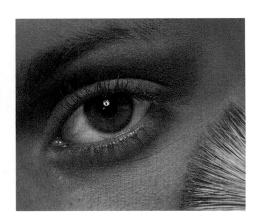

△ **8** Now that you've completed your eyeshadow, flick away the powder from under your eyes.

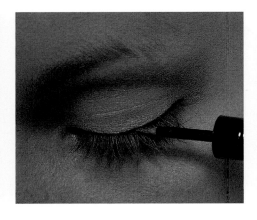

△ **9** Looking down into a mirror and keeping your hand as steady as possible, apply liquid eyeliner along your eyelid.

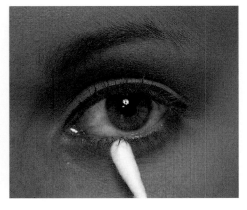

△ **10** Use a clean cotton bud (swab) to work some brown eyeshadow under your lower lashes to add some subtle definition.

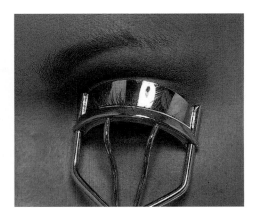

△ **11** Squeeze your lashes with eyelash curlers to make them bend, before applying mascara. This will "open up" the eye area.

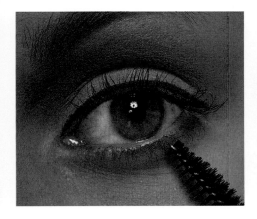

△ **12** Apply mascara to your upper lashes and then use the tip of the mascara wand to coat your lower lashes.

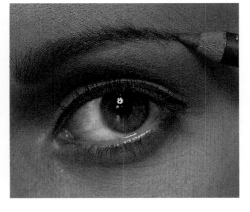

△ **13** Stroke your eyebrows with pencil to shape them and fill in any patches.

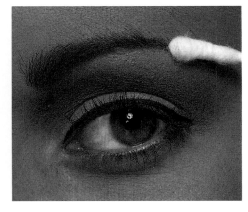

△ **14** Smooth over the top with a cotton bud to soften the eyebrow pencil line.

Lipstick colour

Lipstick has been around for about 5,000 years, and women have always loved using it. It is the easiest and quickest way to give your face a focus and an instant splash of colour.

a lick of colour

Lipsticks in a bullet form are the most popular way to use lip colour. The more pigment a lipstick has, the longer it'll last on your lips. The best way to apply lipstick is with a lip brush.

Another way of applying a touch of colour is with a lip gloss. This can be used alone to give your lips an attractive sheen, or applied over the top of lipstick to catch the light.

Lip liners are used to provide an outline to your lips before applying lipstick. You can also use them over your entire lip for a dark, matte effect. However, you may need to add a touch of lipsalve (balm) over the top to prevent drying out this delicate area of skin. It is particularly important because this area of skin is prone to developing fine lines.

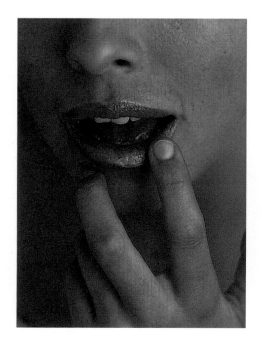

△ **Tinted lip gloss helps to keep lips soft and supple and gives your lips a hint of colour. Use it on its own, or under or over your lipstick.**

step-by-step to perfect lips

Follow this simple guide to apply a perfect layer of luscious colour to your lips.

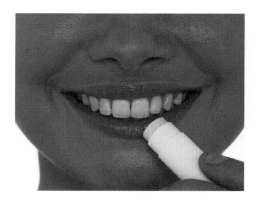

△ **1** Ensure your lips are soft and supple by smoothing over some lipsalve before you start.

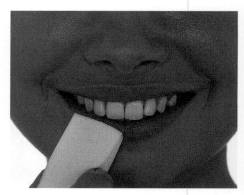

△ **2** Prime your lips with foundation, using a make-up sponge so you reach every crevice on the surface.

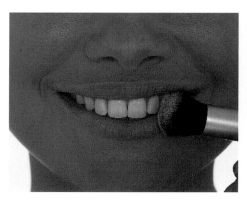

△ **3** Lightly dust over the top of the foundation with your usual face powder, to ensure your lipstick will stay put for longer.

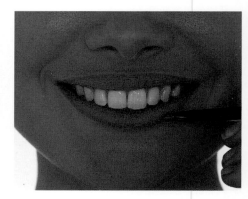

△ **4** Rest your elbow on a firm surface and draw an outline with a lip pencil. Start with a Cupid's bow on the upper lip, then draw an outline on your lower lip.

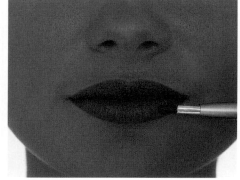

△ **5** Use a lip brush to fill the outline with lipstick; this helps get a more precise definition. Open your mouth to brush the colour into the corners of your lips.

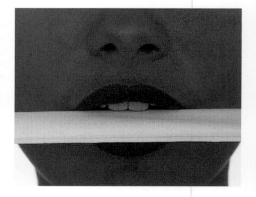

△ **6** You'll make your lipstick last longer if you blot over the surface with a tissue. It'll also give an attractive, semi-matte finish to your lips.

SPECIAL INGREDIENTS

Today's lipsticks offer more than just a pigment to add colour to your lips. In just the same way as technology has been used in skincare products, lipsticks often contain other specially developed ingredients so that they provide optimum care for the delicate skin on your lips. Here are some of the extra ingredients that may be included in your lipstick:

• Vegetable wax to make your lipstick easier to apply smoothly, and to give your lips a natural soft sheen.
• Liposomes containing active moisturizing ingredients, to keep your lips soft.
• Chamomile to soothe and heal the skin on your lips.
• Shea butter to deep-moisturize your lips, especially in extremes of weather and wind, which can have drastic effects.
• Silicas to help give your lipstick a slightly matte effect.
• UV filters to protect your lips from the aging effects of the sun's rays.
• Vitamin E to help heal any cuts, and protect your lips against the fine lines associated with aging.

lavender lip balm

ingredients

• 5ml/1 tsp beeswax
• 5ml/1 tsp cocoa butter
• 5ml/1 tsp wheatgerm oil
• 5ml/1 tsp almond oil
• 3 drops lavender essential oil

Put all the ingredients, except the lavender oil, in a small bowl. Then set the bowl over a pan of simmering water and keep stirring the mixture until the wax has melted. Remember that beeswax has a high melting point so you will need to be patient. Remove from the heat and allow the mixture to cool for a few minutes before adding the lavender oil. Pour into a small jar and leave to set.

▷ **This sweet-scented lavender lip balm is a natural way to soothe and condition your lips.**

Lipstick colour coding

Believe it or not, everyone can wear red lipstick. The key to success is to choose just the right shade for your colouring.

COLOURING	CHOOSE
Blonde hair, cool skin	If you're daring enough you can wear any bright red shade, such as crimson or fire-engine red. Any bold shade will look really effective and striking on you.
Blonde hair, warm skin	Lovely pink-reds look great with your colouring. They're delicate enough not to look too harsh, while the pinky undertones complement the warmth of your skin.
Dark hair, cool skin	Rich blue reds, such as wine, burgundy and blood-red, look wonderful on your China-doll features. The contrast of dark hair, pale skin and red lips is really stunning!
Dark hair, warm skin	Rich brick reds and ruby jewel-like shades suit you. Their warmth is very flattering to your complexion, while the intensity of colour looks great against your hair.
Red hair, cool skin	A delicate orange-red, a paler version of the one mentioned above, will add a splash of colour without overpowering you.
Red hair, warm skin	Warm, fiery reds with brown undertones will complement your rich hair colour and rosy skin.
Dark hair, olive skin	Rich red with orange undertones will flatter your skin. Go for a bold colour, as you can carry it off.
Black hair, brown skin	Berry reds and burgundy reds look wonderful on your skin.

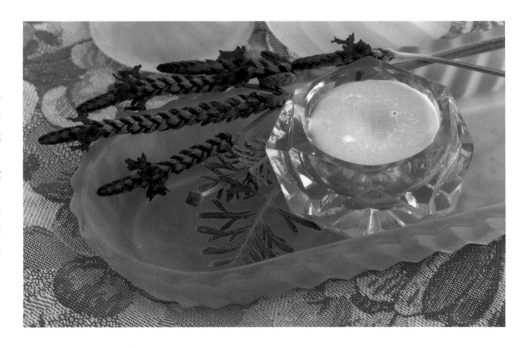

Beautiful nails

Regular care and a little manual labour is all it takes to have nails that you will want to show off, rather than ones you want to hide away.

laying the foundations for healthy nails

There's no point in slicking your nails with colour if they're not in good condition to start with. Following this advice will ensure that they're ultra-tough.

filing know-how

Keep your nails slightly square or oval – not pointed – to prevent them from breaking. Filing low into the corners and sides can weaken nails. File gently in one long stroke, from the side to the centre of the nail. The classic length that suits most hands is just over the fingertip.

condition-plus

Smooth your nails every evening with a nourishing oil or conditioning cream. This helps seal moisture into your nails to prevent flaking and splitting. A tiny drop of olive oil is a great cheap alternative.

cuticle care

Go carefully with tough or overgrown cuticles. Most manicurists are against cutting them with scissors, as this can lead to infection. Instead, soak your nails in warm soapy water to soften the cuticles. Then

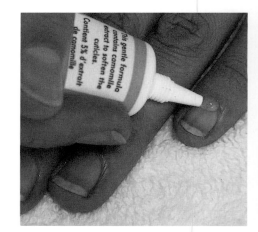

△ **Soften cuticles with a cream or gel before pushing them back.**

smooth them with a little cuticle softening cream or gel, before gently pushing them back with a manicure hoof stick or clean cotton bud (swab). You can then gently scrub away the flakes of dead skin that are still clinging to the nail bed.

colour coding

• If you have long, elegant fingers you can carry off any shade, including the dramatic deep reds, russets and burgundies. Short nails look best with pale or beige-toned polish.

• Pale colours also suit broad nails, but you can make them look narrower by leaving a little space at the sides of each nail unpainted.

• If you love barely-there shades for the daytime, but prefer something more exotic at night, try a pale pearlized polish – the shimmer will be caught by the evening light.

• If you find strong colours too bold on your fingers, try painting your toenails instead. A glimpse of colour in open-toed shoes or on bare feet can look sophisticated. You can create a great look by mixing a little dark red and black nail polish before applying.

• Coral polish and pearlized formulations work very well against a tanned skin.

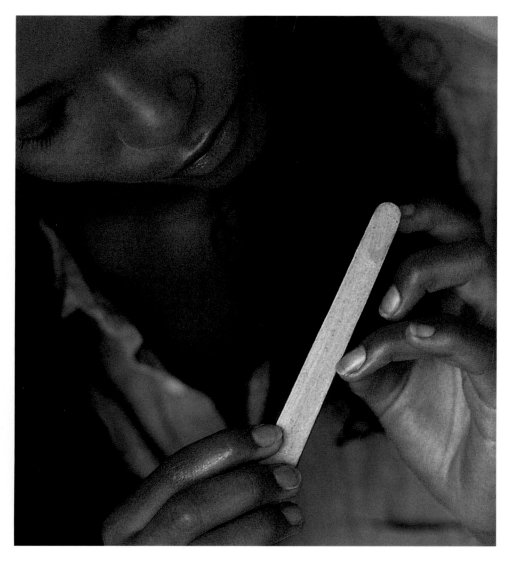

◁ **Fingernails should be filed regularly. To minimize breakage, file them straight across with a soft emery board.**

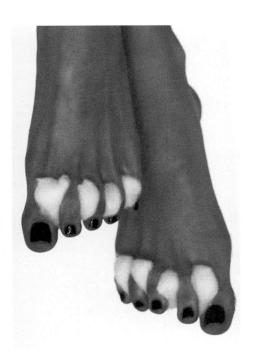

◁ **Use pieces of cotton wool (cotton) between your toes, to keep them apart while you are painting them.**

the French manicure

This is a popular look because it makes all lengths of nail look clean and healthy. It combines white tips with a pink polish over the entire nail. It is suitable for all occasions, from an ultra-natural to a glamorous look. It does take a little practice at first, but it's worth persevering. There are also special kits that contain all you need to get it right.

> **BEAUTIFUL NAIL TIP**
> The key to this look is to be very patient! It is important that you wait for each coat to dry thoroughly before applying the next one. If you rush the stages and apply the coats too quickly, the manicure will not be perfect because you are sure to end up with smudges and a rather messy finish.

top 10 nail tips

1 Avoid using acetone nail polish removers, as these can strip your nails of essential moisture. Choose the conditioning variety of nail polish remover instead.

2 Apply hand cream every time you wash your hands. The oils in the cream will seal moisture into your skin.

3 The most common cause of soft nails is exposure to water, so wear rubber gloves when doing the dishes.

4 If you have very weak nails, try painting your base coat and nail polish under the tip of your nails to give them extra strength.

5 Dry wet nails in an instant by plunging them into ice-cold water.

6 To repair a split nail, tear a little paper from a teabag or coffee filter paper and glue it over the tear with nail glue. Once it's dry, buff until smooth, and then apply your polish on top.

7 If you're planning to do some gardening or messy work, drag your nails over a bar of soap. The undersides of your nails will fill up with soap, and dirt won't be able to get in.

8 Clean ink and stains from your fingertips by using a toothbrush and toothpaste on the affected areas.

9 Never file your nails immediately after a bath, as this is when they're at their weakest and most likely to split.

10 Use a cotton bud with a pointed end to clean under your nails – it's gentler than scrubbing with a nail brush.

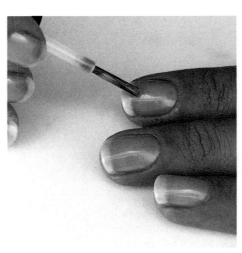

△ **1** Apply a clear base coat to protect your nails and help to prevent chipping.

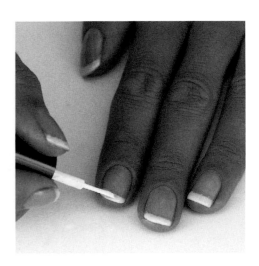

△ **2** Apply two thin coats of white polish to the tips of your nails. Try to apply it in one long stroke, working from one side of your nail to the other.

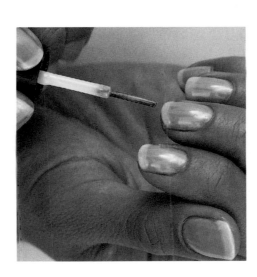

△ **3** Allow the white polish to dry completely, then apply a coat of pink polish over the entire nail. If you like a very natural finish, apply just one coat of pink polish; if you prefer a bolder effect, apply two coats.

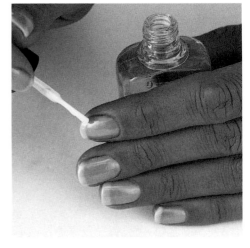

△ **4** Apply a clear top coat over the entire nail for added protection.

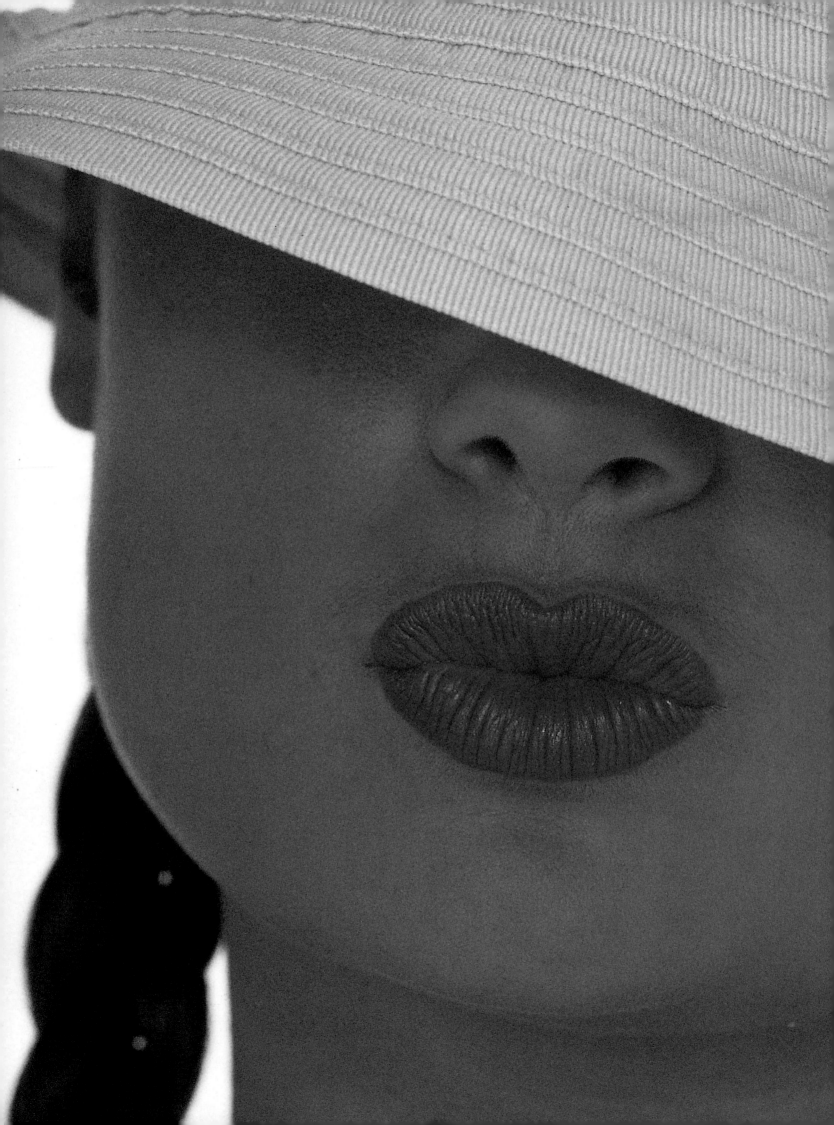

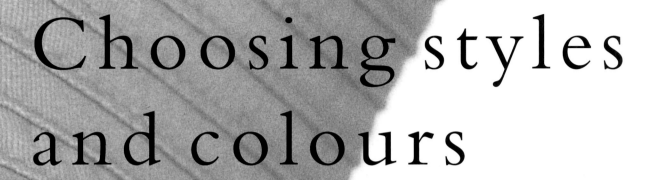

Choosing styles and colours

Every woman can use make-up to enhance her looks, but individual make-up needs will differ from woman to woman. This chapter offers fresh and inspiring ideas to help you find a look to suit you.

Cool skin, blonde hair

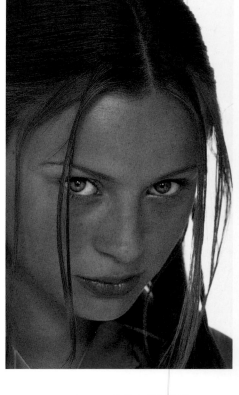

With your porcelain complexion and pale hair, you should opt for baby pastel tones with sheer formulations and a hint of shimmer. This flatters your colouring with a light, fresh make-up look, without overpowering it.

this look suits you if ...

• You have pale blonde to mousey or mid-blonde hair. It also suits women with white or steel-grey hair.
• Your eyes are blue, grey, hazel or green.
• You have pale skin, including whiter-than-white, ivory or a pinky "English rose" style of complexion.

▷ **These subtle pastels and shimmering shades flatter your cool, pale colouring for a soft yet vibrant look.**

EYESHADOW TIPS
• If you're over 35 or unsure about wearing blue eyeshadow, swap it for a cool grey shade. This will create the same soft effect, but it's slightly more subtle.
• Shimmery eyeshadow can highlight crêpey eyelids, so you may prefer to use a matte ivory shadow instead.

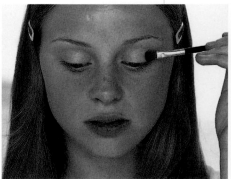

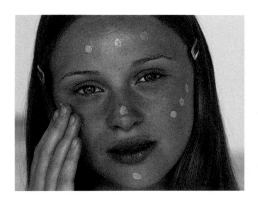

△**1** Your delicate skin doesn't need heavy coverage, so use a light tinted moisturizer. Dot it on to your nose, cheeks, forehead and chin, then blend it in with your fingertips.

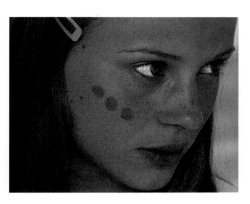

△ **2** Cool pink cream blusher will give your skin a soft glow. Dot on to your cheeks, then blend in with your fingertips. You can either skip powder to leave your skin with a dewy glow, or dust a little over your face. However, use a gentle touch, as you want to let your natural skin tone shine through.

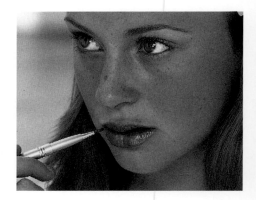

△**3** Take some baby blue eyeshadow on to an eyeshadow brush and sweep it evenly over your entire eyelid. Stroke the brush gently over your eyelid a few times until you've swept away any obvious edges to the colour. Also work a little eyeshadow under your lower lashes.

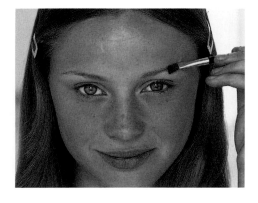

△ **4** Sweep a shimmery ivory shadow from the crease of your eyelid up towards the brow bone. Finish with two coats of brown/black mascara.

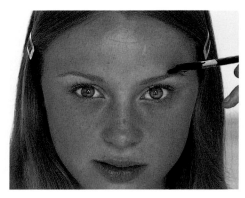

△ **5** Stroke your eyebrows into shape with an eyebrow brush. This will also flick away any powder that's got caught in the hairs.

△ **6** Cool pink lipstick should be applied with a lip brush. If you like, you can slick a little lipgloss or lip balm on top for a sexy shimmer.

Warm skin, blonde hair

Although you have a warm skin tone, your overall look is quite delicate. This means you should opt for tawny, neutral shades of make-up, and apply them with a light touch so you enhance your basic colouring.

this look suits you if …

• You have golden, warm blonde or dark blonde hair. This look also suits women with greying hair that has warm or yellow undertones.

• Your eyes are brown, blue, hazel or green.

• You have a warm skin tone that can develop a light, golden tan.

• Your skin tone and blonde hair mean your colouring is quite delicate. If so, you need to choose make-up shades that are not too intense, such as those shown here.

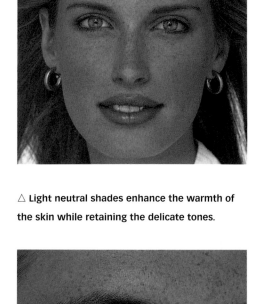

△ **Light neutral shades enhance the warmth of the skin while retaining the delicate tones.**

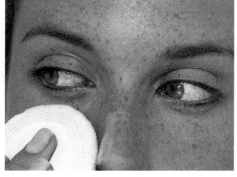

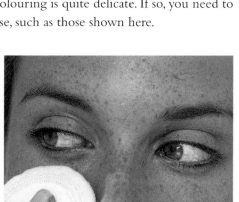

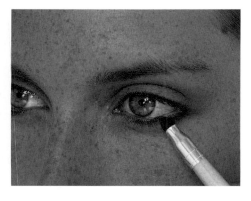

△ **1** After applying a light tinted moisturizer, stroke concealer on to problem areas. Blondes tend to have fine skin, often prone to surface thread veins. Cover these effectively with concealer, applied with a clean cotton bud (swab).

△ **2** Dip a powder puff into loose powder and lightly press over the areas of your face that are prone to oiliness. This will absorb excess oil throughout the day, and leave your skin beautifully matte. Dust off any excess powder with a clean powder brush.

△ **3** Sweep peach eyeshadow over your entire eyelid. It will blend with your natural skin tone, but give a clean, wide-eyed look to your make-up.

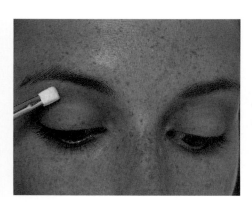

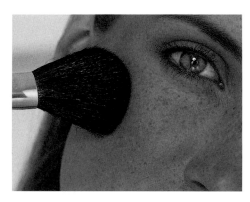

△ **4** Use an eyeshadow brush to work a tiny amount of soft brown eyeshadow into the crease of your eyelid to give depth and definition to your eyes. Sweep it towards the outer corner of your eyes too.

△ **5** Using the same brown eyeshadow, work a little underneath your lower lashes. This gives a softer effect than traditional kohl pencil or eyeliner, and is particularly suitable for those with pale or blonde hair who often can't carry off very strong eye make-up. Finish with two coats of brown/black mascara.

△ **6** Apply a barely-there shade of nude lipstick with a lipbrush. Then apply a tawny blusher, sweeping it a little at a time over your cheeks, forehead and chin. You can even dust a little over the tip of your nose! The advantage of applying blusher after you've completed your make-up is that you can assess exactly how much you need.

Cool skin, dark hair

If you are a pale-skinned brunette you will look fabulous with strong, cool shades of cosmetics. The density of colour provides a striking contrast to your ivory skin tone, while the coolness blends beautifully with your natural look.

this look suits you if...

• Your hair is mid-brown to dark brown in colour.

• Your eyes are brown, blue, hazel, grey or green.

• You have a cool, China-doll skin tone that tans slowly in the sun.

MAKE-UP TIPS

• To stop your mascara from clogging, wiggle the mascara wand slightly from side to side as you pull it through your lashes.

• If you find cream blusher hard to apply, you can opt for the powder variety, applying it after face powder.

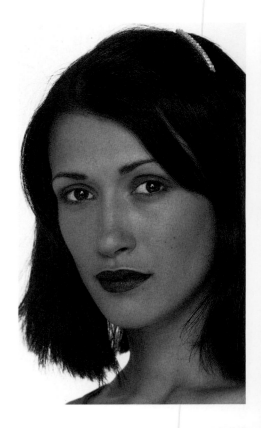

▷ **Strong, dense shades enhance dark hair and cool skin tones.**

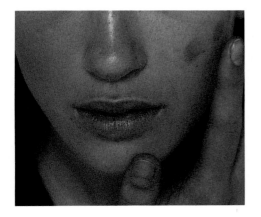

△ **1** Apply foundation or tinted moisturizer. If using foundation, it's likely you'll need the palest of shades. Blend in a few dots of tawny cream blusher, and finish with a dusting of loose powder.

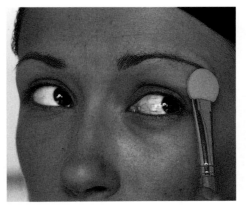

△ **2** Smudge a cool ivory shadow over your eyelids, right up to your eyebrows. Stroke over it with a cotton bud (swab) to blend it if you find it gathers in creases close to your upper eyelashes.

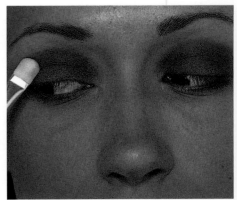

△ **3** Add extra definition with a touch of taupe or khaki eyeshadow on your eyelids. This shade works beautifully on your cool colouring, and emphasizes the colour of your eyes.

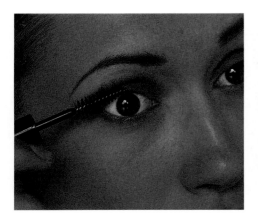

△ **4** Now move on to your eyelashes. You need to apply two thin coats of black mascara to create an effective frame to your eyes.

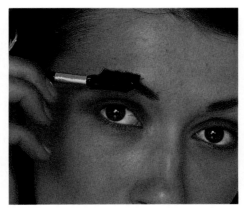

△ **5** Slick your eyebrows into place with an eyebrow brush. If they tend to look untidy, hold them in place by spritzing the brush with a little hairspray first.

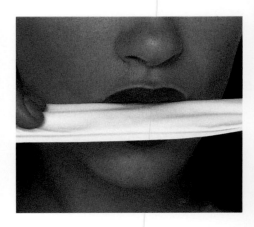

△ **6** Choose a clear shade of berry lipstick to give your look a polished finish. Blot after one coat with a tissue, then re-apply for a longer-lasting finish.

Warm skin, dark hair

Your skin tone can carry off burnished browns, warm reds and earthy shades beautifully. They'll complement your complexion and emphasize your features.

this look suits you if ...

• You have mid- to dark brown hair.
• Your eyes are brown, dark blue, grey, hazel or green.
• You have a warm skin tone that usually tans quite well. Even if it is pale in winter, your skin still has a yellow undertone.

▷ **A flaming red lipstick combines powerfully with the burnished browns to create a warm, sophisticated look.**

POWDER TIP
Carry a powder compact with you during the day to blot break-through shine on nose, forehead and chin.

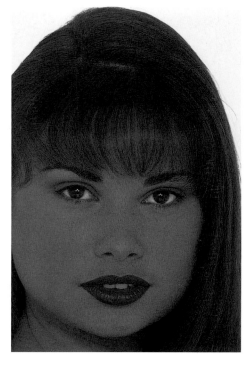

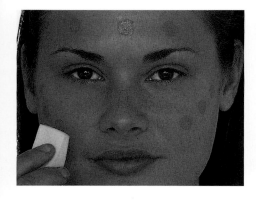

△ **1** Dot liquid foundation on to your skin and blend in with a damp cosmetic sponge. Blend the colour into your neckline for a natural effect. Then apply concealer to any blemishes that need it.

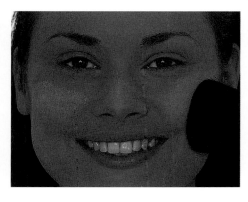

△ **2** Pat your face with translucent loose powder, then brush off the excess with a large, soft brush.

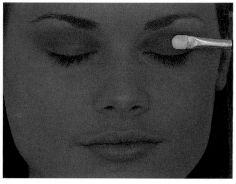

△ **3** Use a sponge-tipped eyeshadow applicator to sweep a red-brown shadow over your entire eyelid. The advantage of the sponge over a brush is that it doesn't tend to flick colour around. Complete your eyes with two thin coats of mascara.

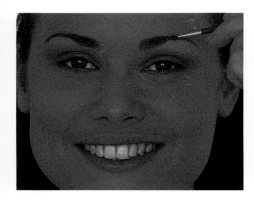

△ **4** Your eyebrows need subtle emphasis for this look. Either pencil them in with soft strokes of brown eyebrow pencil, or use a brown eyeshadow for a softer effect. Whichever method you use, brush them with an eyebrow brush to blend the strokes and slick the hairs in place.

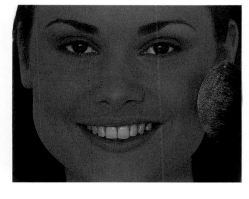

△ **5** Opt for a warm, tawny brown shade of powder blusher, dusted over your cheeks and up towards your temples. As this colour is quite strong, you may need to tone it down a little afterwards by dusting lightly over the top with translucent loose powder.

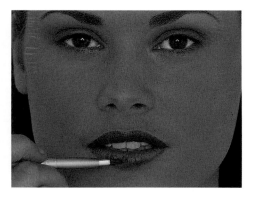

△ **6** A fiery red lipstick balances the overall look. Take care to use a lip brush to ensure you fill in every tiny crease and crevice on the lip surface – this will help your lipstick colour stay put for longer as well as creating a perfect finish.

Cool skin, red hair

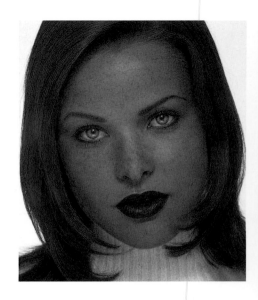

Redheads with cool skin tones often stick to soft colours, but you can experiment with brighter colours to contrast with your wonderful colouring. Greens give an exciting dimension to your eyes, and strong earthy shades supercharge your lips.

this look suits you if ...

• You have strawberry blonde or pale red hair, and these rules apply even if the colour has faded.
• Your eyes are blue, grey, hazel or green.
• You have pale skin, ranging from ivory to a pink-toned complexion.

FRECKLE TIP

If you have freckles, don't fall into the trap of trying to cover them with dark-toned foundation. Instead, match your foundation to your skin tone to avoid a mask-like effect.

△ **A rich burnished red lipstick adds a touch of drama to this look while soft greens enhance the striking colour of the eyes.**

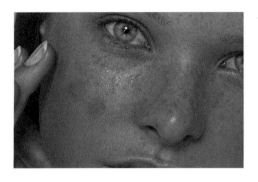

△ **1** Apply foundation and concealer, then dot a peachy shade of cream blusher on to your cheekbones. Unlike powder blusher, you can blend the cream variety with your fingertips, as the warmth from your skin will help smooth it in evenly. Apply a little cream blusher at a time. Finish with a dusting of translucent powder.

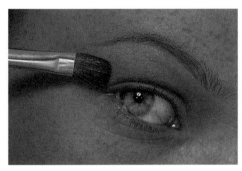

△ **2** A neutral, peach-toned eyeshadow swept over your eyelids will emphasize your eye colour without fighting with it. Ensure you take care to work it close to your eyelashes, to create a balanced effect.

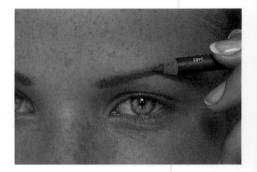

△ **3** Redheads usually have fair eyebrows, so don't forget to emphasize them to create a frame to your eyes. Otherwise the rest of your make-up will look unbalanced as the focus will be placed on your forehead. Opt for a very pale eyebrow pencil, in a subtle grey-brown tone. Stroke it through your eyebrows, taking care to fill any bald spots. Then soften the lines by brushing through with an eyebrow comb.

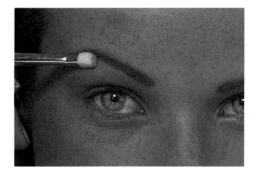

△ **4** Brush a hint of gold, shimmery eyeshadow into the arch under your eyebrows to give your eyes an extra dimension and bring them subtly into focus. This is a particularly good way to bring out gold flecks or warmth in the iris of your irises.

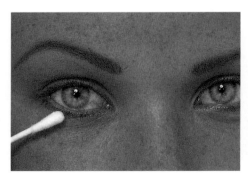

△ **5** Green eyeliner looks great but don't smudge it under your lower lashes as this will drag your features down. Work it along the upper lashes and into the eye corners. Then smudge with a cotton bud (swab) to give a soft finish. Brush with translucent powder to ensure it stays put. Finish with two coats of brown mascara.

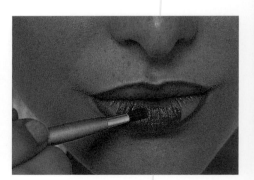

△ **6** Burnished orange lipstick complements this look. Begin by outlining your lips with a toning lip liner to prevent the colour from bleeding. Then use a lipbrush to fill in with the lipstick.

Warm skin, red hair

Your vibrant Pre-Raphaelite colouring is suited to bold shades of wine, purple and brown. These deep, blue-toned colours look fabulous with your warm skin and hair tones, and can make you look truly stunning.

this look suits you if ...

• You have medium to dark red hair. This look may also suit brunettes who have a lot of red tones to their hair.
• Your eyes are blue, grey, hazel, brown or green.
• You have a medium to warm skin tone.
• Your skin takes on a golden colour in the summer, although you're unlikely to get a deep tan. It's quite likely that you have freckles.

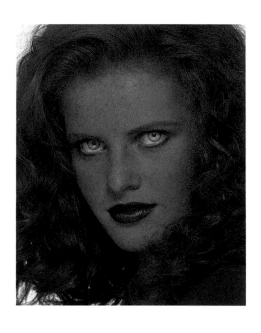

△ **Fiery hair and warm skin tones gain added vibrancy from purples, plums and browns.**

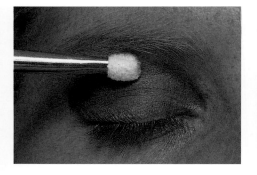

△ **1** After applying foundation, concealer and powder, smooth a wine shade of shadow over your entire eyelid. Using a sponge-tipped eyeshadow applicator will give you more control when applying this colour. You may find it easier to blend in if you sweep some translucent powder over your eyelids first, to create a smooth base on which to work.

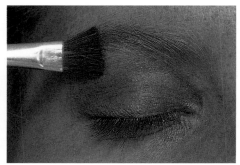

△ **2** Use a pale mauve eyeshadow over your brow bone to balance your eye make-up. Blend it into the crease, to soften any harsh edges of the wine-toned eyeshadow. Take time at this stage for a professional-looking finish.

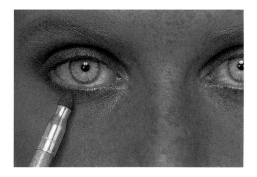

△ **3** Smudge a little of the wine-toned eyeshadow under your lower lashes as well. This will give a modern look to your eye make-up, and give a softer effect than kohl pencil. Ensure you also work it into the outer corners of your eyes, sweeping it slightly upwards to give your eyes a lift. Then finish with two coats of brown mascara. Take care to take the mascara right to the roots of your lashes, especially if they're pale.

△ **4** Use a soft brown eyeshadow to give your eyebrows subtle emphasis, using either a small brush or a cotton bud (swab). Brush the eyebrows through afterwards with an eyebrow comb for a soft finish.

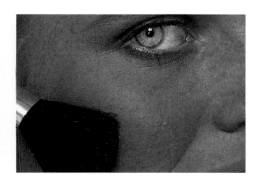

△ **5** Choose a brown-toned blusher or bronzing powder to give your skin warmth. Dust it on with a large blusher brush, blending it towards your hairline for a natural glow. The key is to use a little at a time, increasing the intensity of colour as you go. Avoid shimmery blushers, as these can give your skin an unnatural-looking sheen.

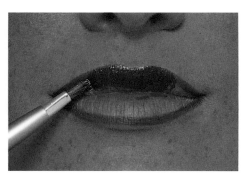

△ **6** You can carry off a deep plum shade of lipstick, outlined with a toning lip pencil. This strong colour needs perfect application to look good, so apply two coats, blotting the first with a tissue. This will also ensure your lipstick stays put for ages, and avoids the need for constant retouching.

Olive skin, dark hair

Your skin tones are easy to complement with rich browns, oranges and a hint of gold or bronze. These shades define your features and work well on your wonderful skin tones.

this look suits you if ...
• You have dark brown to black hair.
• Your eyes are brown, hazel or green.
• Your olive skin tans beautifully, or you have Asian or Indian colouring.

▷ **Shimmery soft orange lipstick and rich golds and browns complement your warm skin-tones.**

LIPSTICK TIP
To create a perfect lip line, stretch your mouth into an "O" shape and fill in the corners with your lip pencil.

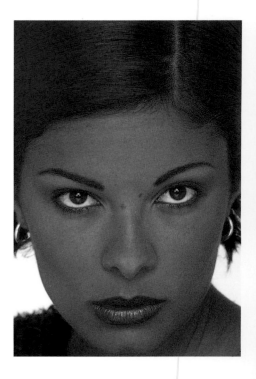

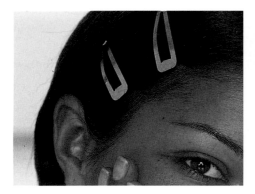

△ **1** Even out minor skin blemishes with a tinted moisturizer, blending it in smoothly with fingertips. If you need more coverage, opt for a liquid or cream foundation. Now apply a concealer and a light dusting of face powder.

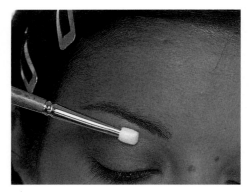

△ **2** After sweeping a golden shadow across your entire eyelid, apply a darker bronze shade into the crease and then apply some carefully under the lower lashes. This gives a wonderfully sultry look to your eyes.

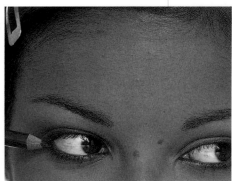

△ **3** Take a warm brown eyeliner and work it along your upper and lower lashes for a strong look that you can carry off beautifully. If you find the effect too harsh, smudge with a clean cotton bud (swab). Apply two coats of black mascara.

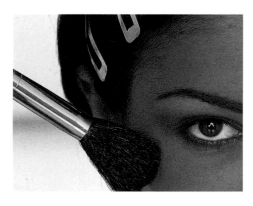

△ **4** A peach-brown powder blusher adds a sunkissed warmth to your cheeks. Apply just a little at a time, increasing the effect as you go.

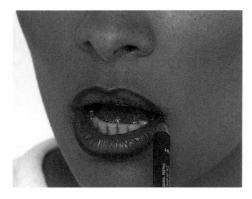

△ **5** Outline your lips with an orange-brown lip pencil. Start at the Cupid's bow on the upper lip, and move outwards. Then complete the other side, and finish with the lower lip.

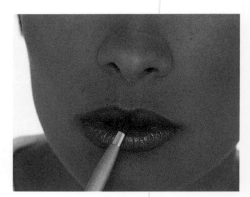

△ **6** To complete the look fill in with a sunny orange shade of lipstick. If you prefer a glamorous, glossy finish, don't blot your lips with a tissue. You can even add a dab of lip balm for extra shine if you wish. But if you prefer a semi-matte look, blot after one coat with a tissue, then re-apply your lipstick for a longer-lasting finish.

Oriental colouring, dark hair

Your black hair and pale – but yellow-toned – skin are best complemented by soft, warm colours. These will define your looks and counteract any sallowness in your complexion.

this look suits you if ...
• You have very dark brown to blue-black hair. It also works if you have grey flecks in your hair.
• Your eyes are hazel or brown.
• You have a pale to medium skin tone. It does tan, although it has a tendency to look quite yellow.

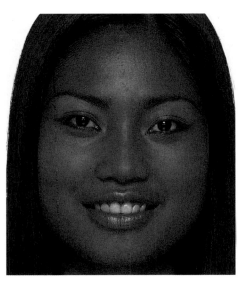

◁ **Baby pink gives your lips a cool, soft look and blue-black eyeliner emphasizes the beautiful shape of your eyes.**

EYELASH TIP
Oriental eyelashes are often poker-straight and so you can really benefit from the use of eyelash curlers.

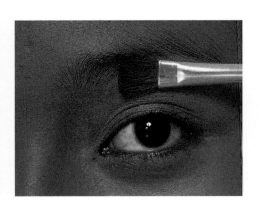

△ **1** After applying foundation, concealer and powder, sweep some lilac eyeshadow over your eyelid. This pale colour is a better option than using darker eyeshadows near the eyes, which have a tendency to make them look deep-set, particularly as your eyelids tend to be quite small.

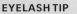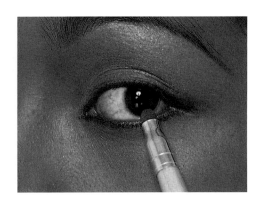

△ **2** Lightly fill in your eyebrows with a dark brown eyeshadow or eyebrow pencil to provide a strong frame to your eyes. This will help balance the eyeliner, which is going to be applied next.

△ **3** A lick of blue-black eyeliner will emphasize your beautifully shaped eyes, and help correct any droopiness. Slick it under the lower lashes and into the outer corners of your eyes to create balance. To prevent the overall look from seeming too harsh, use a cotton bud (swab) to soften the eyeliner slightly.

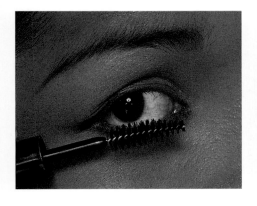

△ **4** Place your eyelashes between the pads of a curler, and gently squeeze for a few seconds. Then apply two coats of black mascara.

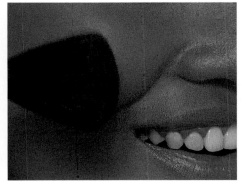

△ **5** A warm pink blusher gives a wonderful boost to your complexion, and brings out its natural glow. Dust it over the plumpest part of your cheeks.

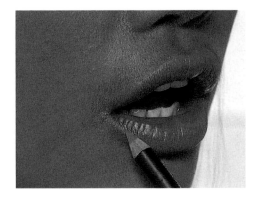

△ **6** A baby pink lipliner and lipstick bring your lips fashionably into focus. The cool blue tone to this shade works very well on your colouring.

Pale black skin, black hair

This make-up combination emphasizes your looks with earthy shades. Your pale black, or brown skin works well with beige, brown and copper colours.

this look suits you if ...
• You have black hair with golden or reddish highlights. It also works if you have grey flecks in your hair.
• You have hazel or brown eyes.
• You have a black skin.

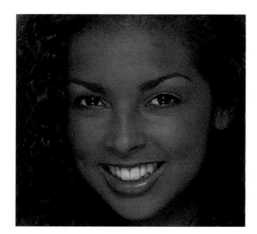

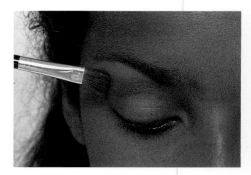

◁ **Ivory-toned eyeshadow and pearly pink-brown lipstick create a pretty contrast with your warm skin tone.**

DARK SKIN TIP
Look at cosmetic ranges especially designed for darker skins for your foundation and powder.

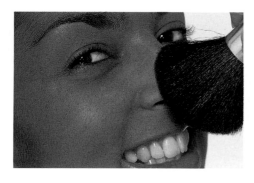

△ **1** After applying foundation, dust on a translucent face powder, ensuring it perfectly matches your skin tone to avoid a chalky-looking complexion. Dust off the excess with a large powder brush, using downward strokes.

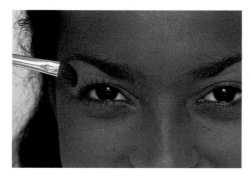

△ **2** Use an eyeshadow brush to dust an ivory-toned shadow over your entire eyelid, creating a contrast with your warm skin tone.

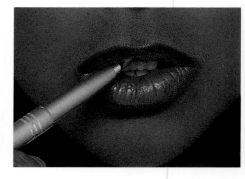

△ **3** Smudge a deep-toned brown eyeshadow into the crease of your eyelid, blending it thoroughly. Also work a little of this colour into the outer corners and underneath your lower lashes, to make your eyes look really striking.

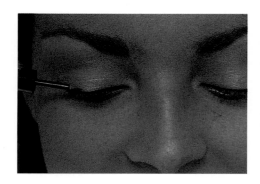

△ **4** Black liquid eyeliner swept along your upper lashes will give a supermodel look to your eyes. A sponge-tipped applicator is easier to use than a brush. Apply the eyeliner while looking down into a mirror, as this stretches any creases out of your eyelids. Rest your elbow on a firm surface. Complete your eyes with two coats of black mascara.

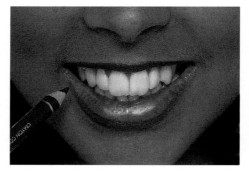

△ **5** Use a brown lipliner pencil to outline your lips. You can use an ordinary brown eyeliner pencil if this is the only thing you have to hand. Blend the line lightly into your lips, using a cotton bud (swab) for a softer effect.

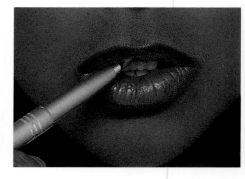

△ **6** A neutral pink-brown lipstick gives a natural-looking sheen to your lips, and instantly updates your look. Apply it with a lip brush for an even finish.

Black skin, black hair

You can experiment with endless colour possibilities as your dark eyes, hair and skin provide the perfect canvas on which to work. The key to success is to choose bold, deep colours as your skin demands these to achieve a wonderful glow.

this look suits you if ...
• You have deep black hair, even if it has flecks of grey.
• You have dark hazel or brown eyes.
• You have a dark black skin.

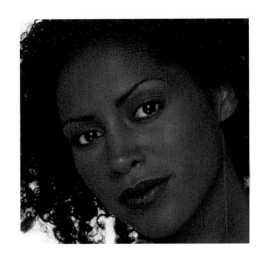

◁ **Soft red lipstick, blackcurrant eyeshadow and tawny blusher combine dramatically with your dark hair and skin.**

MAKE-UP TIP
While dramatic colours suit your skin tone and colouring perfectly, be sure to apply them with a light touch to get a fresh and vibrant look.

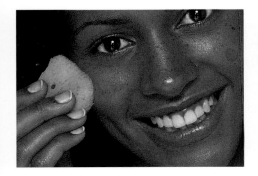

△ **1** Take care to find a foundation that matches your skin tone exactly. Apply it with a sponge so it blends in perfectly. Dampen the sponge with water first to give it extra "slip", and to prevent the sponge from absorbing too much expensive foundation. Blend in thoroughly along your jaw and hairline to avoid tidemarks. Finally, set with a light dusting of translucent loose powder.

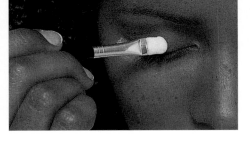

△ **2** Next, sweep a dark blackcurrant eyeshadow over your eyelids. Dust a little loose powder under your eyes first to catch any falling specks of this dark shade, and prevent it from ruining your completed foundation.

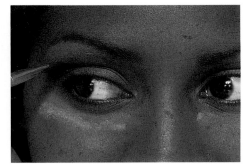

△ **3** Apply a dark charcoal eyeshadow into the crease of your eyelid using an eyeshadow brush. Only take a little colour at a time on to the brush to prevent it from spilling on to your eyelid. If necessary, tap the brush on the back of your hand first to shake away any excess.

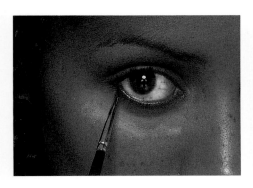

△ **4** Use an eyeliner brush to work some of this charcoal shade under your lower lashes, as this is the ideal colour with which to outline your eyes. Hold the mirror slightly above your eyeliner so that you can achieve an accurate liner effect. Finish with two coats of black mascara.

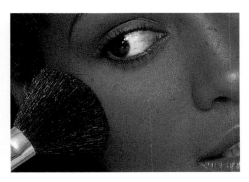

△ **5** A tawny-brown shade of blusher complements your skin beautifully. With a large round brush, dust it over the apples of your cheeks, working it lightly out towards your hairline.

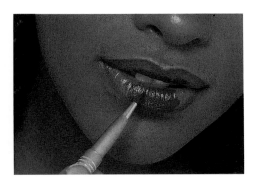

△ **6** After outlining your lips with a toning lip pencil, fill in with a dark plum shade of lipstick, using a lip brush for extra definition.

Look younger in six steps

It is best to avoid fashion extremes and bright colours when you're over 40. Younger skins can get away with garish make-up, but it emphasizes fine lines and wrinkles on most women. Flatter your looks with subtle colours and throw away bright eyeshadows and neon lipsticks. If you don't know where to start, make an appointment for a free makeover. You'll be able to see which shades suit you, before you buy.

▷ **The latest foundations and concealers contain hundreds of light-reflective particles and these bounce light away from your skin. This gives it the illusion of added vitality, and helps disguise problem areas such as fine lines and under-eye shadows.**

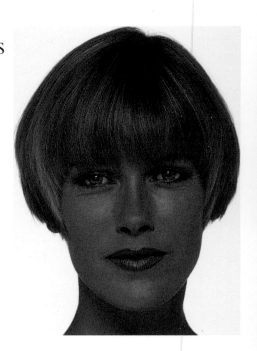

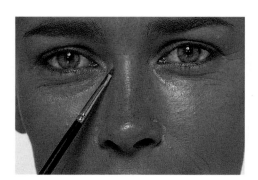

△ **1** Apply your foundation with a damp sponge, blending away any harsh edges to avoid tell-tale tidemarks. This is the stage at which to apply concealer, dotting it on to under-eye shadows, blemishes and thread veins with a brush. Apply a tiny amount at a time, and blend it in thoroughly.

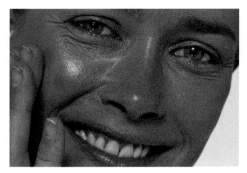

△ **2** Use half as much blusher and twice as much blending. Cream blusher gives your skin a soft glow. Dot the blusher on and blend with your fingertips. Set foundation and blusher with translucent powder, but remember that too much powder will settle into fine lines and wrinkles, and emphasize them. The best way to apply powder is only to blot the areas that need it, then brush away the excess with a large powder brush, stroking downwards.

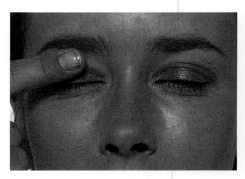

△ **3** Many women don't feel confident about applying eyeshadow properly. One of the most effective is an eyeshadow formulation that is easy to apply – cream-to-powder eyeshadow. It applies as a smooth cream, and dries quickly to a super-soft powder finish. Opt for a subtle shade such as mid-brown, grey or taupe.

A good tip if your eyes look rather droopy is to blend eyeshadow upwards and outwards at the outer corners. Remember to blend it in well.

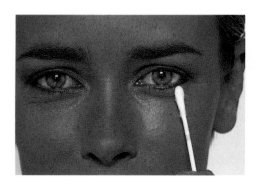

△ **4** Harsh lines of colour close to your eyes can be hard and unflattering. You'll emphasize your eyes much better if you smudge a little neutral-toned powder eyeshadow under your lower lashes with a clean cotton bud (swab).

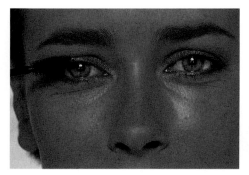

△ **5** Most women's colouring fades slightly over the years. This means that the black mascara you're used to wearing can now look too obvious and harsh. Try switching to a lighter shade for a more flattering effect. Apply two thin coats, allowing time for the first to dry thoroughly before you apply the second.

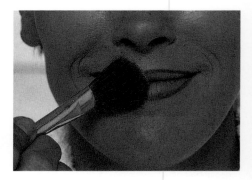

△ **6** If lipstick tends to "bleed" into the lines around your mouth, use a toning lipliner first. Keep it firm to give a precise line, yet soft so as not to drag the skin. Outline your top lip first, working outwards from the centre. Dust your lips with loose powder to set the lipliner, before applying a glossy, moisturizing lipstick.

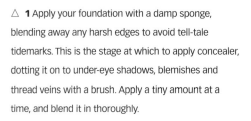

Classic chic

Whatever your age or colouring, this cool, sophisticated, classic look is very easy to apply and will always make a pleasing impact. Whether you are going to an important meeting or getting ready for an interview for a dream job, this simple but striking make-up combination will ensure that you feel completely confident about the way you look.

▷ Red is a lipstick classic, but the range of reds available is truly astonishing. It is simply a matter of experimenting with different tones and shades to find the perfect red for you.

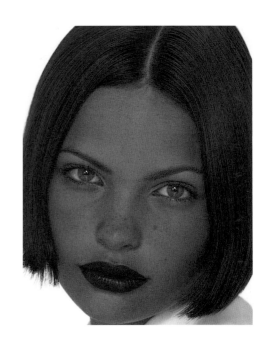

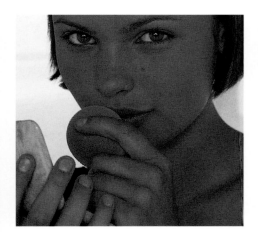

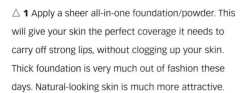

△ **1** Apply a sheer all-in-one foundation/powder. This will give your skin the perfect coverage it needs to carry off strong lips, without clogging up your skin. Thick foundation is very much out of fashion these days. Natural-looking skin is much more attractive.

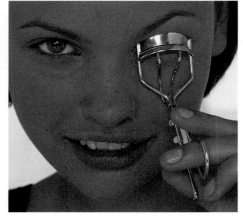

△ **2** The eye make-up for this look is very understated. So, use an eyelash curler to open up your eyes and give them a fresh look.

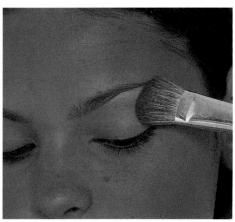

△ **3** Sweep pale ivory eyeshadow across your entire eyelid using a blender brush. Then complete your eyes with two thin coats of brown/black or black mascara.

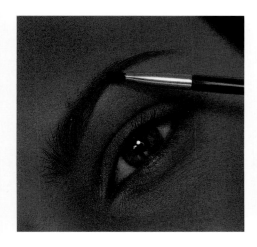

△ **4** Well-groomed eyebrows are essential. Brush them against the growth to remove any stray flecks of powder or foundation. Then lightly fill in any gaps with a toning eyeshadow. This gives a softer, more natural effect than a pencil.

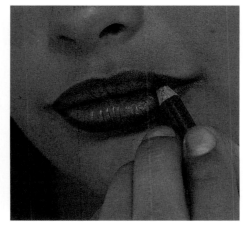

△ **5** Your lips are the focus of this chic look. To ensure that you create a perfect outline, use a toning red lip pencil. Rest your elbow on a hard surface when using the pencil to prevent your hand from wobbling.

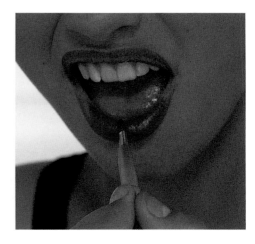

△ **6** Use a lip brush to fill in with a bold shade of red lipstick. Apply one coat, blot with a tissue, then reapply for a long-lasting finish.

Country girl

Having fun with your make-up and experimenting with different styles is the best way to discover what is right for you. Why not try a sunkissed, outdoor look – a summery make-up combination that creates a muted, natural look, complete with fake freckles!

▷ **Natural lipstick, light touches of mascara and eyeshadow and a hint of shimmery blusher will give you a glowing, wholesome look that is perfect for the outdoor days of summer.**

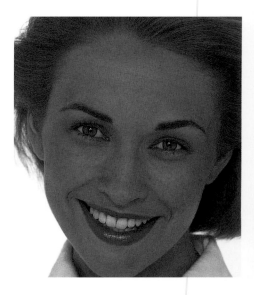

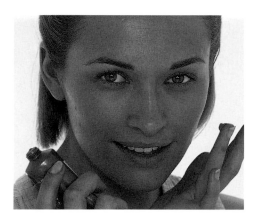

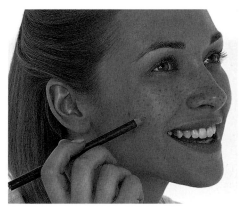

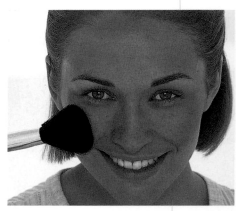

△ **1** You need to avoid heavy foundations when you're outside, so tinted moisturizer is the perfect solution. It'll both nourish your skin and lightly cover any minor blemishes. Apply with your fingertips for ease.

△ **2** If you already have freckles, don't try to hide them – they're perfect for a fresh-air look. If you don't have them, then fake them! Use an eyebrow pencil rather than an eyeliner pencil as it has a harder consistency and is less likely to melt on the skin. Use a mid-brown shade, and dot on the freckles, concentrating them on the nose and cheeks. Be extra creative and apply different sizes of freckles for a realistic look.

△ **3** A bronzing powder rather than a blusher will give your skin a sunkissed outdoor look. Choose one with minimum pearl or shimmer. Apply it to the plumpest part of your cheeks, where the sun would naturally catch your face. Dust the bronzing powder over your temples, too.

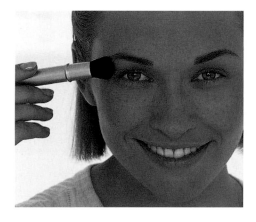

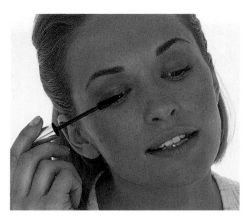

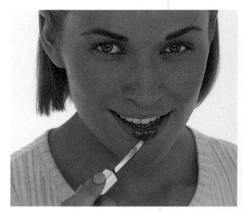

△ **4** Swap to an eyeshadow blending brush to gently sweep some of the bronzing powder over your eyelids. Natural colours like brown work best for this look. Remove any harsh edges with a clean cotton bud (swab).

△ **5** Keep mascara to a minimum. Choose a natural-looking brown or brown/black shade, and apply just one coat. The waterproof type is great for hot days and sudden downpours but remember you'll need a suitable eye make-up remover, too.

△ **6** Don't overpower this subtle look with bold lipstick. Opt for a muted brown-pink shade that's close to your natural lip colour, or use a softly tinted lipgloss for a natural sheen.

City chic

This super-successful look is perfect for work and in the city. Simple, immaculately applied colours can help you put together a polished working image. This stylish, balanced look will help you to feel super-confident, whatever the day at the office brings.

▷ **These clever make-up moves create a simple, stylish look to keep you feeling super-cool throughout the working day.**

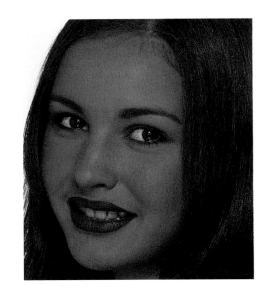

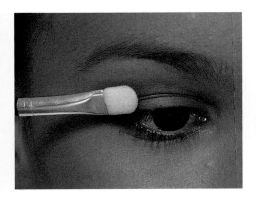

△ **1** After applying a light foundation and dusting your skin with powder to blot out shine, sweep your eyelids with a mid-grey eyeshadow. Use a matte powder formulation as this tends not to crease as much during the day. Use a sponge-tipped applicator to make the eyeshadow easier to apply.

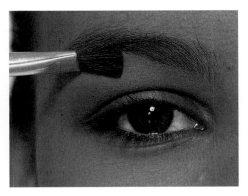

△ **2** Use a beige highlighting eyeshadow over your brow bone to soften the edges of the grey shadow and to bring your eyes into focus. Take care not to leave flecks of powder in your eyebrow hairs – if necessary, flick them away with an eyebrow brush. Finish with two coats of mascara – blondes should use brown or brown/black mascara, while other colourings can opt for black.

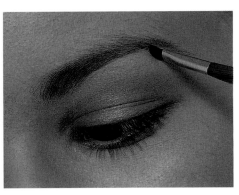

△ **3** Brush your eyebrows with brown eyeshadow to fill in any gaps. This helps to create a strong frame to your make-up look.

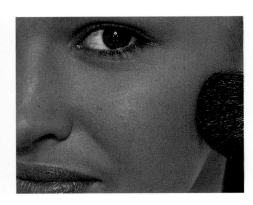
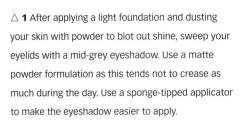

△ **4** A soft pink shade of blusher will give your skin a rosy glow, and neatly co-ordinate the rest of your make-up. It will also give pale work-a-day faces an immediate lift!

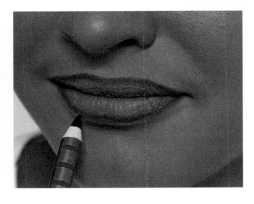

△ **5** Try soft blackcurrant shades as these can work beautifully on your lips, and make a welcome alternative to red. Start by using a lipliner to outline, ensuring you take it well into the outer corners. If you create any wobbly edges, whisk over the top with a clean cotton bud (swab) dipped in a little cleansing lotion. Then powder and try again!

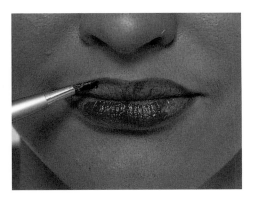

△ **6** Fill in your lips with a matching shade of blackcurrant lipstick. Blot your lips with a tissue afterwards for a semi-matte finish that's perfect for a day at the office.

Quick-fix evening make-up

Follow these six quick steps to achieve a striking, elegant look in just five minutes. When you are in a hurry, there is no time to experiment with new ideas, so the key to a successful quick-fix is to choose simple styles, applied with the minimum of fuss … so here you have straightforward steps to a stunning look!

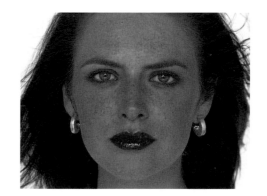

◁ When you don't have much spare time, but want to look presentable fast, try this quick and simple make-up combination for evening sophistication.

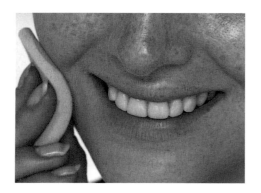

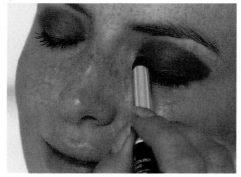

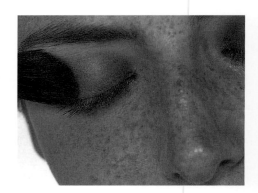

△ **five minutes to go …**

1 The all-in-one foundation/powder formulations give your skin the medium coverage it needs for this look in half the normal time. Also, take it over your lips and eyelids as this will make the rest of your make-up easier to apply and ensure it lasts the whole evening.

△ **four minutes to go …**

2 Cream eyeshadow applied straight from the stick is quick and easy to apply. Opt for a brown shade as it'll bring out the colour of your eyes, and give them a sexy, sultry finish. Slick it over your entire eyelid, right up to the crease of the eye socket.

△ **three and a half minutes to go …**

3 A swift way to blend in your eyeshadow is to brush over the top with a layer of translucent loose powder. This will tone down the colour and blend away any harsh edges.

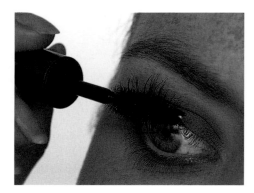

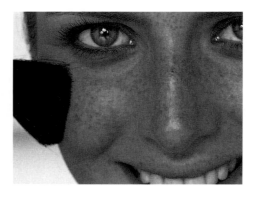

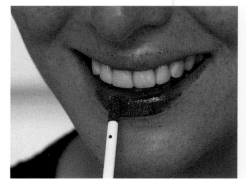

△ **two and a half minutes to go …**

4 Apply a coat of mascara to your lashes, taking care to colour your lower lashes as well as your upper ones. Use the tip of the mascara wand to coat the lower lashes, as this will prevent it from clogging on the hairs – and prevent you from spending valuable time having to use an eyelash comb.

△ **one and a half minutes to go …**

5 A warm berry red blusher will give your skin a fabulous flush. Apply it with a blusher brush, sweeping it from your cheeks up towards your eyes to give your face a lift.

△ **thirty seconds to go …**

6 Choose a berry shade of lip gloss to add instant bold colour to your lips, sweeping it straight on with the sponge-tipped applicator. Cover your lower lip first, then press your lips together to transfer some of the colour on to your upper lip. Touch up any areas you've missed with the applicator, and you're ready to go!

Go for glamour

There's usually one time when you want to make a special effort with your make-up and pull out all the stops, and that is the big night out!

Here's how to create this stunning look in six simple steps. Just follow the step-by-step instructions to create a sultry mixture of dark and light tones.

▷ **Smoky dark-brown eyeshadow, black eyeliner to make sure the focus is on the eyes, and a soft, neutral shade on the lips combine to create a fabulously sultry effect.**

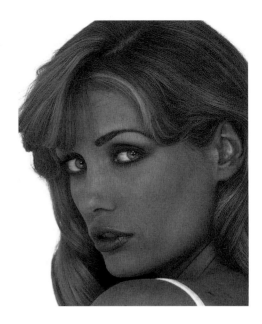

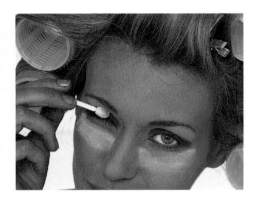

△ **1** This is a sophisticated look, with the focus very much on the eyes. Once you've applied foundation, concealer and powder, you're ready to start work on your eye make-up. Sweep a smoky dark brown eyeshadow over your entire eyelid and blend it carefully into the crease. A simple sponge applicator is less likely to flick colour away than a brush, but still take the precaution of sweeping a line of loose powder under your eyes to catch any falling specks of dark shadow.

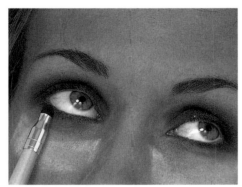

△ **2** Apply a little of the same eyeshadow under your lower lashes to accentuate the shape of your eyes. This will give a balanced look to your eye make-up, and provide a smooth base on which to apply your eyeliner at the next stage. The emphasis is on glamour and impact!

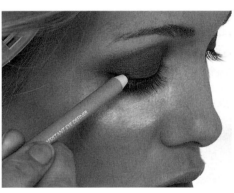

△ **3** Although black eyeliner is usually too severe for harsh daylight, it's perfect for this look, which is designed to be seen in softer, sexier light! Using a pencil, carefully draw a fine line above and below your eyelashes. If you find it hard to create a steady line, try drawing a series of tiny dots, then blend them together with a clean cotton bud (swab).

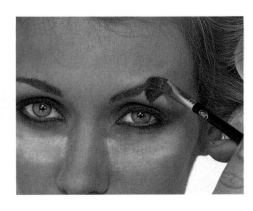

△ **4** To contrast with the dark, smoky look on your eyelids, sweep a pearly ivory shadow over your brow bones for a wide-eyed look. Apply a little at a time, building up the effect gradually. Complete the look with two coats of black mascara.

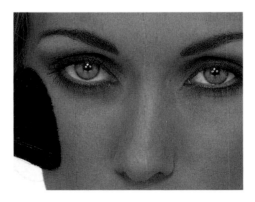

△ **5** Tawny blusher or a bronzing powder is ideal for this look, as the natural colour won't compete with the rest of your make-up. Sweep it smoothly over your cheekbones, taking care to blend away the edges into your hairline.

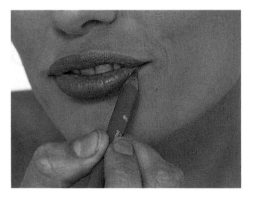

△ **6** Keeping the lips neutral gives this look its real impact, and updates it. Opt for a pinkish-beige shade of lip pencil and smudge it over your entire mouth for a matte, understated effect.

50 effective beauty tips

When you don't have time for trial and error, you need beauty tips that really work. Here are 50 of the most effective.

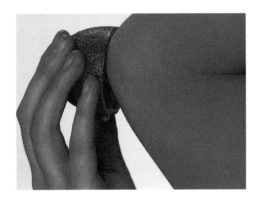

△ **1** Brighten grey elbows by rubbing them with half a fresh lemon – it has a natural bleaching effect. Moisturize afterwards to counteract the drying effects of the juice.

2 Turn foundation into a tinted moisturizer by mixing a few drops of it with a little moisturizer on the back of your hand before applying. It's perfect for summer.

3 Carry a spray of mineral water in your handbag to freshen up your foundation while you're out and about.

4 Sleeping on your back helps stop wrinkles, according to recent research. It's certainly worth a try!

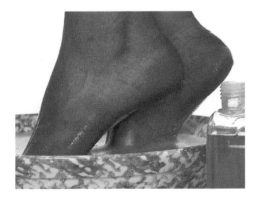

△ **5** Dunk feet into a bowl containing warm water and 45ml/3 tbsp Epsom salts to help ease swollen ankles.

6 If you have very soft nails, file them while the polish is still on, which will prevent them from cracking.

7 If you find eyebrow tweezing painful, hold an ice cube over the area first to numb it before you start.

8 Warm up your looks by dusting a little blusher over your temples, chin and the tip of your nose as well as your cheeks.

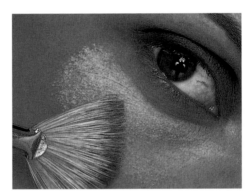

△ **9** Sweep a little loose powder under your eyes when applying dark eyeshadow to catch falling specks and prevent them from staining your skin.

10 Make your lips appear larger by wearing a bright, light lipstick. Make them appear smaller by wearing a dark or muted coloured lipstick.

11 Soak nails in a bowl of olive oil once a week to strengthen them.

12 If you haven't got time for a full make-up, but want to look great, paint on a bright red lipstick – it's a happy, glamorous colour that can immediately brighten your face.

13 If you don't have a different coloured blusher for your cheeks, simply use an ordinary face powder a couple of shades darker than your usual one to slim round cheeks.

14 Add a drop of witch hazel – available from all good pharmacists – to turn ordinary foundation into a medicated one – it's great for oily or blemish-prone skins.

15 Mascara your lashes before applying false ones to help them stick properly.

16 If you look tired, blend a little concealer just away from the outer corner of your eye – it makes you look as though you had a good night's sleep!

17 Go lightly with powder on wrinkles around the eyes – too much will settle into them and emphasize them.

18 When plucking your eyebrows, coat the hairs you want to remove with concealer – it'll help you visualize exactly the shape of brow you're after.

19 Never apply your make-up before blow-drying your hair – the heat from the dryer can make you perspire and cause your make-up to smudge.

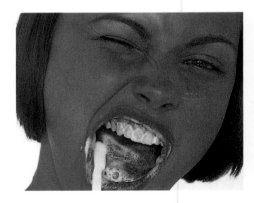

△ **20** Keep your smile looking its best by changing your toothbrush once the bristles begin to splay. This means at least every three months. You should brush for at least two minutes, both morning and evening.

21 Powder eyeshadow can be made to look more intense by dipping your eyeshadow brush in water first.

22 Keep lashes supple by brushing them with petroleum jelly before going to bed.

23 Apply cream blusher in light downward movements, to prevent it from creasing and specks of colour from catching in the fine hairs on your face.

24 If mascara tends to clog on your lower lashes, try using a small thin brush to paint colour on to individual lashes.

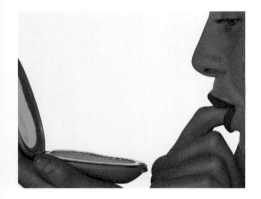

△ 25 To prevent lipstick getting on your teeth, after applying it put your finger in your mouth, purse your lips and pull it out.

26 Give moisturizer time to sink in before you start applying your make-up – it'll help your make-up go on more easily.

27 To make your eyes sparkle, try outlining them just inside your lower eyelashes with a soft white cosmetic pencil.

28 Apply a dot of lipgloss in the centre of your lower lip for a sophisticated look.

29 Hide cracked or chipped nails under stick-on false ones.

30 If your eyeliner is too hard and drags your skin, hold it next to a light bulb for a few seconds before applying.

31 If you find your lashes clog with mascara, try rolling the brush in a tissue first to blot off the excess, leaving a light, manageable film on the bristles.

32 If you're unsure where to apply blusher, gently pinch your cheeks, and if you like the effect, apply blusher in the same area for a natural look.

33 If you're near-sighted, glasses make your eyes look smaller. So, opt for bolder shadows and lots of mascara to enhance them. If you're far-sighted, lenses make your eyes look bigger and make-up more prominent. So, opt for more muted colours.

34 A little foundation lightly rubbed in your eyebrows and brushed with an old toothbrush will instantly lighten them.

35 Coloured mascara can look super-effective if applied with a light hand. Start by coating your lashes with two coats of black mascara. Once the lashes are dry, slick a little coloured mascara – try blue, violet or green – on the underside of your upper lashes. Each time you blink, your eyelashes will reveal a dash of unexpected colour.

36 If you use hypo-allergenic make-up for your sensitive skin, remember to use hypo-allergenic nail polish, too – you constantly touch your face with your hands and can easily trigger a reaction.

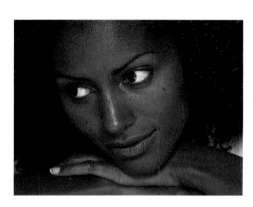

△ 37 For a longer-lasting blusher on hot days, apply cream and powder. Apply the cream formulation, set it with translucent powder then dust with powder blush.

38 Let nails breathe when applying polish by leaving a tiny gap at the base of the nail where the cuticle meets the nail – this is where the new nail cells are growing.

39 Make over-prominent eyes appear smaller with a wide coat of liquid liner.

40 Calm an angry red blemish by holding an ice cube over it for a few seconds to cool and soothe the skin. Then apply your medicated concealer.

41 If you've run out of loose powder it is just as effective to use a dusting of unperfumed talcum powder.

42 Use a little green eyeshadow on red eyelids to mask the ruddiness.

43 If you've run out of liquid eyeliner, dip a thin brush into your mascara.

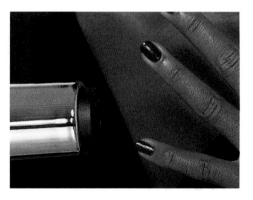

△ 44 If you need to dry your nail polish extra quickly, you can blast your nails with a cold jet of air from your hairdryer to speed up the process.

45 Use a toothpick or dental floss regularly to clean between your teeth. This ensures your teeth are completely clean and cuts down the risk of cavities.

46 Apply foundation/powder with a damp sponge for thicker opaque coverage.

47 Run your freshly sharpened eyeliner pencil across a tissue before you use it. This will round off any sharp edges and remove small particles of wood.

48 If you have obvious under-eye shadows, cover them with a light coat of blue cream eyeshadow before applying your concealer.

49 Remove any excess mascara by placing a folded tissue between your upper and lower lashes and then blinking two or three times.

50 Get together friends and take turns to make each other up – it's good fun, you'll get feedback from your friends, and it's a fantastic way to experiment and find yourself a new look.

50 budget beauty tips

If you can't afford top-of-the-range, expensive beauty products, here are 50 fabulous tips to help you follow a successful beauty regime on a tight budget.

1 Cotton wool (cotton) balls soak up liquids such as toner, so dampen them with water first. Squeeze out the excess, then use as usual.

2 A drop of remover added to a bottle of dried-up nail polish will revive it in a few seconds. Shake well to encourage it to mix in thoroughly.

3 Stand a dried-up mascara in a glass of warm water to bring it back to life.

4 Keep new soaps from getting soft by storing them in a warm cupboard. This helps dry the moisture out, which makes them harder and longer-lasting.

5 To get the last drop from almost-empty bottles, store them upside-down overnight. You'll reap the rewards!

6 Don't rip the cellophane off translucent powder – prick a few holes in it instead – it'll stop you spilling and wasting it.

7 Keep perfume strips from magazines in case you need an instant freshen-up.

8 Sachets in magazines make ideal travel packs for weekends away.

9 Look out for "3 for the price of 2" offers on your favourite products.

10 Turn ordinary mascara into the lash-lengthening variety by dusting eyelashes with a little translucent powder first.

11 Rub a dab of petroleum jelly around the neck of a new nail-polish bottle, and it should be easy to open for the entire life of the product.

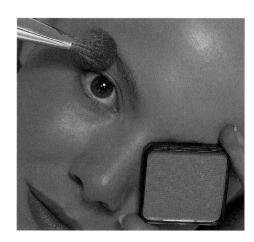

△ **12** Dust blusher over your eyelids as an instant subtle eyeshadow. It's quick to apply, and will give a balanced look to your make-up.

13 One-length hair with no layers is the easiest and cheapest hairstyle to maintain as it doesn't require as many visits to the hairdresser to keep it looking good.

14 Swap commercial face scrubs for a handful of oatmeal massaged directly on to your skin – smooth soft skin naturally.

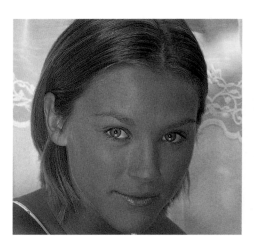

△ **15** If you've run out of blusher, dot a little pink lipstick on to your cheeks and blend well with your fingertips.

16 Don't use too much toothpaste – it's the brushing action that gets teeth really clean. A pea-sized blob is enough.

17 Pick the largest-sized products you can afford – it's much cheaper that way.

18 Don't shop for beauty goodies just in glitzy department stores and fancy pharmacies. These days, your local supermarket can offer a good range.

19 If you're happy to forgo a fancy label, look out for great value own-label product ranges at drug store chains.

20 Sometimes you're just as well off with cheap alternatives. Indulge yourself with the products that are really worth it! For instance, buy cheap and cheerful lip liners, then show off with a fancy lipstick. As well as looking good, expensive lipsticks tend to contain more pigment than cheaper ones – which means they look better and last even longer.

21 Buy cheap but effective moisturizers instead of expensive fragranced ones. This will mean you can save your money to splash out on your favourite perfume.

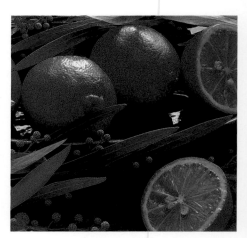

△ **22** A cheap way to boost the shine of dark hair is to rinse it with diluted vinegar. Blonde hair benefits from lemon juice being applied in the same way. Both act by sealing down the outer cuticles of the hair, which helps it to reflect the light more effectively.

23 It used to be that only the pricier ranges offered hi-tech products. However, these days more companies are offering state-of-the-art products – at budget prices. This means you'll get all the benefits without spending a fortune. For instance, there are now affordable skin creams that contain the anti-ageing alpha-hydroxy ingredients at a third or quarter of the price of prestige brands.

24 Many of the more expensive prestige make-up, skincare and fragrance companies offer sample products at their counters. It's always worth asking, especially if you're already buying something from them.

25 There's a great trend at the moment for 2-in-1 products. They're worth trying out, because they can save you money – as you buy only one product that does two jobs. The types of products included are shower gels that are also body scrubs and hair shampoos with built-in conditioners.

26 If you want to indulge in some new make-up, then ask for a makeover at a cosmetic counter. It can be the best way to see how the colours and formulations look on your skin before you buy anything – and can also mean you'll look great for an evening out!

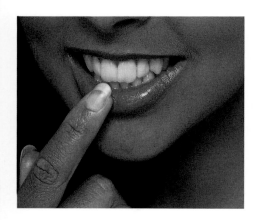

△ 27 Turn lipstick into lip gloss with a coat of lip balm after applying colour.

28 De-fuzz using a razor with replaceable blades – it works out much cheaper in the end than buying disposable razors.

29 Don't throw away an item of make-up just because the colour's not in fashion at the moment – you might like it again in a few months, or be able to blend it with something.

30 Make cheap nail polish last longer by sealing it with a clear top coat.

31 Pure glycerine is an extremely cheap and effective moisturizer when you don't have much to spend.

32 Store your make-up and fragrance in a cool dark place to extend their life span.

33 Double up your lip liner to fill in your lips as well as outline them.

34 Prise eyeshadows out of their cases, and stick into an old paint-box or lid to create a make-up artist's colour palette. It ensures you use the products you've got because you can see them all at a glance.

35 Add a few drops of your favourite *eau de toilette* to some olive oil, and use as a scented bath oil as a cheap treat.

36 Neutral make-up colours are a better investment because they are more versatile.

37 Eyeshadow doubles up as eyeliner, if applied with a cotton bud (swab). Dampen the end of the bud first to get a cleaner line under the eye.

38 If you're choosing a new fragrance, buy the weaker and cheaper *eau de toilette* before splashing out on stronger and more expensive perfume.

39 Check out model nights at your local hairdressers when trainees will style your hair for a fraction of the normal price.

40 Mix different colour lipsticks on the back of your hand with a brush, to create new shades for free!

41 When you're out of toothpaste, brush with bicarbonate of soda – it'll make them extra white, too.

42 Put your lip and eye pencils in the refrigerator before sharpening, as this means they're less likely to break.

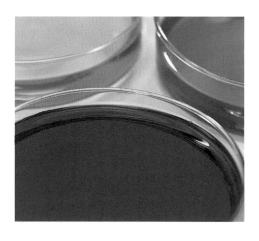

△ 43 A drop of olive oil rubbed nightly into your nails will help them grow long and strong, and is cheaper than shop-bought manicure oils.

44 Make powder eyeshadows last and stay crease-free by dusting eyelids with translucent powder. This keeps make-up looking fresher for longer.

45 Sharpen dull eyebrow tweezers by rubbing sandpaper along the tips.

46 Add a drop of water to the remains of a foundation to use every last dot.

47 Keep the plastic seals or paper discs that come with products and replace after use. It helps prevent air from getting into the products and bacteria from breeding – so your product stays fresher for longer.

48 Spritz your hair lightly with water and blow dry again to revive products already in the hair and revitalize your style.

49 A cup of bicarbonate of soda in your bath is a cheap and cheerful water softener.

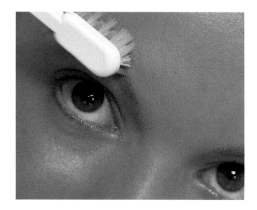

△ 50 Use an old clean toothbrush to slick unruly eyebrows into shape.

Your top 10 make-up questions answered

1 blush baby

Q *"Can I reshape my face using blusher?"*

A The best way to apply blusher is to smile, find the apples of your cheeks, and blend the colour upwards. For special occasions, try using your normal blusher, combined with a barely-there highlighter colour and a colour that is slightly darker than your usual blusher, to reshape your face. Check your face shape and try the following techniques:

• Slim a round face by blending your usual blusher upwards from your cheeks into your hairline. Then highlight along your cheekbones, and use the shader in the hollows of your cheeks.

• Soften a square face by concentrating your blusher in a circle on the rounded parts of your cheeks. Apply shader into the hollows of your cheeks, and also lightly on the square edges of your chin. Lightly dust highlighter on to the bridge of your nose and across the tip of your chin.

• Balance a heart-shaped face by dusting your blusher slightly lower than your cheekbones into the actual hollows of your cheeks. Dust some highlighter on to the tip of your chin, and apply shader to your temples, making sure that you blend it well into your hairline.

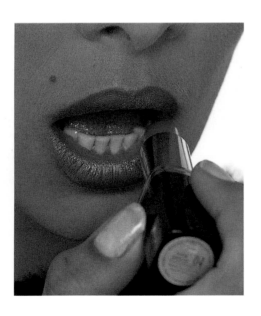

2 long-lasting lipstick

Q *"Is there any way to make my lipstick stay put all day?"*

A Unfortunately there's no such thing as a 24-hour lipstick, no matter what some cosmetic manufacturers claim. The longest-lasting lipsticks are those with the thickest, driest textures, although this can mean they leave your lips feeling quite dry, especially if you use them day in, day out. However, you can look for lipstick sealers, which are clear gels that you paint over your lips after you've applied your lipstick. Once they're dry, these lipstick sealers help your lipstick stay put at least past your first coffee of the day.

3 over-plucked brows

Q *"I plucked my eyebrows very thin last year. Now I'd like to grow them back. How can I do it successfully?"*

A Choose a natural-looking brown eyeshadow. Apply it lightly and evenly with a firm-bristled eyebrow brush, using short sharp strokes across the brow. As the hairs that grow back are often unruly, a light coat of clear mascara can be applied to help keep them in place.

Try to ignore the periodic fashions for highly plucked eyebrows. The fashions don't last for long – but eyebrows can take ages to grow back! It's better to stick with your natural eyebrow shape, just removing stray hairs from underneath the arch and between the brows.

4 covering birthmarks

Q *"Can you recommend something that will cover my birthmark, even when I go swimming?"*

A You need a specialized foundation that will give ultimate coverage, look opaque and be waterproof. Look for a specialized range of camouflage creams tailor-made to

◁ **A good quality lipstick will keep your lips feeling and looking good all day long.**

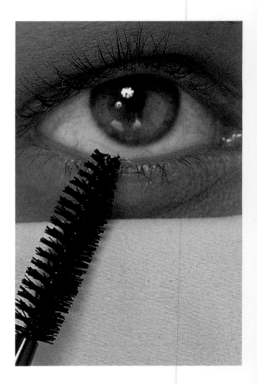

△ **Avoid mascara smudges by holding a piece of tissue underneath your lower lashes while you are applying your mascara.**

cover skin imperfections, such as scars and port wine stains, as well as birthmarks. The formulation means they are applied differently to ordinary foundation. They're applied with fingertips using a "dab, pat" motion. They're available from make-up suppliers and some dermatologists.

5 spider veins

Q *"What can I do about facial spider veins?"*

A Spider or thread veins, known as "telangiectases", are a common beauty problem. An electrolysist qualified in diathermy, or a dermatologist, can treat them by inserting a fine needle into the vein. The heat from the needle coagulates the blood in the vein, rendering it inactive. The number of treatments depends on the size of the area to be treated, and the number of spider veins.

You can also cover the veins with a light covering of concealer, applied with a fine brush and set with a dusting of powder.

▷ Generally most women can wear any colour, but the important thing is to find the shade that suits your colouring.

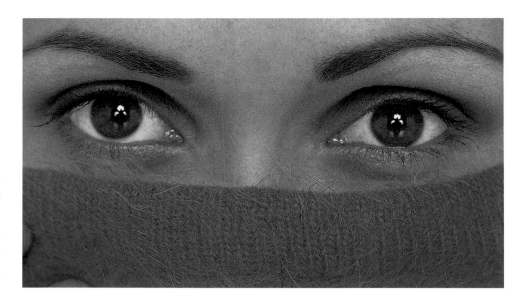

6 mascara matters

Q *"My mascara always seems to run on to my skin and leaves me with 'panda eyes'. What can I do?"*

A Using a waterproof variety of mascara should help if you're prone to this problem, or you can "seal" your normal mascara with a coat of clear mascara.

Alternatively, dip a cotton bud (swab) in eye make-up remover for fast touch-ups before the mascara can dry on your skin. Another, more long-term, solution is to have your eyelashes permanently dyed regularly at a reputable beauty salon.

7 smoother lips

Q *"Lipstick always looks awful on my mouth because my lips are so flaky, and it's impossible to create a smooth finish. Is there a solution?"*

A Slick your lips with a thick coat of petroleum jelly, and leave for 10 minutes to give it a chance to soften any hard flakes of skin. Then cover your index finger with a damp flannel and gently massage your lips. This removes the petroleum jelly and the flakes of dead skin should come off with it, leaving your lips supple and smooth.

▽ Applying your lipstick with a brush will make it much easier to achieve a perfectly smooth finish.

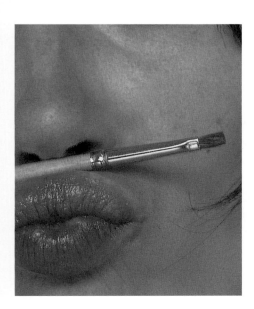

8 colour coding

Q *"Are there colours that some people can never wear?"*

A As a general rule, everyone can wear every colour. However, if you want to wear a particular colour, you should choose the particular shade of it very carefully. For instance, everyone can wear red lipstick, but in different shades. A pale-skinned blonde will suit a soft pink-red, whereas a warm-toned redhead will be able to carry off an orange-based fiery shade of the colour.

In the same way, a blue-eyed, cool-skinned blonde can carry off a pale pastel, baby-blue eyeshadow, whereas her brunette colleague will look much better wearing a darker version to complement her skin tone.

▽ Rolling a nail varnish bottle between your hands to mix it up ensures it is smooth to apply.

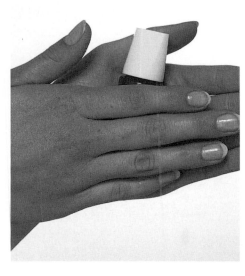

9 problem polish

Q *"I always have bottles of nail varnish that I can't use because they're either dried up, or full of bubbles so they don't go on smoothly. What can I do?"*

A There are some simple solutions to your problem. Dried-up polish can be revived by stirring in a few drops of polish remover before using. You can help prevent it from thickening in the first place by storing it in the refrigerator, as the cold temperature will stem evaporation and stop it changing in texture.

Bubbles of air in the polish will ruin its finish, as it won't create an even surface. You can prevent this by rolling the bottle between the palms of your hands to mix it up before using, rather than shaking it vigorously – as it is this that creates the bubbles in the first place.

10 the changing face of foundation

Q *"I have difficulty keeping up with the changing colour of my skin in the summer, as I gradually get a tan. It's so expensive constantly buying new foundations!"*

A Stick with the colour that suits you when you're at your palest in the middle of winter. Then, also buy a small tube of dark foundation designed for black skins. Blend just a drop or two into your ordinary foundation on the back of your hand before applying, to darken it so that it matches your tan. This means you can change your foundation as often as you need to, without having to spend a fortune on different shades.

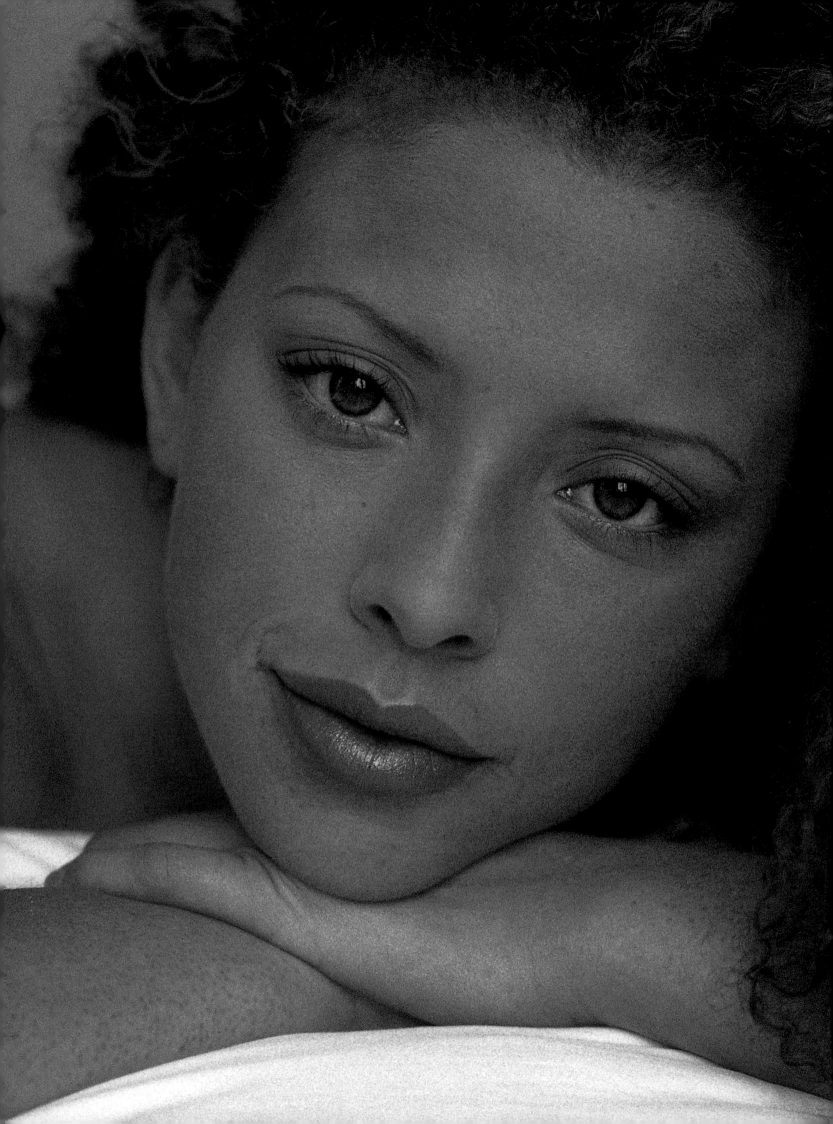

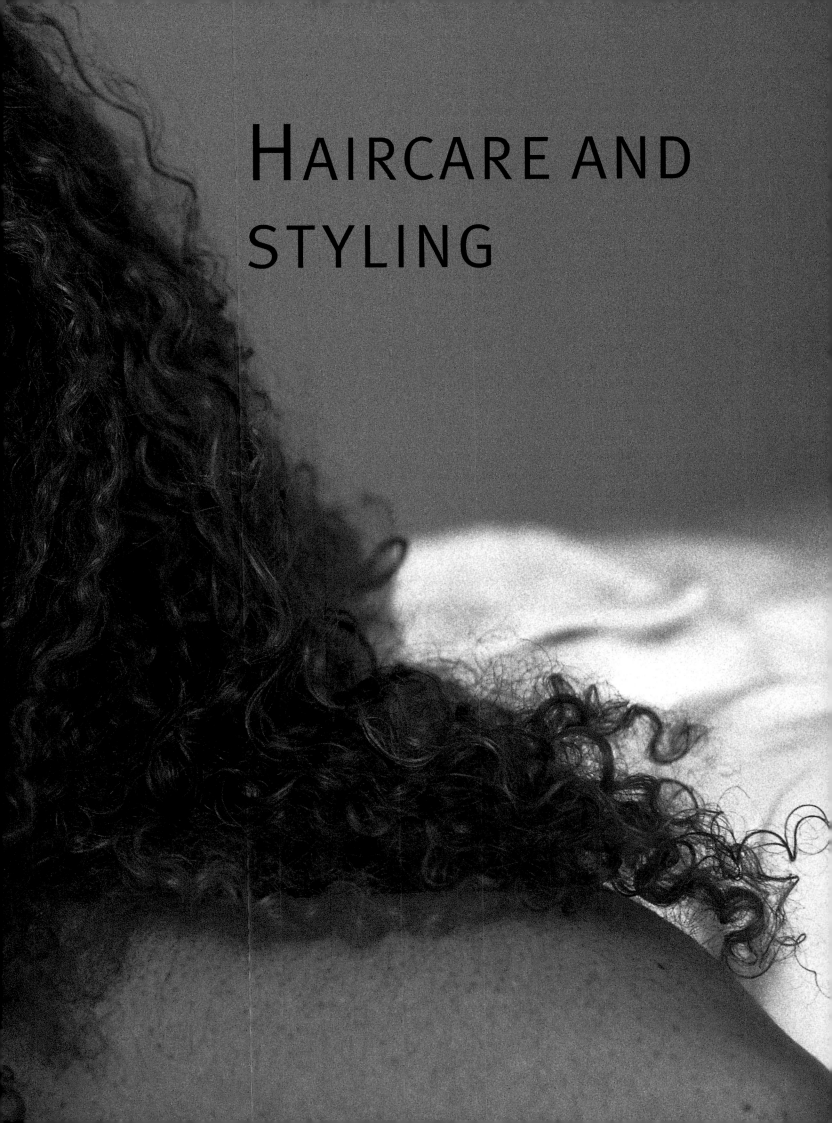

HAIRCARE AND STYLING

The structure of hair

A human hair consists mainly of a protein called keratin. It also contains some moisture and the trace metals and minerals found in the rest of the body. The visible part of the hair, called the shaft, is composed of dead tissue: the only living part of the hair is its root, the dermal papilla, which lies snugly below the surface of the scalp in a tube-like depression known as the follicle. The dermal papilla is made up of cells that are fed by the bloodstream.

Each hair consists of three layers. The outer layer, or cuticle, is the hair's protective shield and has tiny overlapping scales, rather like tiles on a roof. When the cuticle scales lie flat and neatly overlap, the hair feels silky-soft and looks glossy. If, however, the cuticle scales have been physically or chemically damaged or broken, the hair will be dull and brittle and will tangle easily.

Under the cuticle lies the cortex, which is made up of fibre-like cells that give hair its strength and elasticity. The cortex also contains the pigment called melanin, which gives hair its natural colour. At the centre of each hair is the medulla, consisting of very soft keratin cells interspersed with spaces. The actual function of the medulla is not known, but some authorities believe that it carries nutrients and other substances to the cortex and cuticle. This could explain why hair is affected so rapidly by changes in health.

Hair's natural shine is supplied by its own conditioner, sebum, an oil composed of waxes and fats and also containing a natural antiseptic that helps fight infection. Sebum is produced by the sebaceous glands present in the dermis. The glands are linked to the hair follicles and release sebum into them. As a lubricant, sebum gives an excellent protective coating to the hair shaft, smoothing the cuticle scales and helping hair retain its natural moisture and elasticity. The smoother the surface of the cuticle, the more light will be reflected from the hair, and therefore the higher will be the gloss. This is why it is more difficult to obtain a sheen on curly hair than on straight hair.

HAIR STRUCTURE

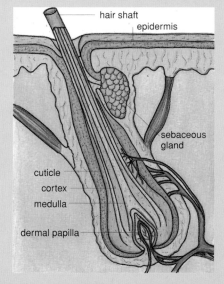

Cross-section of a human hair.

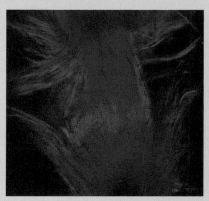

△ **Pictures of a human hair magnified 200 times. A strand of hair in good condition is smooth, but if it has been damaged the outer layer is frayed and broken.**

Under some circumstances, for example excessive hormonal activity, the sebaceous glands produce too much sebum, and the result is oily hair. Conversely, if too little sebum is produced, the hair will be dry.

the growth cycle

The only living part of hair is underneath the scalp – when the hair has grown through the scalp it is dead tissue. Hair has three stages of growth: the anagen phase when it actively grows; the catagen, or transitional, phase when the hair stops growing but cellular activity continues in the papilla; and the telogen, or resting, phase when growth stops completely. During the telogen phase there is no further growth or activity at the papilla; eventually the old hair is pushed out by the new growth and the cycle begins again. The anagen phase continues for a period of two to four years, the catagen phase for only about 15–20 days, and the telogen phase for 90–120 days. At any given time, about 93 per cent of an individual's hair is in the anagen phase, 1 per cent is in the catagen phase and 6 per cent is in the telogen phase. Scalp hair, which reacts to hormonal stimuli like the hair on the rest of the body, is genetically programmed to repeat its growth cycle 24–25 times in the average person's lifetime.

FACT FILE
- Hair grows an average of 12mm/½in per month.
- A single strand lives for up to seven years.
- If a person never had their hair cut it would grow to a length of about 107cm/42in before falling out.
- Women have more hair than men.
- Hair grows faster in the summer and during sleep.
- Hair grows fastest between the ages of 16 and 24.
- Between the ages of 40 and 50 women tend to lose about 20 per cent of their hair.
- Hair becomes drier with age.

the importance of diet

What you eat is soon reflected in the health of your hair. Like the rest of the body, the hair depends on a good diet to ensure it is supplied with all the necessary nutrients for sustained growth and health. Regular exercise is also important as it promotes good blood circulation, which in turn ensures that vital oxygen and nutrients are transported to the hair root via the blood. Poor eating habits and lack of exercise are soon reflected in the state of the hair; even a minor case of ill-health will usually make it look limp and lacklustre.

An adequate supply of protein in the diet is essential. Good sources include lean meat, poultry, fish, cheese and eggs as well as nuts, seeds and pulses. Fish, seaweed, almonds, brazil nuts, yoghurt and cottage cheese all help to give hair strength and a natural shine.

Wholegrain foods and those with natural oils are highly recommended for the formation of keratin, the major component of hair. Seeds are a rich source of vitamins and minerals as well as protein. Try to eat at least three pieces of fruit a day – it is packed with fibre, vitamins and minerals. Avoid saturated fat, which is found in red meat, fried foods and dairy products. Choose skimmed or semi-skimmed (low-fat) milk rather than the whole varieties, and low-fat cheese and yogurt instead of whole cheese and cream. Use vegetable oils such as sunflower, safflower and olive oil instead of animal fats. These foods all provide nutrients that are essential for luxuriant hair.

If you eat a balanced diet with plenty of fresh ingredients you shouldn't need to take any supplementary vitamins to promote healthy hair growth.

colour

Hair colour is closely related to skin colour, which is governed by the same type of pigment, melanin. The number of melanin granules in the cortex of the hair, and the shape of the granules, determines a person's natural hair colour. In the majority of cases the melanin granules are elongated in shape. People who have a large number of elongated melanin granules in the cortex have black hair, those with slightly fewer elongated granules have brown hair, and people with even fewer will be blonde. In

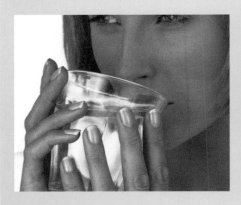

△ **Drink plenty of water every day to keep your hair healthy.**

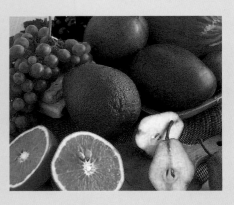

△ **Eating 2 or 3 pieces of fruit a day provides your hair with vital vitamins and minerals.**

other people the melanin granules are spherical or oval in shape rather than elongated, and this makes the hair appear red.

Spherical or oval granules sometimes appear in combination with a moderate amount of the elongated ones, and then the person will have rich, reddish-brown tinges. If, however, spherical granules occur in combination with a large number of elongated granules then the blackness of the hair will almost mask the redness, although it will still be present to give a subtle tinge to the hair and differentiate it from pure black.

Hair darkens with age, but at some stage in the middle years of life the pigment formation slows down and silvery-grey hairs begin to appear. Gradually, the production of melanin ceases, and all the hair becomes colourless – or what is generally termed grey.

When melanin granules are completely lacking from birth, as in albinos, the hair has no colour and is pure white.

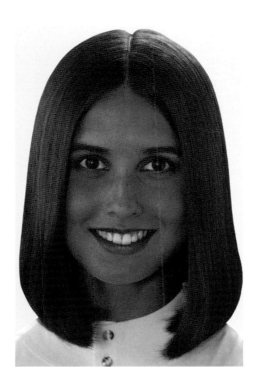

◁ **The colour of your hair is determined by the amount of pigment in the hair and also by the shape of the pigment granules. People with dark hair have larger quantities of pigment than people with blonde hair. In both brunettes and blondes the pigment granules are elongated in shape; red hair results from the presence of oval granules.**

Hair analysis – texture and type

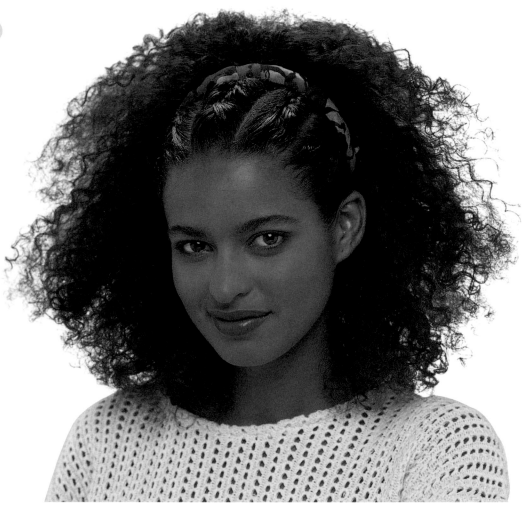

◁ **Hair with a very curly texture needs intensive moisturizing treatments to keep the spring in the curl. On this type of hair always use a wide-toothed comb, never a brush, which will make the hair frizz. Leave-in conditioners are good for curly hair as they help to give curl separation. To revitalize curls, mist with water and scrunch with the hands.**

HAIR FACT FILE
- Healthy hair is highly elastic and can stretch 20 or 30 per cent before snapping.
- Chinese circus acrobats have been known to perform tricks while suspended by their hair.
- A human hair is stronger than copper wire of the same thickness.
- The combined strength of a headful of human hair is capable of supporting a weight equivalent to that of 99 people.

The texture of your hair is determined by the size and shape of the hair follicle, which is a genetic trait controlled by hormones and related to age and racial characteristics.

Whether hair is curly, wavy or straight depends on two things: its shape as it grows out of the follicle, and the distribution of keratin-producing cells at the roots. When viewed in cross section, straight hair tends to be round, wavy hair tends to be oval, and curly hair kidney-shaped. Straight hair is formed by roots that produce the same number of keratin cells all around the follicle. In wavy and curly hair, the production of keratin cells is uneven, so that at any given time there are more cells on one side of the oval-shaped follicle than on the other. Furthermore, the production of excess cells alternates between the sides. This causes the developing hair to grow first

in one direction and then in the other. The result is wavy or curly hair.

The natural colour of the hair also affects the texture. Natural blondes have finer hair than brunettes, while redheads have the thickest hair.

Generally speaking, hair can be divided into three categories: fine, medium, and coarse and thick. Fine hair can be strong or weak; however, because of its texture, all fine

hair has the same characteristic – it lacks volume. As the name suggests, medium hair is neither too thick nor too thin, and is strong and elastic. Thick and coarse hair is abundant and heavy, with a tendency to grow outwards from the scalp as well as downwards. It often lacks elasticity and is frizzy.

A single head of hair may consist of several different textures. For example, fine hair is often found on the temples, and the hairline at the front and on the nape of the head, while the texture over the rest of the head may be medium or even coarse.

ETHNIC DIFFERENCES

Generally, people from Scandinavia have thin, straight, baby-fine hair, and mid-European populations have hair that is neither too fine nor too coarse. People native to the Indian subcontinent have thick-textured tresses while Middle-Eastern populations have strong hair. In very general terms, the further east you travel the coarser hair becomes. The hair of Chinese and Japanese people is usually extremely straight; and that of Latin-speaking and North African peoples can be very frizzy and thick.

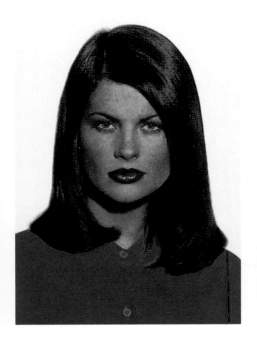

△ Thick straight hair can be made sleeker if you remember always to blow-dry downwards. This encourages the cuticles to lie flat and reflect the light.

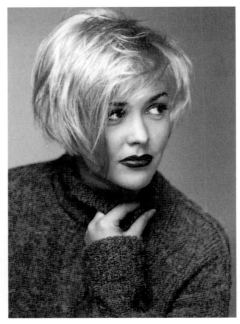

△ Fine hair needs regular expert cutting to maximize the volume. Here, gel spray was used to give lift at the roots and the hair was then blow-dried.

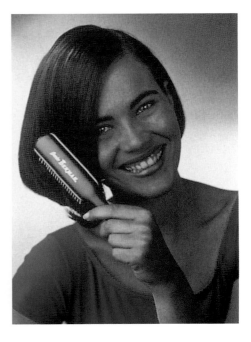

△ Normal hair generally holds a style well. It is usually very easy to look after and responds well to regular brushing, smoothing and polishing.

normal, dry or oily?

Hair type is determined by the hair's natural condition – that is, the amount of sebum the body produces. Treatments such as perming, colouring and heat styling will also have an effect on hair type. Natural hair types and those produced by applying treatments are described here, with advice on haircare where appropriate.

dry hair

It can look dull, feels dry and tangles easily. It is difficult to brush, particularly when it is wet. It is often quite thick at the roots but thinner, and sometimes split, at the ends.
Causes Excessive shampooing, over-use of heat-styling equipment, misuse of colour or perms, damage from the sun, or harsh weather conditions. Each of these factors depletes the moisture content of hair, so that it loses its elasticity, bounce and suppleness. Dryness can also be the result of a sebum deficiency on the hair's surface, caused by a decrease in or absence of sebaceous gland secretions.
Solutions Use a nourishing shampoo and an intensive conditioner. Dry hair naturally.

normal hair

It is neither oily nor dry, has not been permed or coloured, holds its style, and looks good most of the time. Normal hair is suited to the daily use of two-in-one conditioning shampoos. These are formulated to provide a two-stage process in one application. When the product is lathered into wet hair the shampoo removes dirt, grease and styling products. At this stage the conditioner remains in the lather. As the hair is rinsed with more water, the grease and dirt are washed away, and the micro-fine conditioning droplets are released on to the hair, leaving it shiny and easy to comb.

oily hair

It looks lank and greasy and needs frequent washing to look good.
Causes Overproduction of sebum as a result of hormone disturbances, stress, hot and humid atmosphere, excessive brushing, or constantly running hands through the hair, perspiration, or a diet rich in saturated fat. The hair becomes oily, sticky and unmanageable in just a few days, or sometimes within hours.
Solutions Use a gentle, non-aggressive shampoo that also gives the hair volume. A light perm will lift the hair at the roots and limit the dispersal of sebum. Rethink your diet: cut out as many dairy fats and greasy foods as you can. Try to eat plenty of fresh food, and drink six to eight glasses of water every day.

combination hair

It is oily at the roots but dry and sometimes split at the ends.
Causes Chemical treatments, using detergent-based shampoos too frequently, overexposure to sunlight, and over-use of heat-styling equipment. Such repeated abuse often provokes a reaction in sebum secretion at the roots and a partial alteration in the scales, which can no longer fulfil their protective role. The hair ends therefore become dry.
Solutions Use products that have only a gentle action on the hair. Excessive use of formulations for oily hair and those for dry hair may contribute to the problem. Ideally, use a product specially designed for combination hair. If this is not possible try using a shampoo for oily hair and finish by applying a conditioner from the middle lengths to the ends of the hair only.

coloured or permed hair

It is very often more porous than untreated hair, so it needs to be treated with gentle cleansers and good conditioners. Colour-care products will help prevent fading by protecting the hair from the damaging rays of sunlight. Products specially designed for permed hair can also help maintain elasticity, giving longer-lasting results.

Times of change

Hair goes through many different stages during a lifetime. Each stage brings with it different requirements in haircare. The most significant stages are described below, together with recommendations for promoting hair health during each phase.

beginnings: the baby and child

A baby's hair characteristics are determined from the very moment of conception. By the 16th week of pregnancy the foetus will be covered with lanugo, a downy body hair that is usually shed before birth. The first hair appears on the head at around 20 weeks' gestation and it is at this time that the pigment melanin, which will determine the colour of the hair, is first produced.

A few weeks after birth, the baby's original hair begins to fall out or is rubbed off. The new hair is quite different from the initial downy mass, so a baby born with blonde wispy curls might have dark straight hair by the age of six months.

GROWING UP

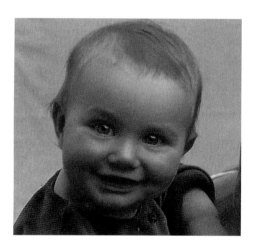

△ A baby's hair is soft and downy at first but it takes on its individual characteristics within six months of birth.

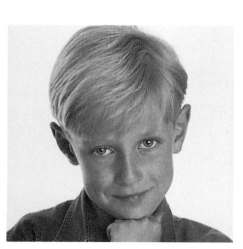

△ Young boys need a hair cut that is easily combed into shape.

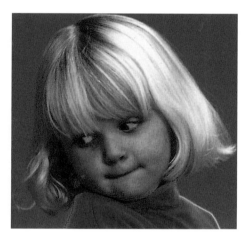

△ The toddler's hair requires a simple cut. At this stage the child is usually taken for her first visit to a salon.

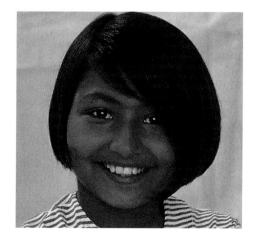

△ Bobs suit most girls and are perfect for straight hair, but need regular trims.

Cradle cap, which appears as thick, yellow scales in patches over the scalp, causes many mothers concern. Cradle cap is the result of a natural build-up of skin cells. It is nothing to worry about and can be gently loosened by rubbing a little baby oil on to the scalp at night and washing it off in the morning. This may need to be repeated for several days until all the loose scales have been lifted and washed away.

Mothers often carefully trim their baby's hair when necessary, and it is not until the child is about two years of age that a visit to a hairdressing salon may be necessary. Children's hair is normally in beautiful condition and is best cut and styled simply.

At the onset of puberty young adults suddenly become much more interested in experimenting with their hair. This is when they may experience oily hair and skin for the first time. A re-evaluation of the shampoos and conditioners currently in use is often necessary to keep hair looking good.

haircare during pregnancy

During pregnancy the hair often looks its best. However after the birth, or after breast-feeding ceases, about 50 per cent of new mothers experience what appears to be excessive hair loss. This is related to the three stages of hair growth (see page 104). During pregnancy and breast-feeding, hormones keep the hair at the growing stage for longer than usual, so it appears thicker and fuller. Some time after the birth – usually about 12 weeks later – this hair enters the resting stage, at the end of which all the hair that has been in the resting phase is shed. What appears to be excessive hair loss is therefore simply a postponement of a natural occurrence, a condition that is known as post-partum alopecia.

A more significant problem that may occur during pregnancy is caused by a depletion in the protein content of the hair. As a result the hair becomes drier and more brittle. Combat this by frequent use of an intensive conditioning treatment.

Avoid perming during pregnancy because the hair is in an altered state and the result can be unpredictable. Try a herbal rinse to give your hair and your spirits a lift.

growing older

With aging the whole body slows down, including the hair follicles, which become less efficient and produce hairs that are finer in diameter and shorter in length. Such shrinkage is gradual and the hair begins to feel slightly thinner, with less volume and density. At the same time the sebaceous glands start to produce less sebum and the hair begins to lose its colour as the production of melanin decreases.

Blonde hair fades, brunettes lose natural highlights, and redheads tone down to brown shades. When melanin production stops altogether the new hair that grows is white, not grey as is commonly perceived. The production of melanin is governed by genetic factors, and the best indication of when an individual's hair will become white is the age at which their parents' hair did. Pigment, apart from giving hair its colour, also helps to soften and make each strand more flexible. This is why white hair tends to become wirier and coarser in texture.

As the texture of the hair changes, it is inclined to pick up dust and smoke from the atmosphere, so that it soon appears to be discoloured and dirty. This is particularly true for those who live in a town or spend time in smoky atmospheres. Cigarette smoke and natural gas from cookers discolour white hair and make it look yellow. Mineral deposits from chlorinated water can give white hair a greenish tinge. Chelating, clarifying or purifying shampoos will help to strip this build-up from the hair.

To counteract dryness associated with aging, use richer shampoos and conditioning products. As well as regular conditioning, weekly intensive treatments are essential to counteract moisture loss.

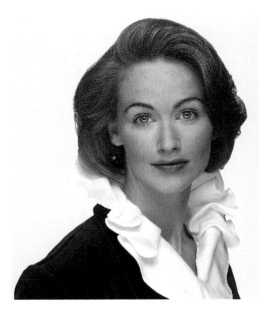

△ **As women grow older the hair becomes thinner. A mid-length to short cut makes the hair less prone to droop.**

AS THE YEARS GO BY

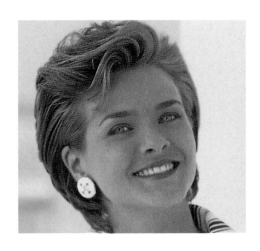

△ **Medium-textured hair that has gone flat and needs a lift can be given height on the crown with a root perm.**

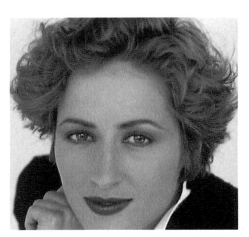

△ **The hair has been cut to create more movement and softness. It was then scrunch-dried and finished with wax.**

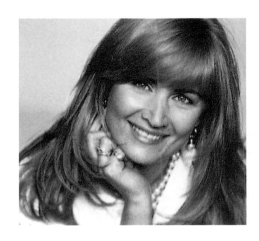

△ **Long hair was softened by feathering the sides and cutting a full fringe (bangs). A semi-permanent colour added gloss.**

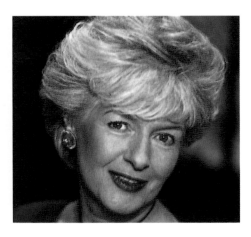

△ **This fine grey hair was highlighted and then toned using a rinse before blow-drying with a round brush.**

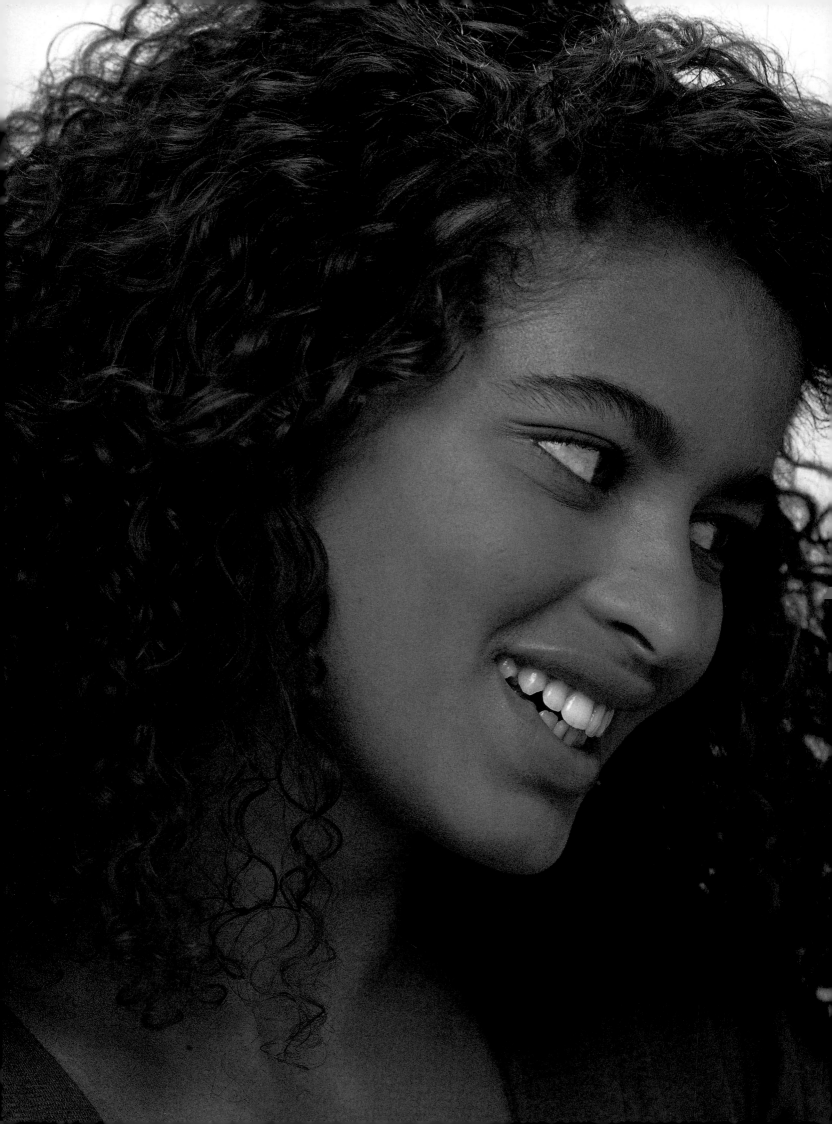

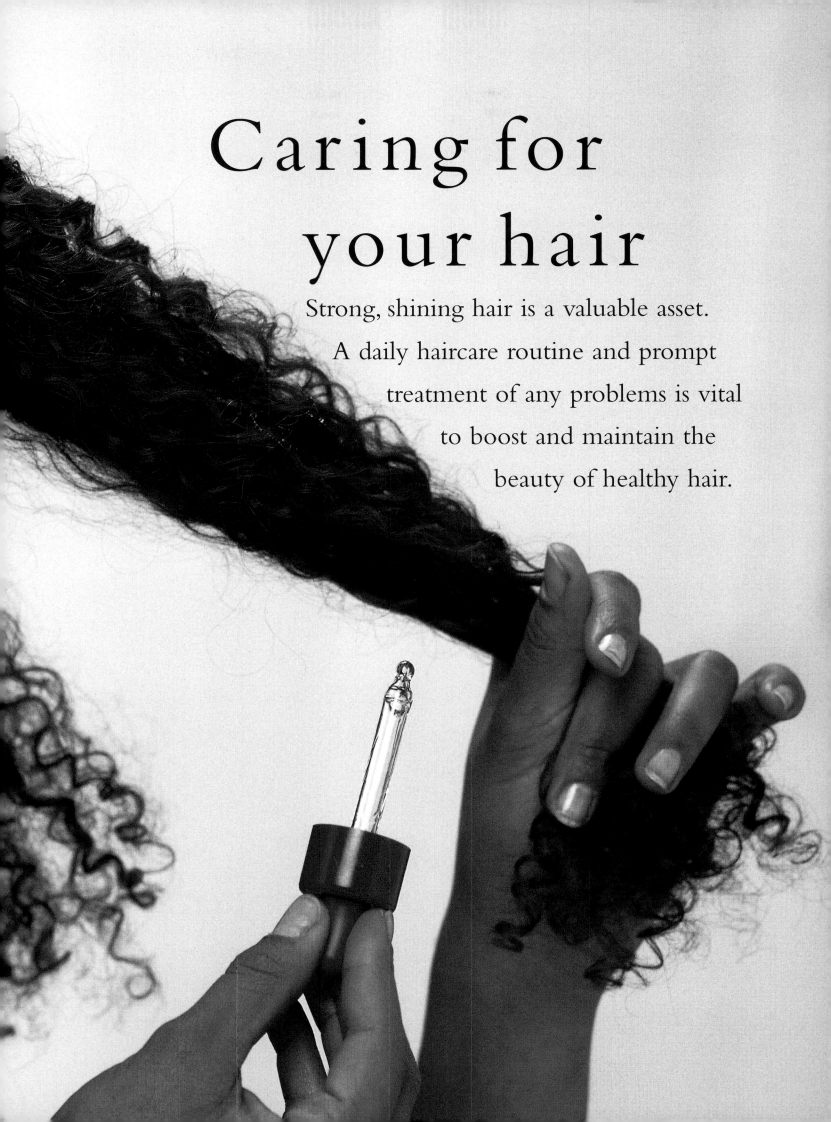

Caring for your hair

Strong, shining hair is a valuable asset.
A daily haircare routine and prompt
treatment of any problems is vital
to boost and maintain the
beauty of healthy hair.

The cut

Hair growth varies over different parts of the head. This is why your cut can appear to be out of shape very quickly. As a general rule, a short precision cut needs trimming every four weeks, a longer style every six to eight weeks. Even if you want to grow your hair long it is essential to have it trimmed regularly – at least every three months – to prevent splitting and keep the ends even.

Hairdressers use a variety of techniques and tools to make hair appear thicker, fuller, straighter or curlier, whatever the desired effect. These techniques and tools are explained below.

Blunt cutting, in which the ends are cut straight across, is often used for hair of one length. The weight and fullness of the hair is distributed around the perimeter of the shape.

Clippers: Used for close-cut styles and sometimes to finish off a cut. Shaved clipper cuts are popular with teenagers.

Graduated hair: This is cut at an angle to give fullness on top and blend the top hair into shorter lengths at the nape.

Layering the hair: This technique evenly distributes the weight and fullness, giving a round appearance to the style.

Slide cutting: (also called slithering or feathering) This thins the hair. Scissors are used in a sliding action, backwards and forwards along the hair length. This technique is often done when the hair is dry.

Razor cutting: Used to create softness, tapering and internal movement so that the hair moves more freely. It can also be used to shorten hair.

Thinning: Either with thinning scissors or a razor, removes bulk and weight without affecting the overall length of the hair.

clever cuts

Fine, thin, flyaway hair can be given volume, bounce and movement by blunt cutting. Mid-length hair can benefit from being lightly layered to give extra volume, while short, thin hair can be blunt cut and the edges graduated to give movement.

Some hairdressers razor cut fine hair to give a thicker and more voluminous effect. It is best not to let fine hair grow too long. As soon as it reaches the shoulders it tends to look wispy and out of control.

Thick and coarse hair can be controlled by reducing the weight to give more style

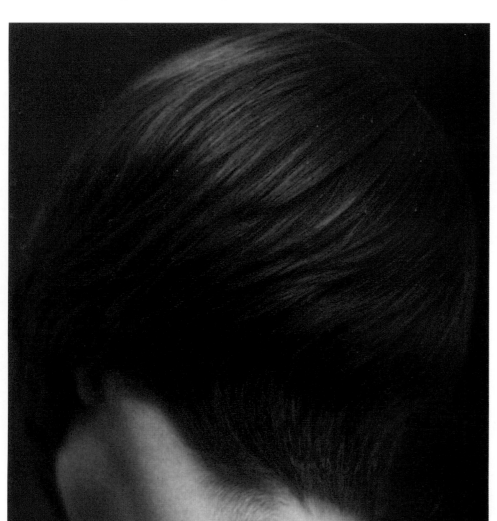

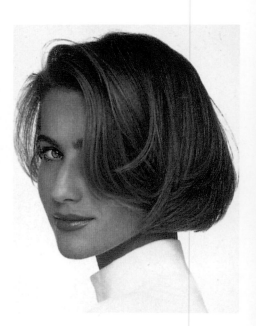

△ For this style the model's straight hair was cut so that it would swing back into shape with every movement of the head. The shine was improved by using a longer-lasting semi-permanent colour.

◁ This heavily layered, graduated bob was cut close into the nape, and then the shape of the hair was emphasized by using a vegetable colour to give tone and shine. The hair was styled by blow-drying.

cutting to add volume and shape

A good stylist can, with technical expertise, make the most of any type of hair, so take time to discuss what you like and dislike about your hair. A good haircut should need the minimum of styling products and drying to achieve the desired result.

and direction. Avoid very short styles because the hair will tend to stick out. Try a layered cut with movement.

Layering also helps achieve height and eliminate weight. On shorter styles the weight can be reduced with thinning scissors expertly used on the ends only.

Sometimes hair grows in different directions, which may cause styling problems. For example, a cowlick is normally found on the front hairline and occurs when the hair grows in a swirl, backwards and then forwards. Clever cutting can redistribute the weight and go some way to solving this problem. A double crown occurs when there are two pivots for natural hair at the top of the head, rather than the usual one. Styles with height at the crown are most suitable here.

To maximize the effect of a widow's peak the hair should be taken in the reverse direction to the growth. This gives the impression of a natural wave.

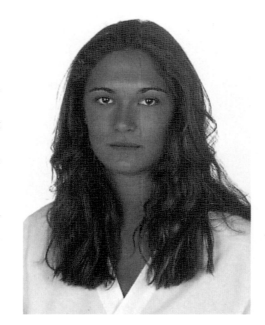

△ **1** Before she had her hair cut, our model's long hair had natural movement but the weight was pulling the hair down and spoiling the shape. For her new style she wanted a shorter, more sophisticated look, and one that would be easy to maintain.

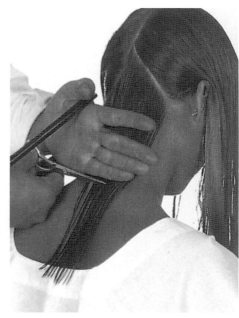

△ **2** First the model's hair was shampooed, conditioned and then combed through to remove any tangles. The stylist was then ready to start cutting. He began by sectioning off the front hair so that the hair at the back could be cut to the required length.

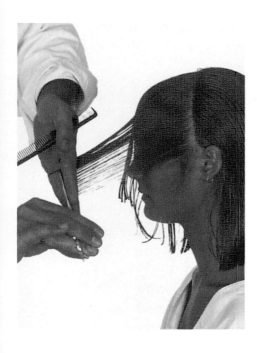

△ **3** Next the front hair was combed forward and cut straight across at an angle. This ensured that when the model's hair was dry it would fall easily into shape.

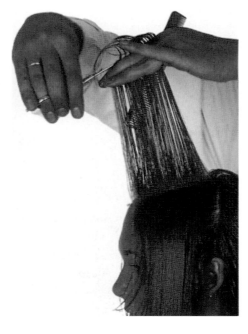

△ **4** The top hair was graduated to help build volume and lift into the style. This versatile cut makes it possible for the hair to be styled either towards the face or towards the back of the head.

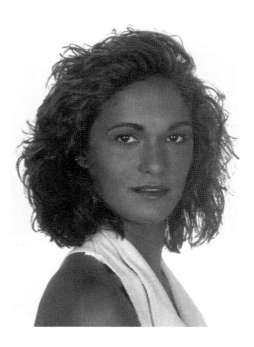

△ **5** To finish, the stylist scrunched the hair, using a blow-dryer and some mousse to encourage the formation of curls. On this type of style a diffuser fitted to the dryer will spread the airflow and give added movement to the hair.

Shampooing

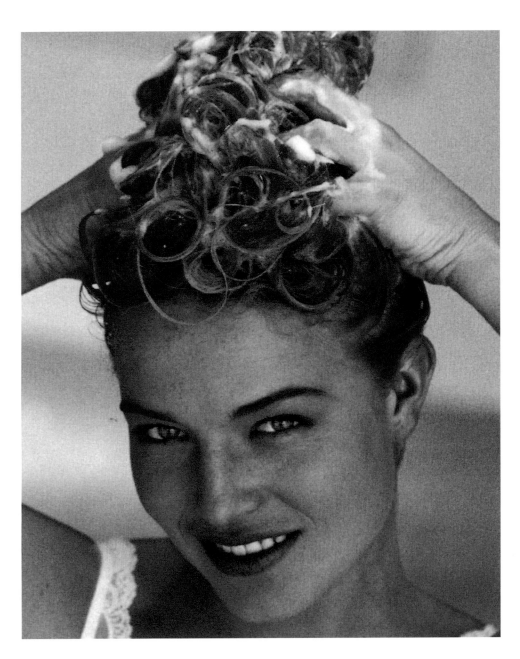

Shampoos are designed to cleanse the hair and scalp thoroughly, removing dirt, grease and grime without stripping away too much of the protective natural sebum. They contain cleansing agents, perfume and preservatives, and some have conditioning properties that can coat the hair shaft to make the hair appear thicker. The conditioning agents also smooth the cuticle scales so the hair doesn't tangle, and help eliminate static electricity from the hair when it dries.

the pH factor

The letters pH relate to the acid/alkaline level of a substance. This level is calculated on a scale of 1 to 14. Numbers below 7 denote acidity, those over 7 indicate alkalinity. The majority of shampoos range between a pH factor of 5 and 7; medicated varieties have a pH of about 7.3, which is near neutral.

Sebum has a pH factor of between 4.5 and 5.5, which is mildly acidic. Bacteria cannot survive in this pH, so it is very important to maintain this protective layer in order to keep the skin, scalp and hair in optimum condition.

◁ **Shampoos are available in different formulas to suit all hair types and conditions. Make sure you choose one that is right for your hair and use it as often as necessary to keep your hair clean. Rinse out the shampoo thoroughly.**

SHAMPOO TIPS

• Use the correct shampoo (and not too much) for your hair type. If in doubt use the mildest shampoo you can buy.

• Don't wash your hair in washing-up liquid, soap or other detergents; they are highly alkaline and will upset your hair's natural pH balance by stripping out the natural oils.

• Read the instructions first. Some shampoos need to be left on the scalp for a few minutes before rinsing.

• If you can, buy small packets of shampoo to test which brand is most suitable for your hair.

• Never wash your hair in the bath; dirty bath water is not conducive to clean hair, and it is difficult to rinse properly without a shower attachment or separate pourer.

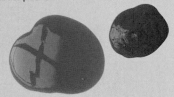

• Always wash your brush and comb when you shampoo your hair.

• Change your shampoo every now and then; hair seems to develop a resistance to certain ingredients after a period of time.

• Don't throw away a shampoo that doesn't lather. The amount of suds is determined by the active level of detergent. Some shampoos have less suds than others but this has no effect on their cleansing ability. In fact, quite often, the more effective the product, the fewer the bubbles.

▷ A head massage reduces scalp tension as well as promoting healthy hair growth. It is also a relaxing and pampering treatment that you can do yourself at home.

Many shampoos are labelled "pH balanced", and this means they have the same acidity level as hair. Individuals with fragile, permed or coloured hair should use a shampoo of this type. However, for strong hair in good condition, a pH balanced shampoo is unnecessary, provided shampooing is followed by conditioning.

shampoo success

Always use a product formulated for your hair type – dry, normal, oily or chemically treated – and before shampooing brush your hair to free any tangles and loosen dirt and dead skin cells. Use lukewarm water, as hot water can be uncomfortable.

Wet the hair, then apply a small amount of shampoo and gently massage into the roots using the pads of your fingertips; never use your nails. Pay special attention to the hairline area, where make-up and dirt can become trapped. Allow the lather to work its way to the ends of the hair. Don't rub vigorously or you will stretch the hair.

When you have finished shampooing, rinse thoroughly until the water runs clean and clear. Repeat the process only if you think your hair needs it, again using only a small amount of shampoo. Finally, blot the hair with a towel to remove excess water before applying conditioner.

massaging the scalp

Massage helps maintain a healthy scalp. It brings extra blood to the tissues, which enhances the delivery of nutrients and oxygen to the hair follicle. It also reduces scalp tension, which can contribute to hair loss, loosens dead skin cells and helps redress the overproduction of sebum, which makes hair oily.

You can give yourself a scalp massage at home. Use warm olive oil if the scalp is dry or tight. Try equal parts of witch hazel and mineral water if you have an oily scalp. For a normal scalp, use equal parts rose and mineral waters.

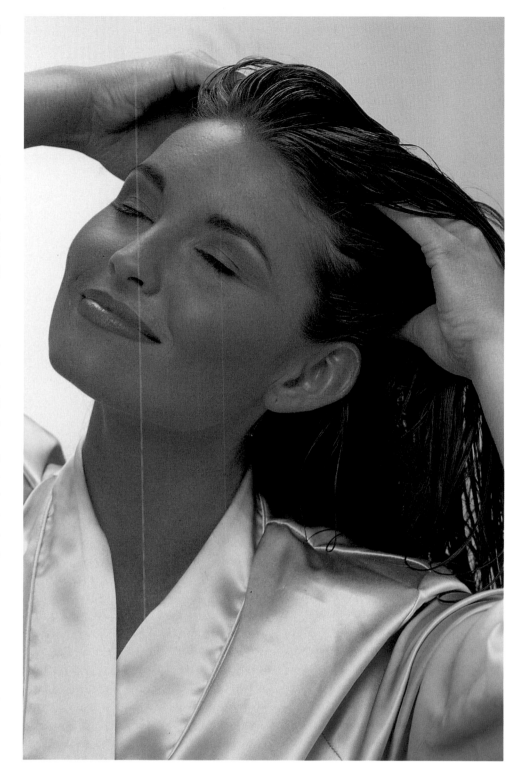

Begin the massage by gently rotating your scalp using the tips of your fingers. Start at the forehead, move to the sides, and work over the crown to the nape of the neck. Then place your fingertips firmly on the scalp without exerting too much pressure. Push the fingers together then pull them apart through the hair in a kneading motion, without lifting or moving them. When you have massaged for about a minute, move to the next section. Continue until your entire scalp and upper neck have been treated.

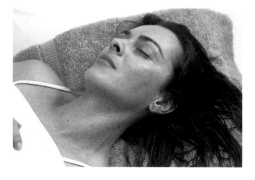

△ For a really deep conditioning treatment, oils can be left on overnight to continue working while you recharge with a restful sleep.

Getting into condition

In an ideal world a regular shampoo would be sufficient to guarantee a glossy head of hair. Unfortunately very few people are able to wash their hair and let the matter rest at that; most need some sort of help just to overcome the effects of modern living, not to mention the occasional problem that needs treatment. Here is a guide to the vast array of products available to get the hair in excellent condition.

the conditioners

Glossy hair has cuticle scales that lie flat and neatly overlap, thus reflecting the light. Perming and colouring, rough handling and heat styling all conspire to lift the cuticles, allowing moisture to be lost from the cortex and making hair dry, lacklustre and prone to knotting and tangling. Severely damaged cuticles break off completely, resulting in thinner hair which eventually breaks.

To put the shine back into hair and restore its natural lustre it may be necessary to use a specific conditioner that meets the hair's requirements. Conditioners, with the exception of hot oils, should be applied to freshly shampooed hair that has been blotted dry with a towel to remove excess moisture.

Today there is a large, and sometimes confusing, number of conditioners on the market. The following list describes those that are widely available:

Basic conditioners: These coat the hair with a fine film, temporarily smoothing down the cuticle and making hair glossier and easier to manage. Leave for a few minutes before rinsing thoroughly.

Conditioning sprays: These are used prior to styling and form a protective barrier against the harmful effects of heat. They are also good for reducing static electricity on flyaway hair.

Hot oils: Used to give an intensive, deep nourishing treatment. To use, place the unopened tube in a cup of hot tap water and leave to heat for one minute. Next, wet the hair and towel it dry before twisting off the

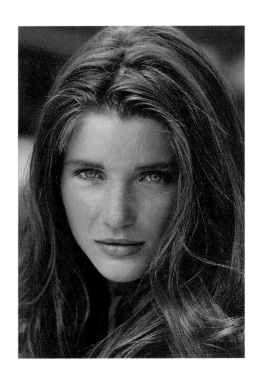

△ **Long hair needs a regular conditioning regime to keep it healthy and shiny.**

tube top. Massage the hot oil evenly into the scalp and through the hair for one to three minutes. For a more intensive treatment cover the head with a shower cap. To finish, rinse the hair and shampoo.

Intensive conditioners: These can help hair to retain its natural moisture balance, replenishing it where necessary. Use this type if the hair is split, dry, frizzy or difficult to manage. Distribute the conditioner evenly through the hair and then allow it to penetrate for two to five minutes, or longer if required. Rinse very thoroughly with lots of fresh, warm water, lifting your hair from the scalp to ensure any residue is washed away.

Leave-in conditioners: Designed to help retain moisture, reduce static and add shine, they are especially good for fine hair as they avoid conditioner overload, which can cause lankness. Convenient and easy to use, they also provide a protective barrier against the effects of heat styling. Apply after shampooing but don't rinse off. These products are ideal for daily use.

Restructants: These penetrate the cortex, helping to repair and strengthen the inner part of damaged hair. They are helpful if the hair is lank and limp and has lost its natural elasticity as a result of chemical treatments or physical damage.

Split end treatments/serums: Used to condition damaged hair. The best course of action for split ends is to have the ends trimmed, but this does not always solve the whole problem because the hair tends to break off and split at different levels. As an intermediate solution, split ends can be temporarily sealed using these specialized conditioners. They should be worked into the ends of newly washed hair so that they surround the hair with a microscopic film that leaves the hair shaft smoother.

Colour/perm conditioners: These are designed for chemically treated hair. After-colour products add a protective film around porous areas of the hair, preventing colour loss. After-perm products help stabilize the hair, thus keeping the bounce in the curl.

problems and solutions

Split ends, dandruff and a dry, itchy scalp are common problems that can detract from otherwise healthy hair. In most cases such problems can be overcome by giving the appropriate treatment.

Dandruff: This consists of scaly particles with an oily sheen that lie close to the hair root. This condition should not be confused with a flaky scalp (see below).

Causes Poor diet, sluggish metabolism, stress, a hormonal imbalance, and sometimes infection. These conditions usually produce increased cell renewal on the scalp, which is often associated with an increase in sebum. The scales will absorb the excess oil, however if the problem remains untreated it will become worse.

Solutions Rethink your diet and lifestyle. Learn relaxation techniques if the problem appears to be caused by stress. Brush the hair

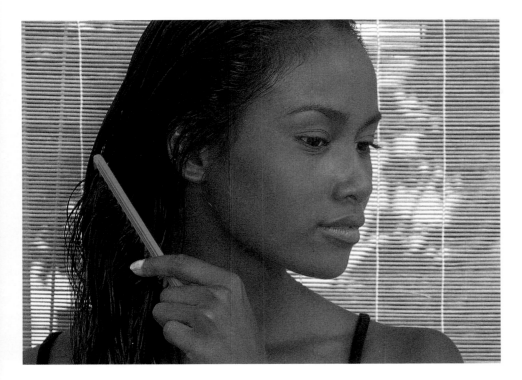

△ **Leaving the oils in your hair after an oil massage is a holistic treatment and helps leave your hair and scalp in excellent condition.**

before shampooing and scrupulously wash combs and brushes. Always choose a mild shampoo with an antidandruff action that gently loosens scales and helps prevent new ones. Follow with a treatment lotion, massaged into the scalp using the fingertips. The treatment must be used regularly if it is to be effective. Avoid excessive use of heat stylers. If the dandruff persists, consult your doctor or trichologist.

Flaky/itchy scalp: This condition produces tiny white pieces of dead skin that flake off the scalp and are usually first noticed on the shoulders. This condition can often be confused with dandruff but the two are not related. Sometimes the scalp is red or itchy and feels tight. The hair usually has a dull appearance.

Causes Hereditary traits, stress, insufficient rinsing of shampoo, lack of sebum, using a harsh shampoo, vitamin imbalance, pollution, air conditioning and central heating.

Solutions Choose a moisturizing shampoo and a conditioner with herbal extracts to help soothe and remoisturize the scalp.

Fine hair: This tends to look flat, and is hard to style because it does not hold a shape.

Causes The texture is hereditary, but the problem is often made worse by using too heavy a conditioner, which weighs the hair down. Excessive use of styling products can have the same effect.

Solutions Wash hair frequently with a mild shampoo and use a light conditioner.

Volumizing shampoos can help give body, and soft perms will make hair appear thicker.

Frizzy hair: This can result from the merest hint of rain or other air moisture being absorbed into the hair. It looks dry, lacks lustre, and is difficult to control.

Causes It can be inherited or it can be caused by rough treatment, such as too much harsh brushing or regularly pulling the hair into rubber bands.

Solutions When washing the hair, massage the shampoo into the roots and allow the lather to work its way to the ends. Apply a conditioner from the mid-lengths of the hair to the ends, or use a leave-in

PROFESSIONAL TIPS
• Blot hair to remove excess moisture before applying conditioner.
• Gently massage conditioner into the hair, or use a wide-toothed comb to distribute it evenly.
• Leave the conditioner on the hair for the time specified – check whether it is a "leave-in" or "rinse-out" variety.
• If necessary, rinse thoroughly.
• Treat wet hair with care; it is much more sensitive and vulnerable than dry hair.
• Avoid rubbing, pulling or stretching wet hair.

conditioner. The hair is often best styled with a gel, and it is most effective if it is applied when the hair is wet. Alternatively, allow the hair to dry naturally and then style it using a wax or pomade. Serums can also help. These are silicone-based products that work by surrounding the cuticle with a transparent microscopic film, which leaves the hair shaft smoother. Serums effectively prevent moisture loss and inhibit the absorption of dampness from the surrounding air.

Split ends: These occur when the cuticle is damaged and the fibres of the cortex unravel. The hair is dry, brittle and prone to tangling, and can split at the end or anywhere along the shaft.

Causes Over-perming or colouring, insufficient conditioning, or too much brushing or backcombing, especially with poor-quality combs or brushes. Careless use of spiky rollers and hair pins, excessive heat styling and not having the hair trimmed regularly can also cause the problem.

Solutions Split ends cannot be repaired; the only long-term solution is to have them snipped off regularly. What is lost in the length will be gained in quality. It may help if you reduce the frequency with which you shampoo, as this in itself is stressful to hair and causes split ends to extend up the hair shaft. Never use a dryer too near the hair, or set it on too high a temperature. Minimize the use of heated appliances. Try conditioners and serums that are designed to seal split ends temporarily and give resistance to further splitting.

Product build-up: This is caused by the residue of styling products and two-in-one shampoo formulation left on the hair shaft.

Causes When these residues combine with mineral deposits in the water a build-up occurs, preventing thorough cleansing and conditioning. The result is hair that is dull and lack lustre; it is often difficult to perm or colour successfully because there is a barrier preventing the chemicals from penetrating the hair shaft. The colour can be patchy and the perm uneven.

Solutions Use one of the stripping, chelating or clarifying shampoos, which are specially designed to strip out product build-up. This is particularly important prior to perming or colouring.

Natural hair treatments

For thousands of years, herbs and plants have been mixed and blended and then used to heal, freshen, pamper and beautify hair. The following are a few age-old haircare recipes that you might like to try at home. Remember to use these treatments immediately after you have made them because they won't keep well.

natural dandruff treatment
Mix a few drops of oil of rosemary with 30ml/2 tbsp olive oil and rub well into the scalp at bedtime. Shampoo and rinse thoroughly in the morning.

easy egg shampoo
In a blender mix together two small (US medium) eggs with 50ml/2fl oz/¼ cup still mineral water and 15ml/1 tbsp cider vinegar or lemon juice. Blend for 30 seconds at low speed. Massage well into the scalp and rinse very thoroughly using lukewarm water (if the water is any hotter the egg will begin to set).

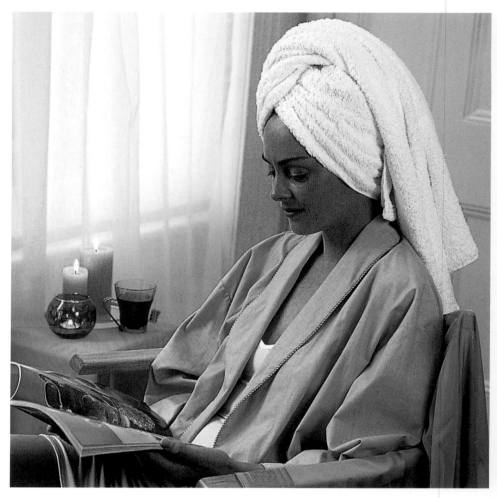

△ Once you have applied a conditioning treatment to your hair, wrap your hair in a warm towel. Then lie back and relax for 20 minutes or so, to allow the treatment plenty of time to work.

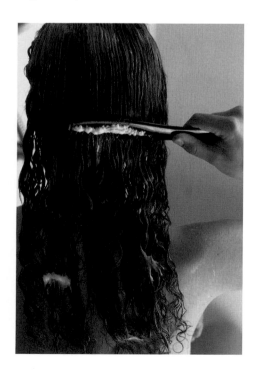

△ Treatments can be applied more thoroughly to the hair by using a wide-toothed comb. This ensures it is applied from root to tip.

herbal shampoo
Crush a few dried bay leaves with a rolling pin, or with a pestle and mortar, and mix with a handful of dried chamomile flowers and one of rosemary. Place in a large jug and pour over 900ml/3½ cups boiling water. Strain after 2–3 minutes and mix in 5ml/ 1 tsp soft or liquid soap. Apply to the hair, massaging well. Rinse thoroughly.

zesty hair cream
Beat 150ml/⅔ cup natural yoghurt with an egg; add 5ml/1 tsp sea kelp powder and 5ml/1 tsp finely grated lemon rind. Mix thoroughly and work into the hair. Cover your hair with a plastic shower cap and leave in place for 40 minutes. Shampoo and rinse.

hair rescuer
For dry, damaged hair, apply this mixture after shampooing. Leave for 5 minutes, then rinse.

ingredients
- 30ml/2 tbsp olive oil
- 30ml/2 tbsp light sesame oil
- 2 eggs
- 30ml/2 tbsp coconut milk
- 30ml/2 tbsp runny honey
- 5ml/1 tsp coconut oil
- blender or food processor
- bottle

Process the ingredients until smooth. Transfer to a bottle. Keep in the fridge and use within 3 days.

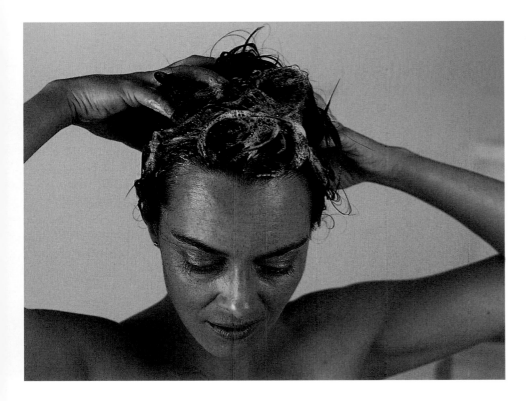

◁ As you apply the treatments, gently massage your scalp for a few minutes to improve circulation and allow the treatment to have the most beneficial effect.

rosemary hair tonic

This hair tonic made from fresh-smelling rosemary can be used as a substitute for mildly medicated shampoos. It is also effective in controlling greasy hair and enhances the shine and natural colour, especially of dark hair. Use this tonic as a final finishing rinse after shampooing, catching it in a bowl and pouring it repeatedly through the hair.

ingredients

- 250ml/8 fl oz/1 cup fresh rosemary tips
- 1.2 litres/2 pints/5 cups bottled water
- pan
- strainer
- funnel
- bottle

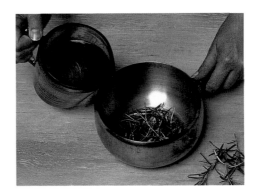

△ **1** Place the rosemary and water in a saucepan and bring to the boil. Simmer for approximately 20 minutes, then allow to cool in the pan.

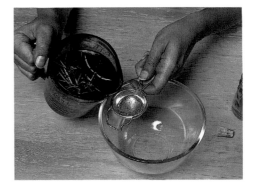

△ **2** Strain the liquid and use a funnel to pour it into a clean bottle. Store in a cool place. Apply as a soothing and invigorating rinse after shampooing.

parsley hair paste

This hair paste stimulates circulation, aids hair growth and leaves hair healthy and glossy.

ingredients

- 1 large handful parsley sprigs
- blender or food processor
- 30ml/2 tbsp water

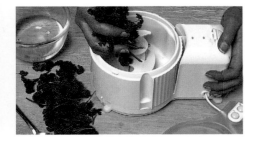

△ **1** Place the parsley in a blender or food processor with the water.

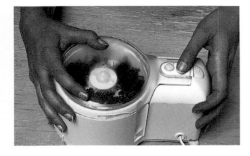

△ **2** Process until the parsley is ground to a smooth green purée. Apply the lotion to your scalp, then wrap a warm towel around your head. Leave for about an hour before washing your hair as usual.

BENEFITS OF NATURAL HAIR TREATMENTS

Commercial haircare products may work to a certain extent; however, a more holistic approach is required if we are to achieve the strong, lustrous hair that most of us long for. Strong hair growth is closely related to our general state of health and also to diet and fitness.

In some cultures people do not shampoo their hair but use other treatments such as oiling or just washing with water. It is true that when left alone the hair reaches a point of homeostasis where it is protected by its natural oils and there is no need for soap. Frequent hair-washing is actually damaging to the hair. It strips it of all its natural oils and dries out the scalp. This stimulates the sebaceous glands to produce more oil to compensate, which then leads to greasy hair and more hair washing.

Hairdryers and heated styling devices also have a damaging and drying-out effect on the hair so it is best to leave it to dry naturally.

Research suggests that there may be some risks associated with using chemical dyes or other products on the hair, as they can be absorbed into the bloodstream through the scalp and could be toxic for the body. There are many plant- or vegetable-based dyes and natural treatments available that do not pose this risk.

hot oil treatment

Any vegetable oil is suitable for conditioning. Just heat the oil until slightly warm. Rub a little into your scalp and then through every part of your hair, massaging gently as you go. Cover your head with a plastic shower cap for 20 minutes; the heat from your head will help the oil penetrate the hair shaft. Shampoo and rinse thoroughly.

intensive conditioning

Warm 15ml/1 tbsp each wheatgerm and olive oil and massage gently into the scalp. Wrap a warm towel around the head and leave for 10 minutes. Then rinse with a basin of water to which you have added the juice of a lemon.

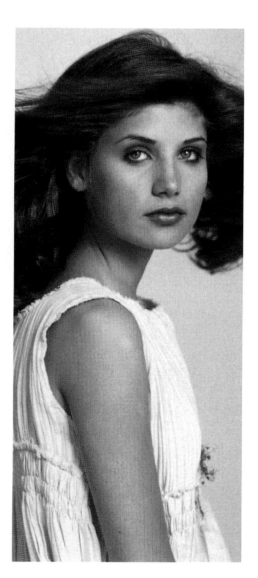

using essential oils

Pure aromatherapy oils can be used for hair-care. The following recipes come from world-famous aromatherapist Robert Tisserand. The number of drops of oil, as listed, should be diluted in 30ml/2 tbsp vegetable oil, which will act as a carrier oil.

Dry hair: rosewood 9, sandalwood 6.
Oily hair: bergamot 9, lavender 6.
Dandruff: eucalyptus 9, rosemary 6.

Mix the required treatment and apply to dry or wet hair. Massage the scalp using the fingertips. Leave for two to five minutes. Shampoo your hair as usual and then rinse thoroughly.

warm oil treatment

These treatments feel better and are more easily absorbed by the scalp. If you apply this treatment once a month, it should improve the texture of your hair and the condition of your scalp.

ingredients

- 90ml/6 tbsp coconut oil
- 3 drops rosemary essential oil
- 2 drops tea tree essential oil
- 2 drops lavender essential oil
- dark-coloured glass bottle with stopper

1 Pour all the ingredients into the bottle and shake gently to mix. Use the oil sparingly on dry hair; the head should not be soaked.
2 Massage the oil in, then cover your head with a warm towel for 20 minutes. Shampoo as normal.

◁ **Natural ingredients such as herbs and essential oils can help you achieve beautifully conditioned hair. Here a hot oil treatment was applied to the model's hair to enhance its shine and condition. Natural oils that are suitable for applying to the hair and scalp include vegetable oils, but rosemary, ylang ylang and lavender essential oils are fragrant alternatives. Use according to the manufacturer's directions.**

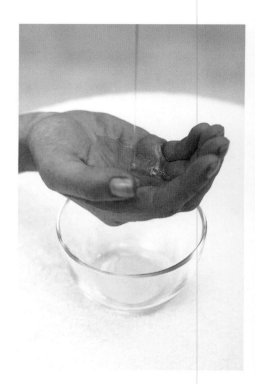

△ **Warm the oil in the palm of your hand or on a radiator before applying it. Heated oil is more easily absorbed by the hair and scalp and is more pleasant to apply.**

HEAD MASSAGE FOR COMMON HAIR PROBLEMS

For a therapeutic head massage, warm the oil in the palm of your hand and apply it to the top of your head. Using the pads of your fingers make circular strokes across your scalp with medium pressure. Work methodically from the front to the back, covering the whole head. When you have finished, cover your head and leave the oils for as long as possible to sink into your hair and scalp.

• **Greasy hair:** Massage stimulates the sebaceous glands to work properly and help prevent the hair follicles from clogging up with sebum. Jojoba oil helps to regulate over-productive sebaceous glands. For hair washing, use mild shampoos and avoid washing too often.

• **Dry hair:** Massage, combined with regular hot-oil treatments, is ideal for conditioning and moisturizing dry hair. Ideally leave the oil in overnight. Avoid hair products that contain isopropyl or ethyl alcohol, which dry the hair.

• **Hair loss:** Massage will have a stimulating effect, speeding up the delivery of nutrients to the roots and hair shaft and encouraging new hair growth.

▷ Many natural hair treatments can be made safely, economically and simply at home. Fresh herbs are most effective and a wide range of beautifully scented herbs are easy to grow in pots and window boxes.

natural hair rinses

Hair rinses are simple to make, use fresh, natural ingredients, and are a pleasantly sweet-scented finishing treatment after you have shampooed your hair.

lemon verbena rinse

This rinse fragrances your hair and stimulates the pores and circulation of the scalp. Lemon verbena is easy to grow in the garden.

Put a handful of lemon verbena leaves in a bowl and pour 250ml/8fl oz/1 cup boiling water over them. Infuse for an hour. Strain and discard the leaves. Pour over your hair after conditioning.

geranium and chamomile condition rinse

Chamomile flowers will not affect the colour of medium to dark hair, but they will help to brighten naturally fair hair. The geranium flowers add a delightful scent.

▽ Use a natural hair rinse after shampooing to treat and gently fragrance your hair.

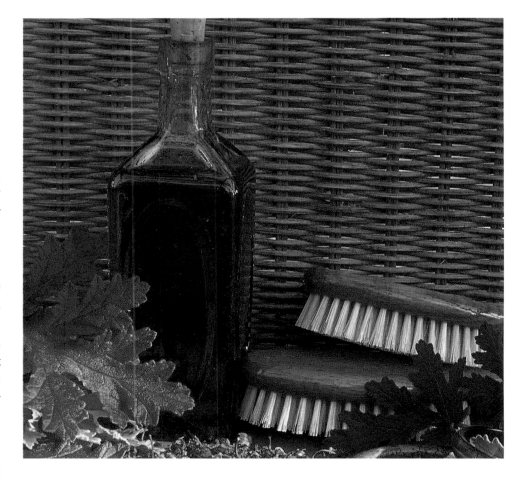

Put 25g/1 oz/^{1}/4 cup of chamomile flowers in a pan with 600ml/1 pint/2^1/2 cups water. Boil and then simmer for 15 minutes. Strain the hot liquid over scented geranium leaves and leave to soak for 30–40 minutes. Strain into a bottle.

cider vinegar rinse

This traditional country treatment will invigorate your scalp and give your hair a deep, natural shine. This recipe makes enough for one treatment. Mix 250ml/8fl oz/1 cup cider with 1 litre/3^3/4 pints/4 cups warm water, and use as a final rinse for your hair. Towel dry, gently comb through and leave to dry naturally.

Other rinses (to use as a finishing treatment after shampooing) can be made up to treat various hair problems. First, make an infusion by placing 30ml/2 tbsp of the fresh herb (see below) in a china or glass bowl. Fresh herbs are best, but if you use dried herbs remember they are stronger so you will need to halve the amount required. Add 475ml/16fl oz/2 cups boiling water, cover and leave to steep for three hours. Strain before using.

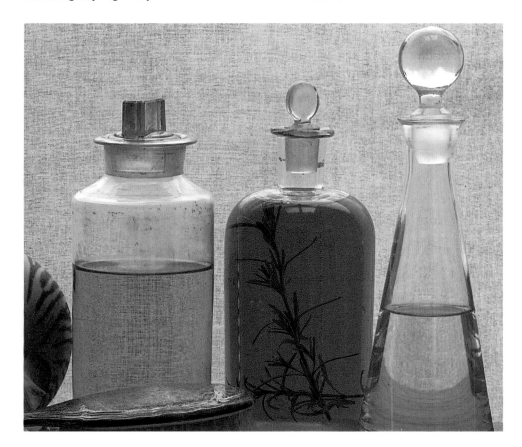

HAIR INFUSIONS

Make infusions with the following herbs for the specific uses as listed:

- Southernwood to combat grease.
- Nettle to stimulate hair growth.
- Rosemary to prevent static.
- Lavender to soothe a tight scalp.

Colouring and bleaching

Hair colourants have never been technically better; nowadays it is a simple matter to add a temporary tone and gloss to the hair or make a more permanent change. And there is a wide variety of home colouring products from which to choose.

the choice

Temporary colours are usually water-based and are applied to pre-shampooed, wet hair. They work by coating the outside, or cuticle layer, of the hair. The colour washes away in the next shampoo. Temporary colours are

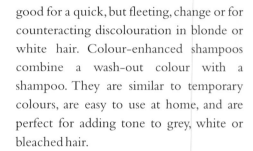

COLOUR FACT FILE
• Colouring swells the hair shaft, making fine hair appear thicker.
• Because colour changes the porosity of the hair it can help combat oiliness.
• Rich tones reflect more light and give hair a thicker appearance.
• Highlights give fine hair extra texture and break up the heaviness of very thick hair.
• Too light a hair colour can make the hair appear thinner.

good for a quick, but fleeting, change or for counteracting discolouration in blonde or white hair. Colour-enhanced shampoos combine a wash-out colour with a shampoo. They are similar to temporary colours, are easy to use at home, and are perfect for adding tone to grey, white or bleached hair.

Semi-permanent colours give a more noticeable effect that lasts for six to eight shampoos. They can only add to, enrich, or darken hair colour, they cannot make it any lighter. Semi-permanent colours penetrate the cuticle and coat the outer edge of the cortex (the inner layer of the hair). The colour fades gradually and is ideal for those who want to experiment with colour but don't want to commit themselves to a more permanent change.

Longer-lasting semi-permanent colours remain in the hair for 12–20 shampoos and are perfect for blending in the first grey hairs. The colour penetrates even deeper into the cortex than in semi-permanent colours. This type is perfect for a more lasting change.

Permanent colours lighten or darken, and effectively cover white. The colour enters the cortex during the development time (around 30 minutes) after which oxygen in the developer swells the pigments in the colourant, and holds them in. The roots may need retouching every six weeks. When retouching it is important to colour only the new hair growth. If the new colour overlaps previously treated hair there will be a build-up of colour from the mid-lengths to the ends, which will make the hair more porous.

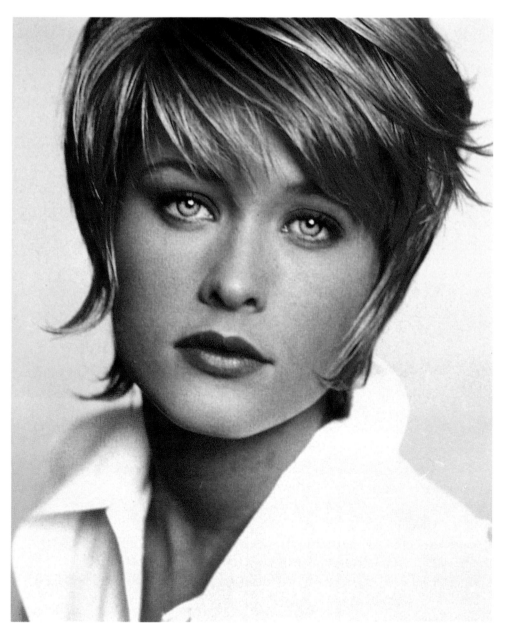

◁ **The model's fine hair was made to look thicker by working fine highlights of different tonal values throughout the hair. The feather cut was then styled forward and blow-dried into shape. A little wax was rubbed between the palms of the hands and applied to the hair with the fingertips to give further definition.**

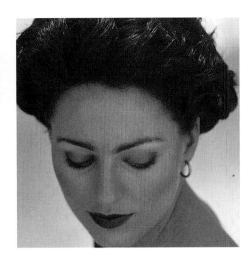

△ These copper tones were achieved by applying a permanent tint; the volume of hair was then increased by using a hot air brush to style the hair away from the face. You can get the same effect by working on one section of the hair at a time. Finish with firm-hold hairspray.

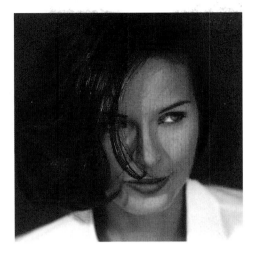

△ Here, reddish hues were created with a longer-lasting semi-permanent colour that added deep tones and luminosity. The hair was blow-dried straight, pointing the nozzle of the dryer downwards in order to polish and encourage the shine.

It is always wise to test the henna you intend to use on a few loose hairs (the ones in your hairbrush will do), noting the length of time it takes to produce the result you want.

Neutral henna can be used to add gloss and lustre to the hair without changing the colour. Mix the henna with water to a stiff paste. Stir in an egg yolk for extra conditioning, plus a little milk to help keep the paste pliable. Apply to the hair and leave for an hour before rinsing. Repeat every two to three months.

natural colouring – chamomile

Chamomile has a gentle lightening effect on hair and is good for sun-streaking blonde and light brown hair. However, it takes several applications and a good deal of time to produce the desired effect. The advantage of chamomile over chemical bleach is that it never gives a brassy or yellow tone. Best for blonde hair, it will also gently lighten red.

To make a chamomile rinse to use after shampooing, add 30m/2 tbsp dried chamomile flowers to 600ml/1 pint/2½ cups boiling water. Simmer for 15 minutes, strain and cool before use. For more positive results add 50g/2oz/1 cup dried chamomile flowers to 250ml/8fl oz/1 cup boiling water and leave to steep for 15 minutes. Cool, simmer and strain. Stir in the juice of a fresh lemon along with 30ml/2 tbsp of a rich conditioner. Comb through the hair and leave to dry – in the sun, if possible. Finally, shampoo and condition your hair as usual.

natural colouring – henna

Vegetable colourants such as henna and chamomile have been used since ancient times to colour hair, and henna was particularly popular with the Ancient Egyptians. Although henna is the most widely used natural dye, others can be extracted from a wide variety of plants, including marigold petals, cloves, rhubarb stalks and even tea leaves. Natural dyes work in much the same way as semi-permanent colourants by staining the outside of the hair. However, results are variable and a residue is

often left behind, making further colouring with permanent tints or bleaches inadvisable.

Henna enhances natural highlights, making colour appear richer. It is available today as a powder, which is mixed with water to form a paste. The colour fades gradually but frequent applications will give a stronger, longer-lasting effect. The result that is achieved when using henna depends on the natural colour of the hair. On brunette or black hair it produces a lovely reddish glow, while lighter hair becomes a beautiful titian. Henna will not lighten, and it is not suitable for use on blonde hair. On hair that is more than 20 per cent grey, white, tinted, bleached or highlighted, the resultant colour will be orange.

The longer the henna is left on the hair, the more intense the result. Timings vary from one to two hours, but some Indian women leave henna on the hair for 24 hours, anointing their heads with oil to keep the paste supple.

The condition of the hair being treated is another factor that effects the intensity. The ends of long hair are always slightly lighter than the roots because they are more exposed to the sun, and henna will emphasize this effect. The resulting colour will be darker on the roots to the mid-lengths and more vibrant from the mid-lengths to the ends.

> **DO'S AND DON'TS**
> • Do rinse henna paste thoroughly, or the hair and scalp will feel gritty.
> • Don't expose hennaed hair to strong sunlight and always rinse salt and chlorine from the hair immediately after swimming.
> • Do use a henna shampoo between colour applications to enhance the tone.
> • Don't use shampoos and conditioners containing henna on blonde hair, grey hair or hair that has been chemically treated.
> • Do use the same henna product each time you apply henna.
> • Don't use compound henna (one that has had metallic salts added); it can cause long-term hair-colouring problems.

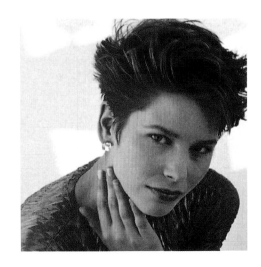

△ Russet tones were further emphasized by weaving a few lighter colours into the front hair. The hair was blow-dried with styling gel to get lift at the roots.

Permanent solutions

Making straight hair curly is not a new idea. Women in Ancient Egypt coated their hair in mud, wound it around wooden rods and then used the heat from the sun to create the curls.

Waves that won't wash out are a more recent innovation. Modern perms were pioneered by A. F. Willat, who invented the "cold permanent wave" technique in 1934. Since then, improved formulations and evermore sophisticated techniques have made perms the most versatile styling option in hairdressing.

how perms work

Perms work by breaking down inner structures (links) in your hair and re-forming them around a curler to give a new shape. Hair should be washed prior to perming as this causes the scales on the cuticles to rise gently, allowing the perming lotion to enter the hair shaft more quickly. The perming lotion alters the keratin and breaks down the sulphur bonds that link the fibre-like cells together in the inner layers of each hair. When these fibres have become loose, they can be formed into a new shape when the hair is stretched over a curler or perming rod.

Once the curlers or rods are in place, more lotion is applied and the perm is left to develop to fix the new shape. The development time varies according to the condition and texture of the hair. When the development is complete, the changed links in the hair are re-formed into their new shape by the application of a second chemical known as the neutralizer. The neutralizer contains an oxidizing agent that is effectively responsible for closing up the broken links and producing the wave or curl – permanently.

The type of curl that is produced depends on a number of factors. The size of the curler is perhaps the most important as this determines the size of the curl. Generally speaking the smaller the curler the smaller and therefore tighter the curl, whereas medium to large curlers tend to give a much

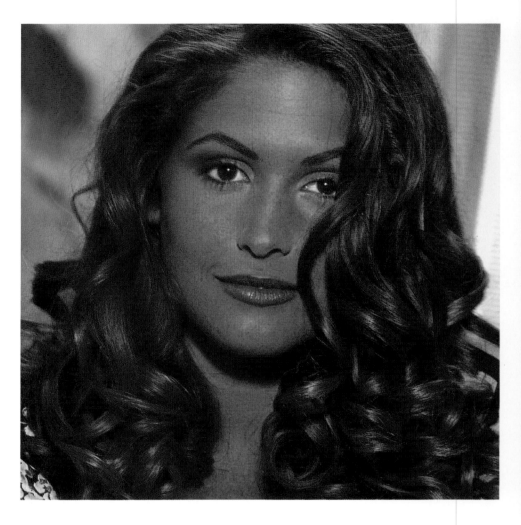

△ **Specialist formulations enable your hairdresser to perm long hair while maintaining it in optimum condition**. Here the hair was wound on to large rods to achieve soft curls.

looser effect. The strength of lotion can also make a difference, as can the texture and type of hair. Hair in good condition takes a perm much better than hair in poor condition, and fine hair curls more easily than coarse hair.

After a perm it takes 48 hours for the keratin in the hair to harden naturally. At this time the hair is vulnerable to damage and must be treated with care. Resist shampooing, brushing or combing, blow-drying or setting, which may cause the perm to drop.

Once hair has been permed it remains curly and shaped the way it has been formed, although new growth will be straight. As time goes by the curl can soften, and if the hair is long its weight may make the curl and the wave appear much looser.

home versus salon

Perming is such a delicate, and potentially hazardous operation that the majority of women prefer to leave it in the hands of experienced professional hairdressers. The advantages of having hair permed in a salon are several. The hair is first analysed to find out whether it is in good enough condition to take a perm; coloured, out-of-condition or over-processed hair may well be damaged even more by a perm. With a perm carried out by a professional there is also a greater variety in the type of curl and texture you can choose – different strengths of lotion and different winding techniques all give a range of curls that are not generally available in home perms.

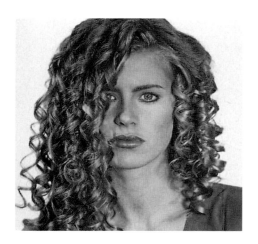

△ Spiral perming gives a ringlet effect on long hair. It is important with hair of this length to re-perm only at the roots when the hair grows, or you may cause damage to previously permed hair.

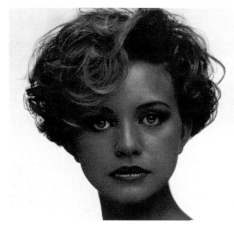

△ A soft perm gives volume to short hair. Set the hair on rollers to achieve the maximum amount of lift, and to give extra height and body to short hair.

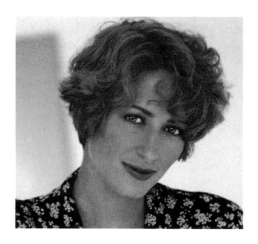

△ Tinted hair can also be permed if the correct formulation is chosen. Your stylist will be able to advise you on the formulation that is most suitable for you.

home rules

If you do use a perm at home, it is essential that you read the instructions that are supplied with the product and that you follow them very carefully. Remember to do a test curl to check whether your hair is suitable, and check to make certain you have enough curlers. You will probably want to enlist the help of a friend, as it is impossible to curl the back sections of your own hair properly, so you will definitely need a helping hand.

Timing is crucial – don't be tempted to remove the lotion before the time given or leave it on longer than directed.

salon perms – the choices

Professional hairdressers can offer a number of different types of perm that are not available for home use:

Acid perms: These produce highly conditioned, flexible curls. Ideally suited to hair that is fine, sensitive, fragile, damaged or tinted, they have a mildly acidic action that minimizes the risk of hair damage.

Alkaline perms: These give strong, firm curl results on normal and resistant hair.

Exothermic perms: For bouncy, resilient curls, "exothermic" refers to the gentle heat that is produced by the chemical reaction that occurs when the lotion is mixed. The heat allows the lotion to penetrate the hair cuticle, which will have the effect of conditioning and strengthening the hair from inside as the lotion moulds the hair into its new shape.

perming techniques

Any of the above types of perm can be used with different techniques to produce a number of results.

Body perms: These are soft, loose perms created using large curlers, or sometimes rollers. They add volume with a hint of wave and movement rather than curls.

Root perms: These add lift and volume to the root area only. They will add height and fullness, and are therefore ideal for short hair that tends to go flat.

POST-PERM TIPS

• Don't wash newly permed hair for 48 hours after processing as any stress can cause curls to relax.

• Use shampoos and conditioners formulated for permed hair. They help retain the correct moisture balance and prolong the perm.

• Always use a wide-toothed comb and work from the ends upwards. Never brush the hair.

• Blot wet hair dry before it is styled to help prevent stretching.

• Avoid using too much heat on permed hair. If possible, wash, condition and then leave it to dry naturally.

• If your perm has lost its bounce, mist with water or try a curl reviver. These are designed to put instant volume and bounce into permed hair. They are also ideal for eliminating frizziness on naturally curly hair.

• Expect your perm to last three to six months, depending on the technique and lotion used.

Pin curl perms: These give soft, natural waves and curls, achieved by perming small sections of hair that have been pinned into pre-formed curls.

Stack perms: This perm gives curl and volume to one-length hair by means of different-sized curlers. The hair on top of the head is left unpermed while the middle and ends have curl and movement.

Spiral perms: These create romantic spiral curls, an effect produced by winding the hair around special long curlers. The mass of curls makes long hair look much thicker.

Spot perms: These give support on the area to which they are applied. For example, if the hair needs lift, the perm is applied just on the crown. They can also be used on the fringe (bangs) or side areas around the face.

Weave perms: These involve perming sections of hair and leaving the rest straight to give a mixture of texture and natural-looking body and bounce, particularly on areas around the face such as the fringe.

regrowth problem

When a perm is growing out, the areas of new growth can be permed if a barrier is created between old and new growth. The barrier can be a special cream or a plastic protector, both of which effectively prevent the perming lotion and neutralizer from touching previously permed areas.

There are also products that facilitate re-perming the length of hair without damaging the structure. These complex solutions are available only from salons.

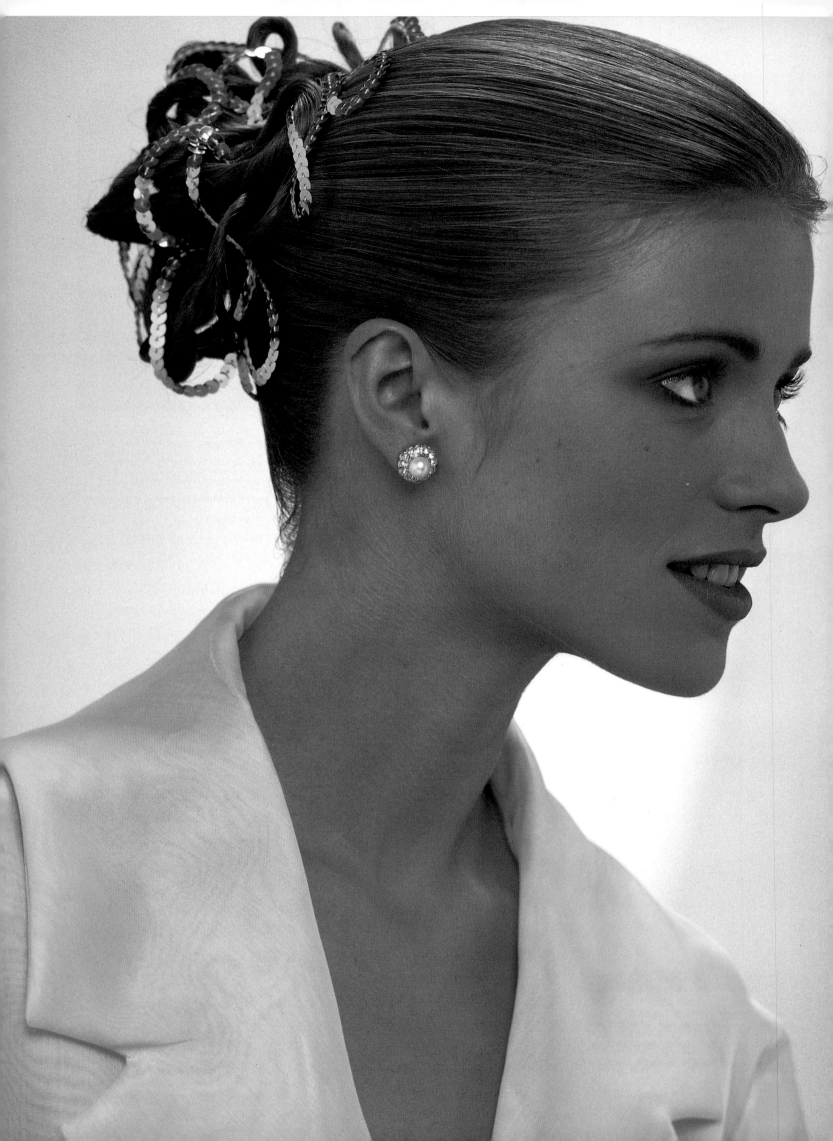

Choosing a style

Successful styling means choosing a hairstyle that suits your looks and lifestyle, and then learning the techniques that will ensure a perfect finish. There is an enormous range of gadgets, hair products and heated styling equipment available, all of which, if used properly, can effect wonderful transformations. The trick is to know what to use and when in order to achieve the desired results. Here we show you how.

Choosing a style to suit your face

Make the most of your looks by choosing a style that maximizes your best features. The first feature you should consider is the shape of your face – is it round, oval, square or long? If you are not sure what shape your face is, the easiest way to find out is to scrape your hair away from your face so that you can see all your features clearly. Stand squarely in front of a mirror and use a lipstick to trace around the outline of your face so that the shape is transferred to the mirror. When you stand back you should be able to see into which of the following categories your face shape falls.

the square face

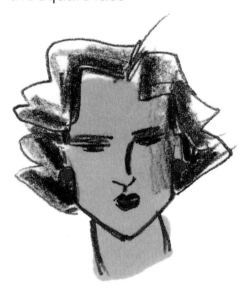

The square face is angular with a broad forehead and a square jawline. To make the best of this shape, choose a hairstyle with long layers, preferably one that features soft waves or curls. This will create a softness that detracts from the hard lines particularly around the jaw. The hair should be parted at the side of the head and any fringe (bangs) combed away from the face.

Styles to avoid: Very severe geometric cuts – they will only have the effect of emphasizing the squareness of your face; long bobs with a heavy fringe; severe styles in which the hair is scraped off the face and with a parting down the centre.

the round face

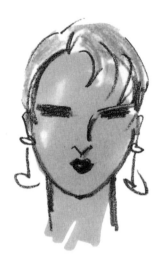

On the round face the distance between the forehead and the chin is about equal to the distance between the cheeks. Choose a style with a short fringe, which lengthens the face, and a short cut, which makes the face look thinner.

Styles to avoid: Curly, because they will draw attention to the roundness; very full, long hair; styles that are pulled right back off the face.

the oval face

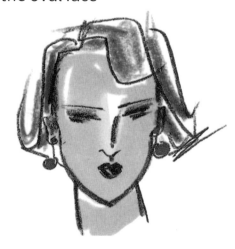

The oval face has wide cheekbones that taper down into a small, often pointed, chin and up to a fairly narrow forehead. This is regarded by many experts as the perfect face shape. If your face is oval in shape then you have the advantage of being able to wear any hairstyle you choose.

the long face

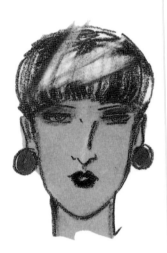

A long face is characterized by a high forehead and long chin, and needs to be given the illusion of width. Soften the effect with short layers, or go for a bob with a fringe to create horizontal lines. Scrunch-dried or curly bobs balance a long face.

Styles to avoid: Styles without a fringe; long, straight, blunt cuts.

the complete you

When choosing a new style you should also take into account your overall body shape. If you are a traditional pear-shape don't go for elfin styles; they will draw attention to the lower half of your body, making your hips look even wider. Petite women should avoid masses of very curly hair as this makes the head appear large and out of proportion with the body.

IF YOU WEAR GLASSES . . .
Try to choose frames and a hairstyle that complement each other. Large spectacles could spoil a neat, feathery cut, and very fine frames could be overpowered by a large, voluminous style. Remember to take your glasses to the salon when having your hair restyled, so that your stylist can take their shape into consideration when deciding on the overall effect.

SPECIFIC PROBLEMS

• Prominent nose: incorporate softness into your style.

• Pointed chin: style hair with width at the jawline.

• Low forehead: choose a style with a wispy fringe, rather than one with a full fringe.

• High forehead: disguise with a fringe.

• Receding chin: select a style that comes to just below chin level, with waves or curls.

• Uneven hairline: fringes should conceal this problem.

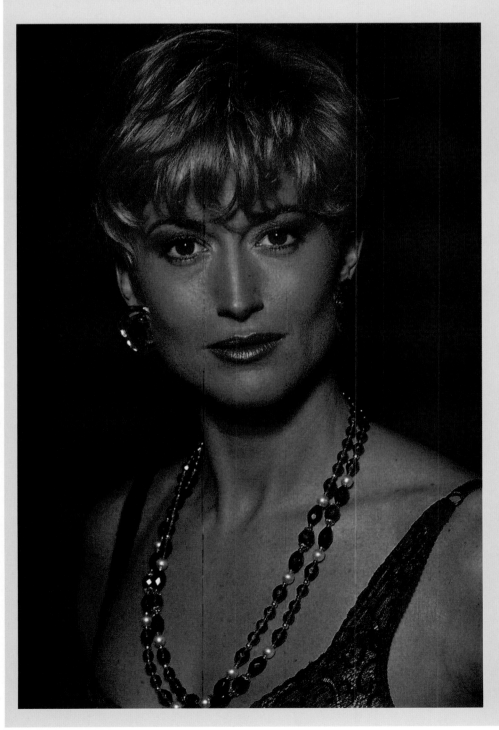

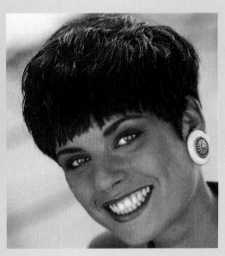

△ A high forehead or uneven hairline can be hidden under a fringe.

◁ A wispy fringe stylishly disguises a low forehead.

▽ Strong features benefit from a soft, full hairstyle.

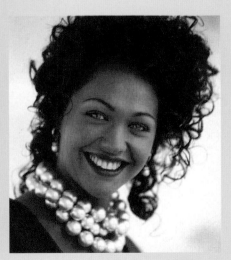

Style gallery, short hair

Short hair is usually easier to maintain but it does need more regular cutting. It can be cut close to the shape of the head, cropped or layered in a variety of styles. Generally a short cut will make the face look thinner.

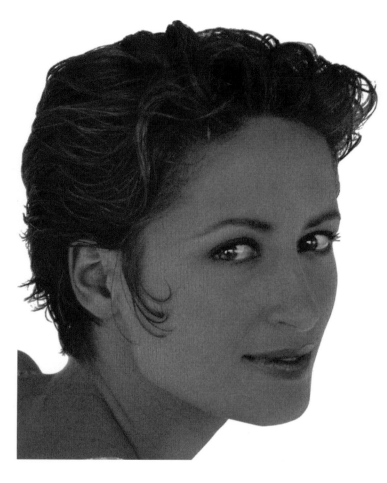

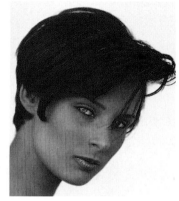

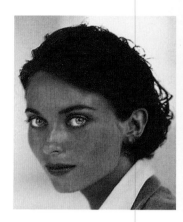

△ Fine, straight hair was lightly layered and cut close into the nape. A root perm provided extra volume at the crown of the head. The hair was then finger-dried using a styling mousse.

△ Naturally wavy hair was cut into a one-length bob and taken behind the ears, using wet-look gel to give definition and accentuate the waves.

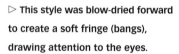

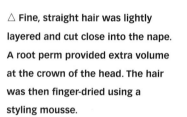

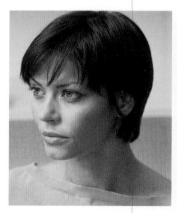

▷ This style was blow-dried forward to create a soft fringe (bangs), drawing attention to the eyes.

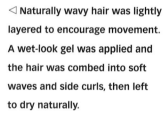

◁ Naturally wavy hair was lightly layered to encourage movement. A wet-look gel was applied and the hair was combed into soft waves and side curls, then left to dry naturally.

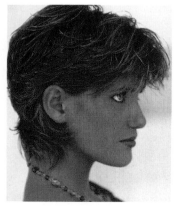

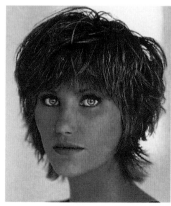

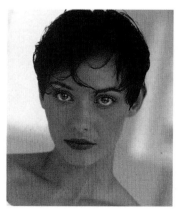

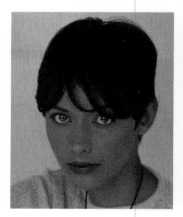

△ Thick hair was feather-cut into layers, with slightly longer lengths left at the nape. The hair was highlighted and then blow-dried into shape using a styling brush.

△ For a different look the hair was combed down over the ears.

△ Fine hair was softly layered and given an application of mousse, then ruffle-dried with the fingers to create just a little lift at the roots.

△ The same haircut was blow-dried forwards using a styling brush.

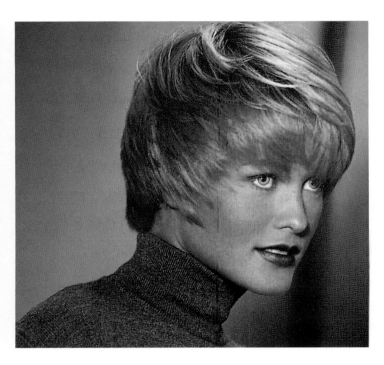

◁ Medium-textured hair was cut into layers of the same length, then blow-dried using a strong-hold mousse to get lift, and finished with a mist of firm-hold hairspray.

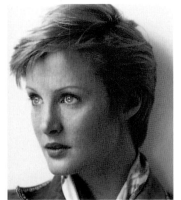

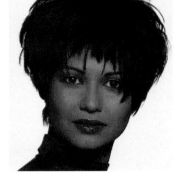

△ Choppy layers give an uneven texture to this thick hair. The hair was blow-dried using mousse and a styling brush to create lift.

△ A root perm helped to give lift at the crown on this short, layered look. Mousse was applied to give extra lift and the hair was blow-dried forwards from the crown.

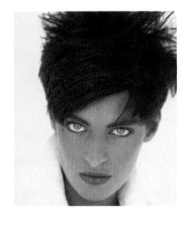

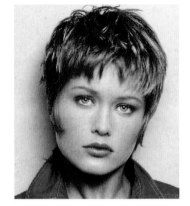

△ A short cut was given extra interest by bleaching the hair honey-blonde. It was then blow-dried into shape and finished using wax to create separation.

△ A short, urchin cut is good for all hair textures. Highlights give extra interest and add thickness to finer hair.

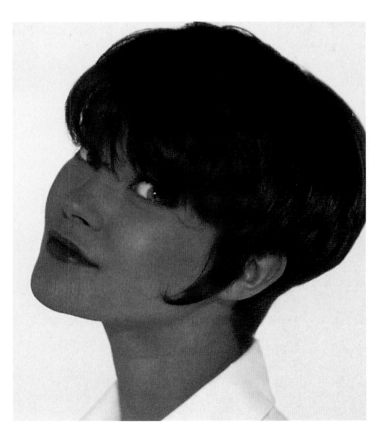

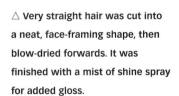

△ Very curly, wiry hair was cropped close to the head, then dressed using just a little wax to give definition and separation.

△ Very straight hair was cut into a neat, face-framing shape, then blow-dried forwards. It was finished with a mist of shine spray for added gloss.

△ Medium-textured hair was graduated to give this head-hugging cut. Mousse was applied from the roots to the ends, then the hair was blow-dried forwards from the crown.

Style gallery, mid-length hair

Hair of medium length has the advantage of being a little more versatile, because it can be worn in a smooth, sleek bob or lightly layered to allow for more variety in styling.

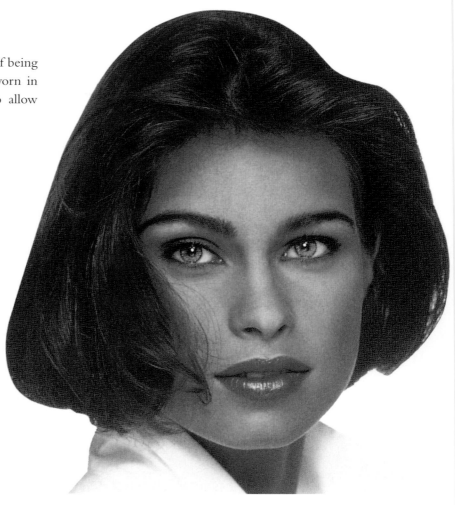

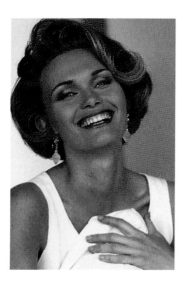

△ Medium-textured hair was cut into a one-length bob. Styling spray was applied to partially dried hair, which was then wound on large rollers and heat set. After the rollers were removed the hair was brushed into shape.

△ Fine mid-length hair can be made to look thicker by blunt cutting just below ear level. This style can be roller-set and brushed through with a bristle brush to smooth, or simply blow-dried with a round brush.

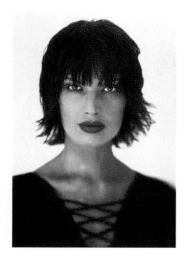

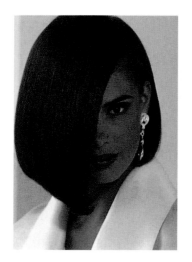

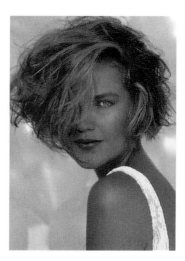

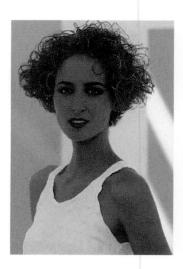

△ Layering gives this 70s-inspired style a fresh look. The hair was misted with styling spray and rough-dried before finishing with a little gloss.

△ This longer, one-length, graduated bob is perfect for thick, straight hair. Add extra shine by using a longer-lasting semi-permanent colour.

△ A mid-length bleached bob was scrunch-dried with mousse to give a tousled look. Use a diffuser to encourage more volume.

△ This layered cut was permed to give plenty of movement. The hair was scrunch-dried and styled, with the head held forward to give maximum volume.

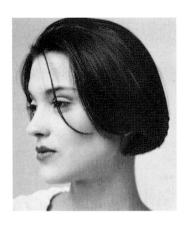

△ A soft body perm gives volume to this one-length bob. The hair was gently dried using mousse for additional lift.

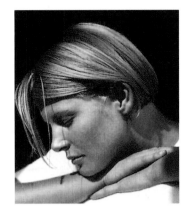

△ Thick, straight hair was heavily highlighted and cut into a blunt, short bob. Either blow-dry or leave to dry naturally.

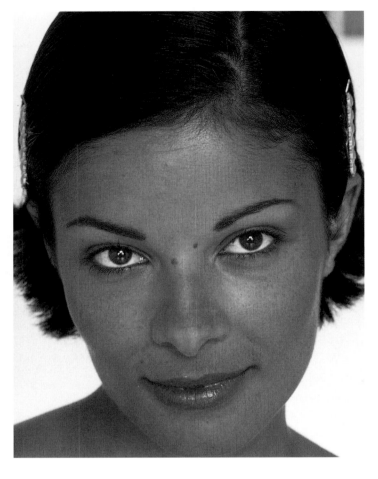

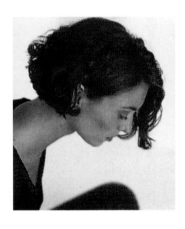

△ Natural movement was encouraged by blunt cutting and leaving the hair to dry naturally. Alternatively, the hair could be dried using a flat diffuser attachment on the dryer.

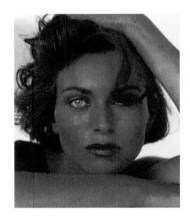

△ The same style was sprayed with styling lotion and set on large rollers. When the rollers were removed the hair was ruffled through with the fingers, not brushed.

△ This fine straight hair has been cut in a simple short bob that is easy to style but can also be left to dry naturally.

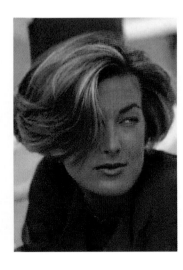

△ A bob was highlighted using a light, golden-blonde colour to give natural, warm lights, then styled and blow-dried using a soft sculpting spray.

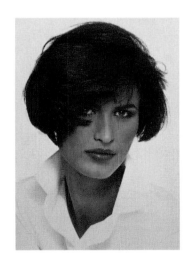

△ A razor-cut bob gives graduation so the hair moves freely. The hair was coloured with a shade of mahogany to give more depth, and then blow-dried using mousse.

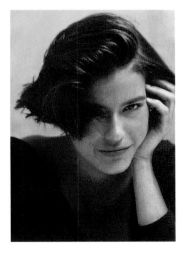

△ Thick hair was cut into a bob, then sprayed with styling lotion before setting on large rollers. After drying, the hair was brushed through to give a smooth style.

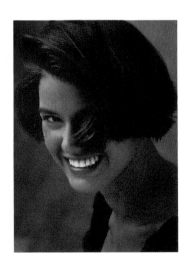

△ The same cut was blow-dried smooth using a styling brush.

Style gallery, long hair

Long locks are particularly versatile and can be transformed into a fabulous range of styles using different techniques. They can be waved, curled, straightened or left to fall free.

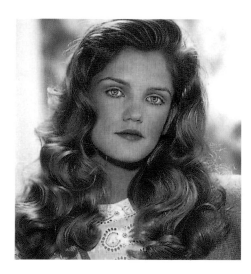

△ Naturally wavy hair was roller-set and heat-dried, then brushed through lightly. A similar look could be achieved with a soft perm.

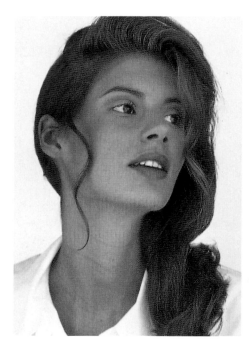

△ After an application of styling spray the hair was set on large rollers. When dry the hair was combed to one side and allowed to fall into soft waves, with a tiny tendril pulled in front of one ear.

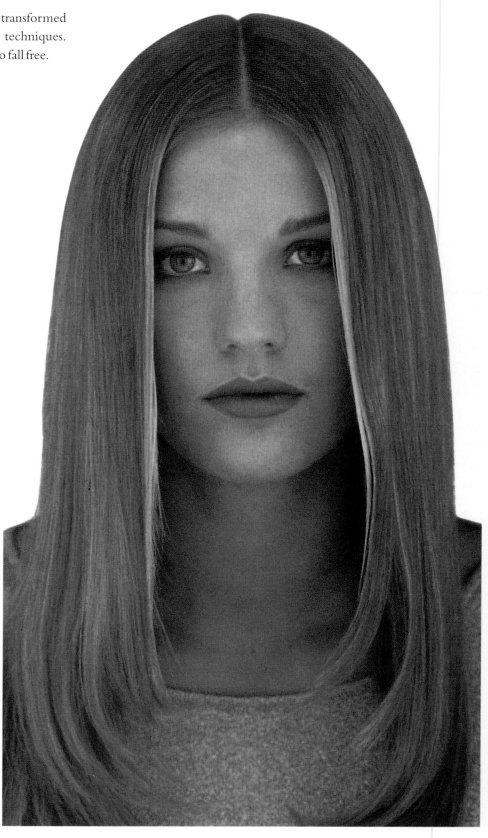

△ Straight hair was graduated at the sides to give interest. It was then shampooed and conditioned, and left to dry naturally.

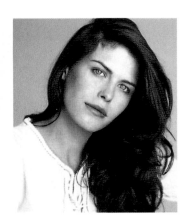

△ A vegetable colour adds depth and makes hair appear even thicker. The hair was then simply styled by blow-drying.

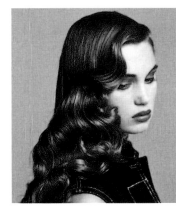

△ Soft, undulating waves were achieved by tonging the hair, then lightly combing it through. Spray shine was applied to the finish.

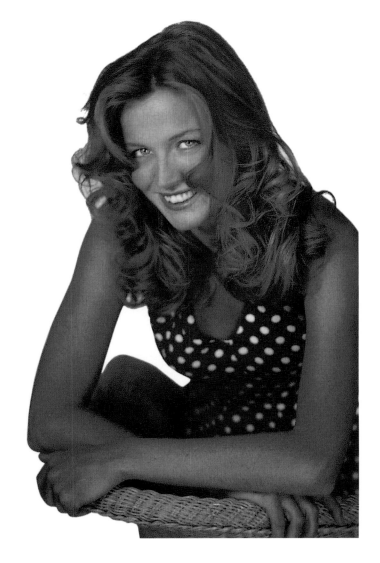

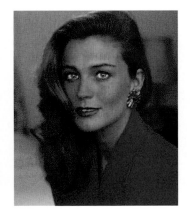

△ Mousse was applied to rough-dried hair, which was then set on heated rollers. The hair was then brushed through into soft waves.

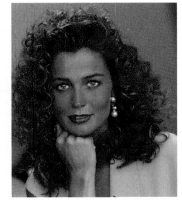

△ This alternative style was achieved by tonging. It could also be set on shapers.

△ Naturally wavy hair was lightly layered, then set on large rollers. When the hair was dry it was brushed lightly to give broken up-waves and curls.

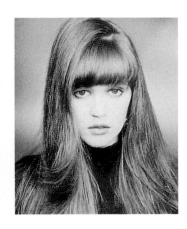

△ Thick hair was cut with graduated sides and a heavy fringe to give this 60s look. The hair can be blow-dried smooth or left to dry naturally.

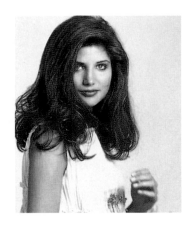

△ Setting lotion was applied to clean hair, which was set on large rollers and heat-dried. When the hair was completely dry the rollers were removed and the hair gently back-combed at the roots to give even more height and fullness.

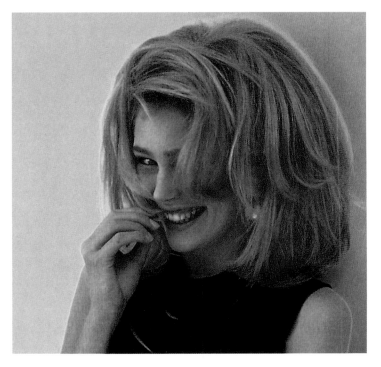

△ A thick graduated cut was given maximum lift by spraying the roots with gel spray and backcombing lightly, then brushing over the top layers.

more sleek looks for long hair

One of the most important aspects of having long hair is keeping it in good condition, sleek and glossy, but once you have cracked that, long locks provide a wealth of opportunities when it comes to impeccable styling and making an impact.

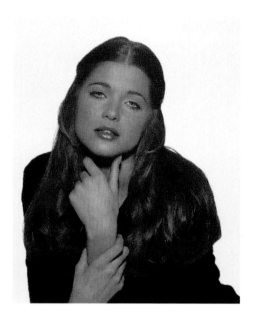

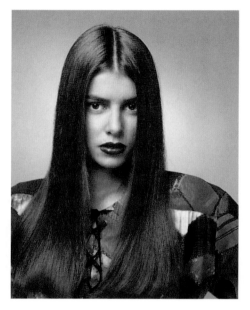

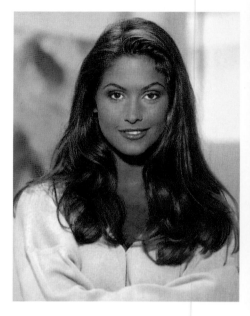

△ The hair was sprayed with styling lotion and set on heated rollers. When it was dry a bristle brush was used to smooth it into waves.

△ Straight hair was blunt-cut at the ends and simply styled from a centre parting.

△ To give one-length hair extra body the head was tipped forwards and the hair misted with sculpting lotion. The roots were scrunched a little with the hands before straightening the head.

take one girl

The following styles illustrate how one-length hair can be transformed using different styling techniques.

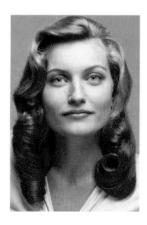

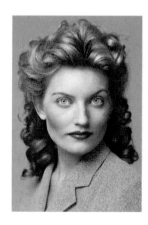

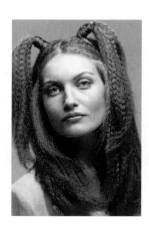

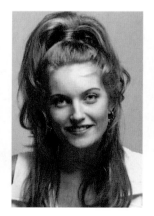

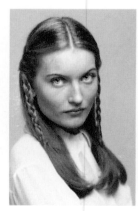

△ **1** Soft waves were created with rollers.

△ **2** The top hair was clipped up and the back hair tonged into tendrils.

△ **3** High bunches were carefully secured and the hair crimped.

△ **4** The top hair was secured on the crown. A band was wrapped with a small piece of hair and the length allowed to fall freely.

△ **5** The hair was clipped back and two simple braids were worked at each side.

Style gallery, long hair for special occasions

These styles will inspire you when you want to transform your long hair for a glamorous party or special event.

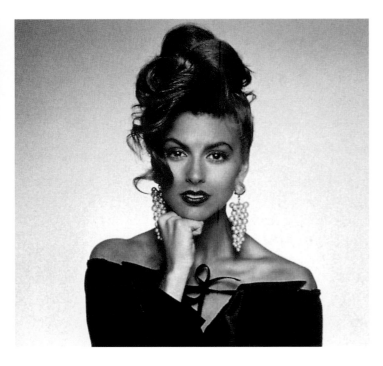

△ The hair was softly scooped into large curls and pinned in place. One tendril was left to fall free to soften the style.

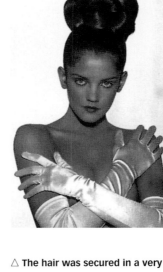

△ The hair was secured in a very high ponytail on the crown, then divided into sections and looped into curls. If your hair isn't long enough for this style, you could use a hairpiece.

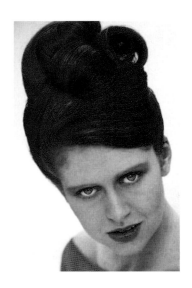

△ Vibrant blonde and copper lights add brilliance to the hair. The front hair was sectioned off and the back hair secured in a high ponytail. The hair was then divided and coiled into loops before pinning in place. The front hair was smoothed over and secured at the back.

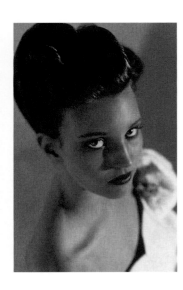

△ The foundation for this style came from a roller-set. The back hair was then formed into a French pleat and the top hair looped, curled and pinned into place.

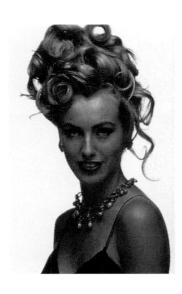

△ Very curly hair was simply twisted up at the back and secured with pins. Curls were allowed to fall down on one side to give a feminine look.

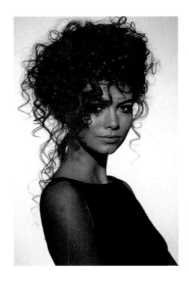

△ Long hair was scooped up, but the essence of this style is to allow lots of strands to fall in soft curls around the face.

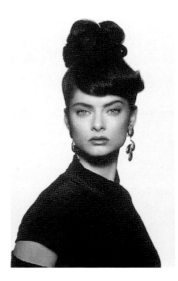

△ A high ponytail forms the basis of this style. The hair was then looped into curls and pinned, and the fringe (bangs) was combed to one side.

Styling tools

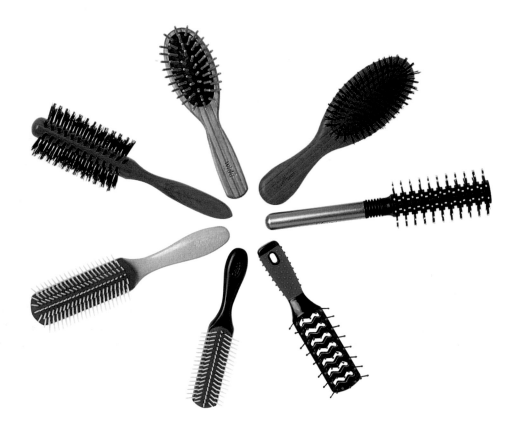

Brushes, combs and pins are the basic tools of styling. The following is a guide to help you choose what is most suitable from the wide range that is available.

brushes

These are made of bristles (sometimes called quills or pins), which may be natural hog bristle, plastic, nylon or wire. The bristles are embedded in a wooden, plastic or moulded rubber base and set in tufts or rows. This allows loose or shed hair to collect in the grooves without interfering with the action of the bristles. The spacing of the tufts plays an important role – generally, the wider the spacing between the rows of bristles, the easier the brush will flow through the hair.

the role of brushing

Brushes help to remove tangles and knots to smooth the hair. The action of brushing from the roots to the ends removes dead skin cells and dirt, and encourages the cuticles to lie flat, thus reflecting the light. Brushing also stimulates the blood supply to the hair follicles, promoting healthy growth.

△ **Choosing the right tools not only makes hairstyling fun, but also makes it much easier.**

natural bristles

These bristles are produced from natural keratin (the same material as hair) and therefore create less friction and wear on the hair. They are good for grooming and polishing, and help to combat static on flyaway hair. However, they will not penetrate wet or thick hair and you must

HAIRBRUSH FASHIONS

In the 17th century it was thought that brushing the hair would rid an individual of the vapours (fainting spells) and women were advised not to groom their hair in the evening, as it could lead to headaches the next day.

Hairbrushes made from hog bristle or hedgehog spines were first introduced in the late Middle Ages. With the invention of nylon in the 1930s designs changed, and now we can choose from an extensive range, each suitable for specific tasks.

CLEANING BRUSHES

All brushes should be cleaned by removing dead hairs and washing in warm, soapy water, then rinsing thoroughly. Natural bristle brushes should be placed bristle-side down and left to dry naturally. If you use a pneumatic brush with a rubber cushion base, block the air hole with a matchstick before washing.

use a softer bristle brush for fine or thinning hair. In addition, the sharp ends can scratch the scalp.

plastic, nylon or wire bristles

These bristles are easily cleaned and heat resistant, so they are good for blow-drying. They are available in a variety of shapes and styles. Cushioned brushes give good flexibility as they glide through the hair, preventing tugging and helping to remove knots. They are also non-static.

A major disadvantage is that the ends can be harsh, so try to choose bristles with rounded or ball tips.

types of brush

Circular or radial brushes: These come in a variety of sizes and are circular or semi-circular in shape. These brushes have either mixed bristles for finishing, a rubber pad with nylon bristles, or metal pins for styling. They are used to tame and control naturally curly, permed and wavy hair and are ideal for blow-drying. The diameter of the brush determines the resulting volume and movement, in much the same way as the size of rollers do.

Flat or half-round brushes: They are ideal for wet or dry hairstyling and blow-drying. Normally they are made of nylon bristles in a rubber base. Some bases slide into position on to the plastic moulded handle. Rubber bases can be removed for cleaning and replacement bristles are sometimes available.

Pneumatic brushes: These have a domed rubber base with bristles set in tufts. They can be plastic, natural bristle, or both.

Vent brushes: All these have hollow centres allowing the air-flow from the dryer to pass through the brush. Special bristle, or pin, patterns are designed to lift and disentangle even wet hair. Vents and tunnel brush heads enable the air to circulate freely through both the brush and the hair so the hair dries faster.

combs

It is advisable to choose good-quality combs with saw-cut teeth. This means that each individual tooth is cut into the comb, so there are no sharp edges that will damage your hair. Avoid cheap plastic combs that are made in a mold and so form lines down the centre of every tooth. They are sharp, and gradually scrape away the cuticle layers of the hair, causing damage and often breakage.

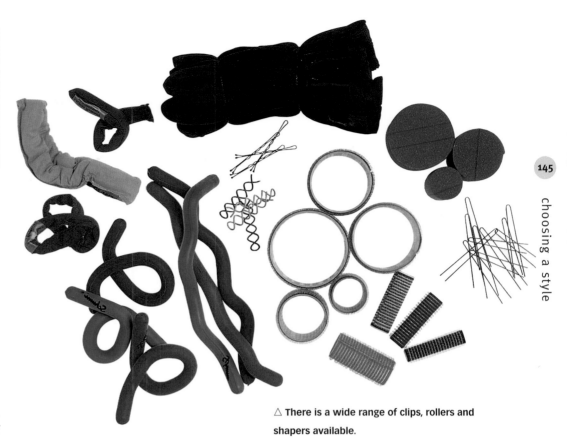

△ **There is a wide range of clips, rollers and shapers available.**

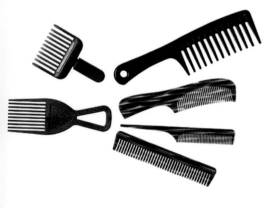

△ **A wide-toothed comb is ideal for disentangling and combing conditioner through the hair. Fine tail-combs are for styling. Afro combs are specially designed for curly hair.**

pins and clips

These are indispensable for sectioning and securing hair during setting, and for putting hair up. Most pins are available with untipped, plain ends, or cushion-tipped ends. Non-reflective finishes are available, so the pins are less noticeable in the hair, and most are made of metal, plastic or stainless steel. Colours include brown, black, grey, blonde, white and silver.

Double-pronged grips: These are most frequently used for making pin or barrel curls. Grips give security to curls, French

pleats and all upswept styles. In North America they are known as "Bobby" pins, in Britain as "Kirbies". To avoid discomfort, position grips in the hair so that the flat edge rests towards the scalp.

Heavy hairpins: Made of strong metal, they are either waved or straight. These are ideal for securing rollers in place and when putting hair up.

Fine hairpins: Used for dressing hair, they are delicate and prone to bend out of shape, so they should be used to secure only small amounts of hair. These pins are easily concealed, especially if you use a matching colour. They are sometimes used to secure pin curls during setting, rather than heavier clips which can leave a mark.

Sectioning clips: These are clips with a single prong, and are longer in length than other clips. They are most often used for holding hair while working on another section, or for securing pin curls.

Twisted pins: Shaped like a screw, they are used to secure chignons and French pleats.

rollers

These invaluable styling tools vary in diameter, length and the material from which they are made. Smooth rollers, that is those without spikes or brushes, will give the sleekest finish, but they are more difficult to

put in. More popular are brush rollers, especially the self-fixing variety that do not need pins or clips.

shapers

These soft styling devices were inspired by the principle of rag-rolling hair. Soft "twist tie" rollers are made from pliable rubber, plastic or cotton fabric and provide one of the more natural ways to curl hair. In the centre of each roller is a tempered wire, which enables it to be bent into shape. The waves or curls that are produced are soft and bouncy and the technique is gentle enough for permed or tinted hair.

To use, section clean, dry hair and pull to a firm tension, "trapping" the end in a roller that you have previously doubled over. Roll down to the roots of the hair and fold over to secure. Leave in for 30–60 minutes without heat, or for 10–15 minutes if you apply heat. If you twist the hair before curling you will achieve a more voluminous style.

Style easy

The combination of practice and the right styling products enables you to achieve a salon finish at home. The products listed below enable you to do it in style.

gels

Sometimes called sculpting lotions and used for precise styling, gels come in varying degrees of viscosity, from a thick jelly to a liquid spray. Use them to lift roots, tame wisps, create tendrils, calm static, heat set and give structure to curls. Wet gel can be used for sculpting styles.

GEL TIP
A gel can be revitalized the following day by running wet fingers through the hair, against the direction of the finished look.

hairspray

Traditionally, hairspray was used to hold a style in place; today, varying degrees of stiffness are available to suit all needs. Use hairspray to keep the hair in place, get curl definition when scrunching, and mist over rollers when setting.

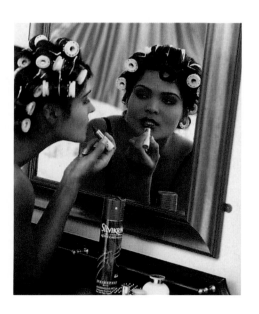

△ **Hairsprays are available in a variety of formulations, including light and firm holds.**

HAIRSPRAY TIPS
• A light application of spray on a hairbrush can be used to tame flyaway ends.
• Use hairspray at the roots and tong or blow-dry the area to get immediate lift.

mousse

The most versatile styling product, mousse comes as a foam and can be used on wet or dry hair. Mousses contain conditioning agents and proteins to nurture and protect the hair. They are available in different strengths, designed to give soft to maximum holding power, and can be used to lift flat roots or smooth frizz. Use when blow-drying, scrunching and diffuser drying.

MOUSSE TIPS
• Make sure you apply mousse from the roots to the ends, not just in a blob on the crown.
• Choose the right type for your hair. Normal is good for a great many styles, but if you want more holding power, don't just use more mousse as it can make hair dull; instead, choose a firm or maximum-hold product.

serums

Used to improve shine and softness by forming a microscopic film on the surface of the hair, serums, glossers, polishes and shine sprays are made from oils or silicones Formulations can vary from light and silky to heavier ones with a distinctly oily feel. They also contain substances designed to smooth the cuticle, encouraging the tiny scales to lie flat and thus reflect the light and make the hair appear shiny. Use these

SERUM TIP
Take care not to use too much serum or you will make your hair oily.

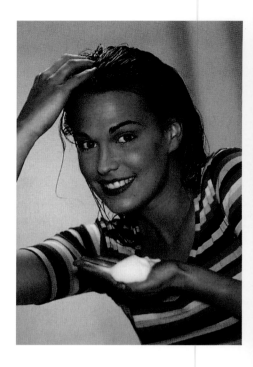

△ **When applying mousse use no more than a "handful", and take care to ensure that you distribute it evenly.**

products to improve the feel of the hair, to combat static, de-frizz, add shine and gloss, and temporarily repair split ends.

styling or setting lotions

Containing flexible resins that form a film on the hair and aid setting, styling lotions protect the hair from heat damage. There are formulations for dry, coloured or sensitized hair; others give volume and additional shine. Use for roller-setting, scrunching, blow-drying and natural drying.

STYLING LOTION TIP
If using a styling lotion for heat-setting look out for formulations that offer thermal protection.

waxes, pomades and creams

These products are made from natural waxes, such as carnauba (produced by a Brazilian palm tree), which are softened with other ingredients such as mineral oils and lanolin to make them pliable. Both soft and hard formulations are available. Some pomades contain vegetable wax and oil to give gloss and sheen. Other formulations produce foam and are water soluble, and leave no residue. Use for dressing the hair and for controlling frizz and static.

Useful appliances

Heated styling appliances allow you to style your hair quickly, efficiently and easily. A wide range of heated appliances is available.

air wavers

Air wavers combine the speed of a blow-dryer with the ease of a styling wand. They operate on the same principle as a blow-dryer, blowing warm air though the shaft. Many wavers are available with a variety of clip-on options, including brushes, prongs and tongs, some with retractable teeth. Use for creating soft waves and volume at the roots.

AIR WAVING TIP

Apply a styling spray or lotion before air waving, and style the hair while it is still damp.

crimpers

These consist of two ridged metal plates that produce uniform patterned crimps in straight lines in the hair. The hair must be straightened first, either by blow-drying or using flat irons. The crimper is then used to give waves or ripples. Some crimpers have reversible or dual-effect styling plates to give different effects.

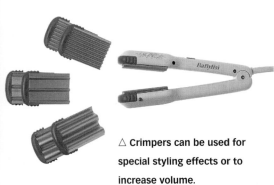

△ Crimpers can be used for special styling effects or to increase volume.

CRIMPING TIPS

• Do not use on damaged, bleached or over-stressed hair.

• Brushing crimped hair gives a softer result.

BLOW-DRYING TIPS

• Always point the airflow down the hair shaft to smooth the cuticle and encourage shine.

• Take care not to hold the dryer too near the scalp; it can cause burns.

• When you have finished blow-drying allow the hair to cool thoroughly, then check that the hair is completely dry. Warm hair often gives the illusion of dryness while it is, in fact, still damp.

• Never use a dryer without its filter in place – hair can easily be drawn into the machine.

blow-dryers

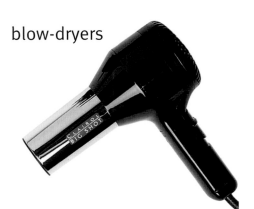

Choose a dryer that has a range of heat and speed settings so that the hair can be power-dried on high heat, finished on a lower heat, and then used with cool air to actually set the style. The average life expectancy of a blow-dryer is usually between 200 and 300 hours.

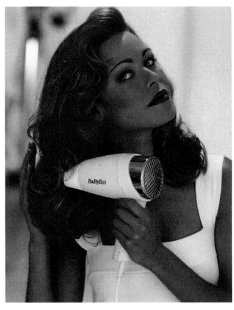

△The blow-dryer is an essential piece of equipment, particularly when you need to dry your hair in a hurry.

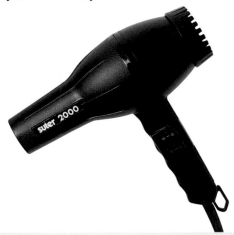

DIFFUSERS AND NOZZLES

Originally, diffusers were intended for drying curly hair slowly, in this way encouraging curl formation for scrunched styles. The diffuser serves to spread the airflow over the hair so the curls are not literally blown away. The prongs on the diffuser head also help to increase volume at the root and give lift. Diffusers with flat heads are designed for gentle drying without ruffling, and are more suitable for shorter styles. The newest type of diffuser has long, straight prongs which are designed to inject volume into straight hair while giving a smooth finish. Nozzles fit over the end of the barrel of the blow-dryer and are used to give precise direction when styling.

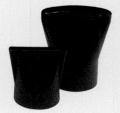

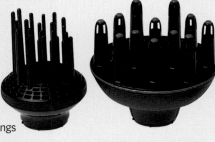

heated rollers

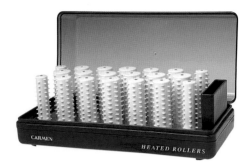

△ Heated rollers are available in sets, normally comprising a selection of 20 or so small, medium and large rollers.

Early heated rollers had spikes, which many women prefer because they have a good grip. New developments include ribbed rubber surfaces, which are designed to be kinder to the hair, curved barrel shapes that follow the form of the head, and clip fasteners.

HEATED ROLLER TIP

Ten minutes is enough time in which to heat up a heated roller-set.

The speed at which the rollers heat up varies, depending on the type of roller. PTC (positive temperature co-efficient) element rollers heat up fastest because they have an element inside each roller, and the heat is transferred directly from the base to the roller. Wax-filled rollers take longer, around 15 minutes, but they retain their temperature over a longer period. All rollers cool down completely in 30 minutes. Use heated rollers for quick sets, to give curl and body. They are ideal for preparing long hair for dressing.

REDUCING STATIC

Heat drying encourages static, causing hair to fly away. You can reduce static by lightly touching your hair, or misting your hairbrush with spray to calm the hair down.

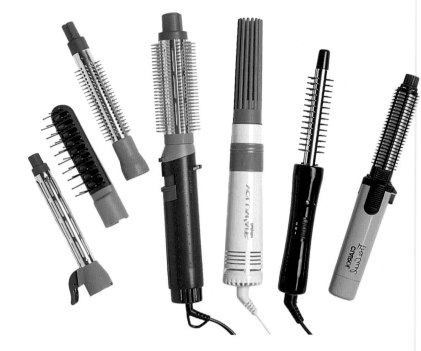

△ Easier to handle than tongs, hot brushes come in a wide range of sizes and are specially designed for creating curls of different sizes. Use for root lift, curl and movement.

hot brushes

The most effective styling technique to use with a hot brush is to wind down the length of the hair, then hold it there for a few seconds until the heat has penetrated through the hair, then gently remove it. Cordless hot brushes, which use batteries to produce heat, are also available and are very convenient for taking on holiday or on business trips.

HOT BRUSH TIP

Take neat, methodical sections when working with a hot brush or the hair may tangle. Use large clips to keep back the rest of your hair.

▽ When using a hot brush make certain you follow the manufacturer's instructions carefully.

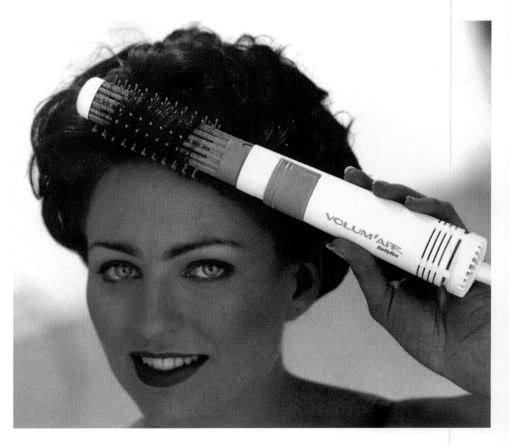

straighteners

Ceramic straighteners are based on the same principle as crimpers but have flat plates to iron out frizz or curl. Use for "pressing" really curly hair. For the best results choose a ceramic rather than a ceramic-coated one. Some ceramic straighteners claim to seal in moisture and natural oils so they won't dry your hair. They smooth the cuticles and leave your hair soft and static-free.

STRAIGHTENING TIPS

• Use a styling spray before straightening.

• Straighteners are designed for occasional, not daily, use because they function at a very high temperature, which can cause damage to the hair.

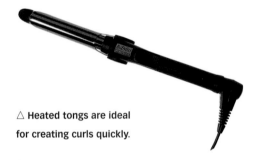

△ **Heated tongs are ideal for creating curls quickly.**

tongs

Styling tongs consist of a barrel, or prong, and a depressor groove. The barrel is round; the depressor is curved to fit around the barrel when the tong is closed. The thickness of the barrel varies, and the size of the tong that is used depends on whether small, medium, or large curls are required.

TONGING TIPS

• Be careful when tonging white or bleached hair as it can discolour.

• Always use tongs on dry, not wet, hair.

• If curling right up to the roots, place a comb between the tongs and the scalp so the comb forms a barrier against the heat.

• Leave tonged curls to cool before styling.

travel dryers

Specially made for taking on holiday, travel dryers are usually miniature versions of standard dryers, and some even have their own small diffusers. Check that the dryer you buy has dual voltage and a travel case.

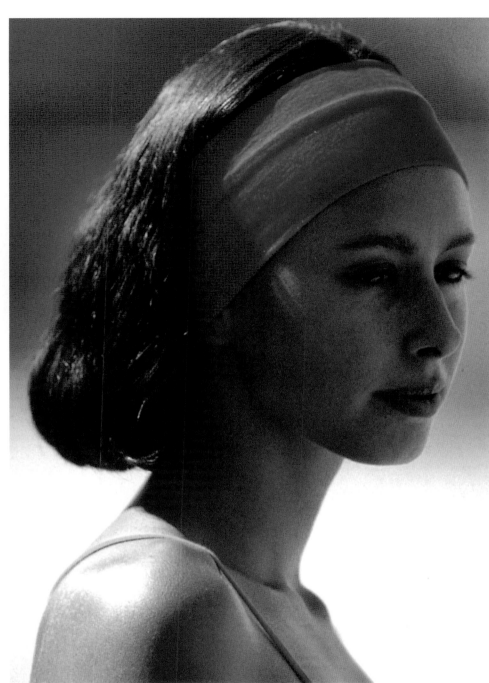

△ **Keep holiday haircare to a minimum by making use of dual-purpose heated appliances. Don't forget to pack a universal plug when travelling abroad.**

SAFETY TIPS

• Equipment should be unplugged when not in use.

• Never use electric equipment with wet hands, and don't use near water.

• Only use one appliance for each socket outlet – adaptors may cause overload.

• The cord should not be wrapped tightly around the equipment; coil it loosely before storing.

• Tongs can be cleaned by wiping with a damp cloth; if necessary use a little alcohol to remove dirt.

• All electrical equipment should be checked periodically to ensure that leads and connections are in good order.

• Untwist the cord on the dryer from time to time.

• Clean filters regularly – a blocked filter means the dryer has to work harder and will eventually overheat and cut out. If the element overheats it can distort the dryer casing.

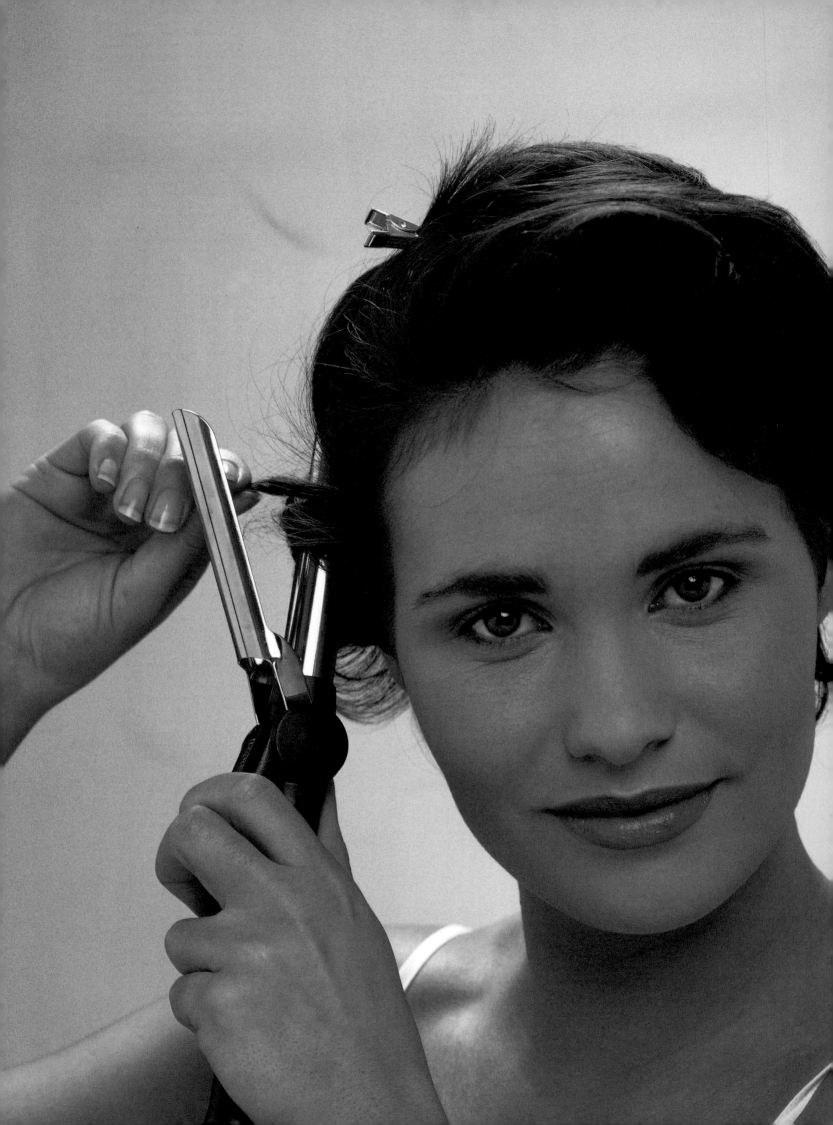

Styling your hair

This section tackles the basics of hair setting and drying techniques. Then you can use these skills to tackle the special projects, which show you how to create braids, chignons, French pleats (rolls), top knots, twists, coils and curls. By following the simple step-by-step pictures, you'll be amazed at how easy it is to transform your hair to suit almost every mood and occasion.

Blow-drying

Follow these simple instructions to achieve the smoothest, sleekest blow-dry ever.

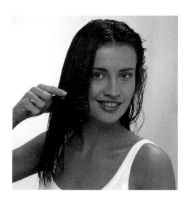

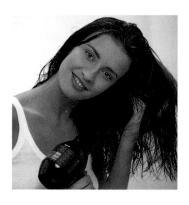

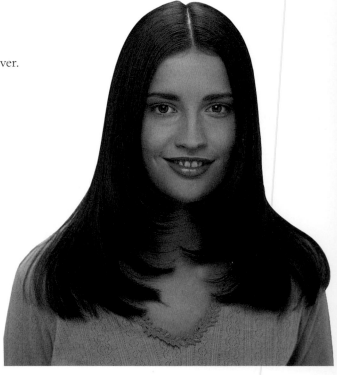

△ **1** Shampoo and condition your hair as usual. Then comb through with a wide-toothed comb to completely remove any tangles.

△ **2** Partially dry your hair, running your fingers through it as you work. This is just to remove the excess moisture.

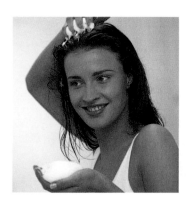

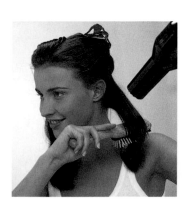

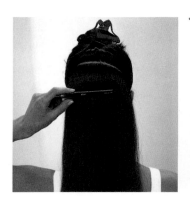

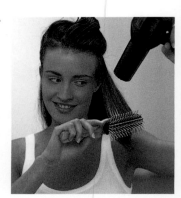

△ **3** Apply a handful of mousse to the palm of your hand. Then using your other hand, spread the mousse through the hair, distributing it evenly from the tips to the ends.

△ **4** Divide your hair into two main sections by clipping the top and sides out of the way. Then, working on the hair that is left free and taking one small section at a time, hold the dryer in one hand and a styling brush in the other. Place the brush underneath the first section of hair, positioning it at the roots. Keeping the tension on the hair taut (but without undue stress), move the brush down towards the ends, directing the airflow from the dryer so that it follows the downwards movement of the brush.

△ **5** Curve the brush under at the ends to achieve a slight bend. Focus on drying the roots first, repeatedly applying the brush to the roots once it has moved down the length of the hair. Continue this until the first section is dry. Repeat step 4 until the whole of the back section is completely dry.

△ **6** Release a section of hair from the top and dry it in the same manner. Continue in this way until you have dried all your hair. Finish by smoothing a few drops of serum through the hair to flatten any flyaway ends.

STYLING CHECKLIST

You will need:

- styling comb
- dryer
- mousse
- clip
- styling brush
- serum

BLOW-DRYING TIPS

- Use the highest heat or speed setting to remove excess moisture, then switch to medium to finish drying.
- Point the airflow downwards. This smoothes the cuticles and makes the hair shine.
- Ensure each section is competely dry before working on the next.

Finger drying

This is a simple and quick method of drying and styling your hair. It relies on the heat released from your hands rather than the heat from a hairdryer. However, finger drying is only really viable for short to mid-length hair.

FINGER-DRYING TIP

Finger-drying is the best way to dry damaged hair, or to encourage waves in naturally curly, short hair.

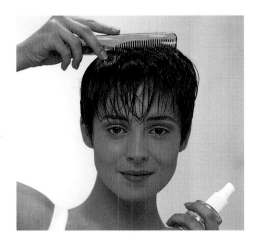

△ **1** Shampoo and condition your hair, then spray with gel and comb through.

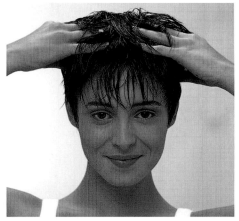

△ **2** Run your fingers rapidly upwards and forwards, from the roots to the ends.

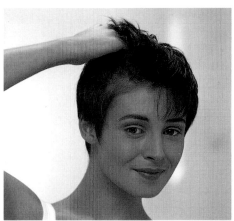

△ **3** Lift up the hair at the crown to give it volume and body at the roots.

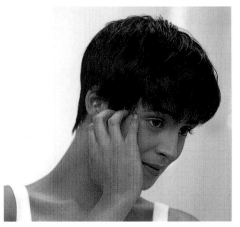

△ **4** Continue lifting as the hair dries. Use your fingertips to flatten the hair at the sides.

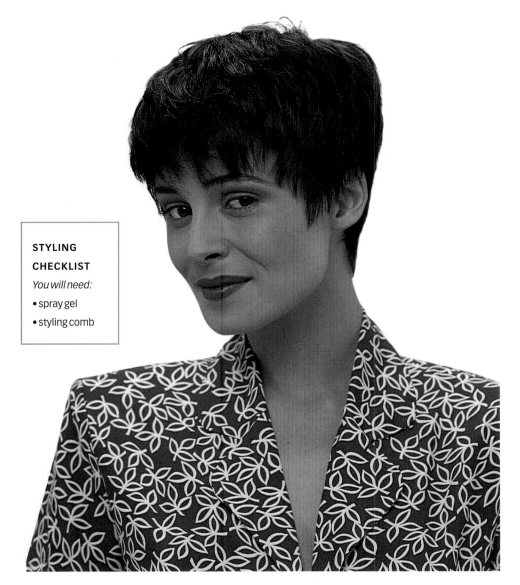

STYLING CHECKLIST

You will need:
- spray gel
- styling comb

Barrel curls

One of the simplest sets is achieved by curling the hair around the fingers and then pinning the curl in place. Barrel curls are a great way to create a natural, soft set.

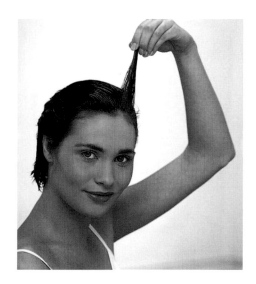

△ **1** Shampoo and condition; apply setting lotion and comb from the roots to the ends. Take a small section of hair (about 2.5cm/1in) and smooth it upwards.

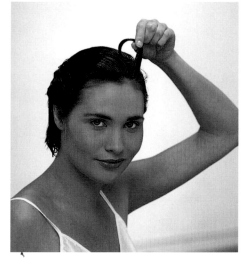

△ **2** Loop the hair into a large curl.

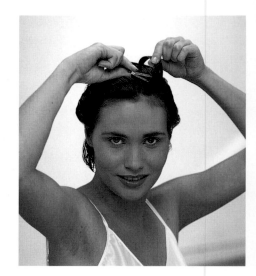

△ **3** Clip in place.

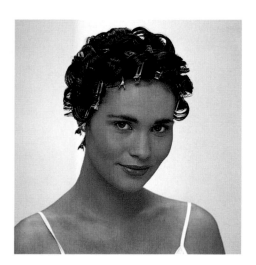

△ **4** Continue to curl the rest of the hair in the same way.

▷ **5** Allow the hair to dry naturally, or with a hood dryer, then carefully remove the clips. To achieve a natural tousled look rake your fingers through your hair. For a smoother finish use a hair brush.

STYLING CHECKLIST

You will need:

- setting lotion
- styling comb
- clips
- hood dryer (optional)

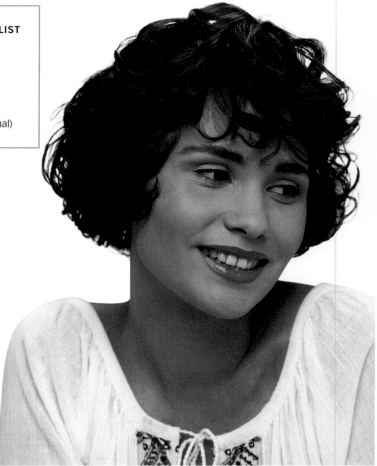

Roll-up

A roller set forms the basis of many styles; it can be used to smooth hair, add waves or soft curls, or provide a foundation for an upswept style.

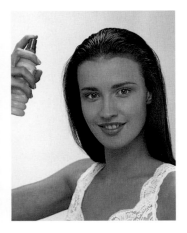

△ **1** Shampoo and condition your hair, then partially dry to remove excess moisture. Mist with a styling spray.

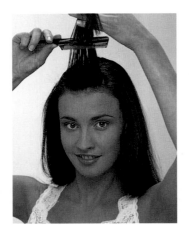

△ **2** For a basic set, take a 5cm/2in section of hair (or a section the same width as your roller) from the centre front and comb it straight up, smoothing out any tangles.

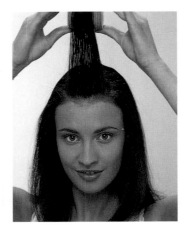

△ **3** Wrap the ends of the sectioned hair around the roller, taking care not to buckle the hair. Then wind the roller down firmly towards the scalp, keeping the tension even.

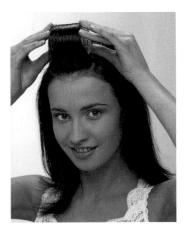

△ **4** Keep winding until the roller sits on the roots of the hair. Self-fixing rollers will stay in place on their own but if you are using brush rollers you will have to fasten them with pins.

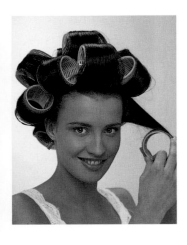

△ **5** Continue around the whole head, always taking the same width of hair. Re-mist the hair with styling spray if it begins to dry out.

▷ **6** Leave the finished set to dry naturally, or dry it with a diffuser attachment on your hand dryer, or with a hood dryer. When using artificial heat sources allow the completely dry hair to become quite cool before you remove the rollers. Brush through the hair following the direction of the set. Mist the brush with hairspray and use to smooth any stray hairs.

STYLING CHECKLIST
You will need:
- styling spray
- tail comb
- self-fixing rollers or brush rollers and pins
- hand or hood dryer (optional)
- hairspray

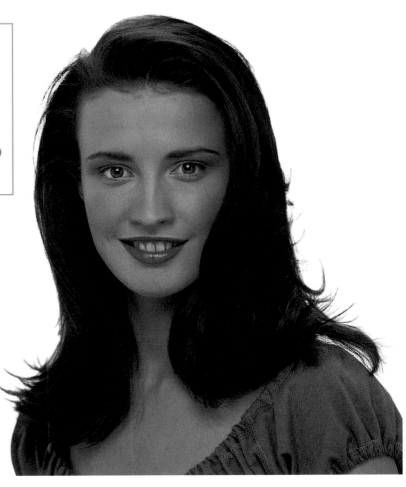

Soft setting

Fabric rollers are the modern version of old-fashioned rags. Apart from being very easy to use they are kind to the hair and give a highly effective set.

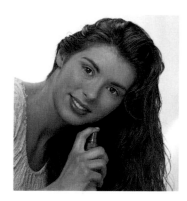

△ **1** Dampen the hair with styling spray, making sure you distribute it evenly from the roots to the ends.

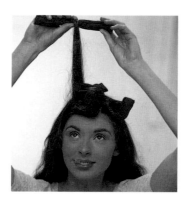

△ **2** Wind sections about 2.5cm/1in wide around fabric rollers. Wind the roller smoothly towards the scalp.

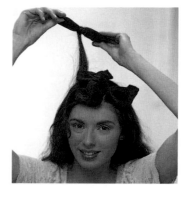

△ **3** Continue winding the roller gently and firmly, taking it right down to the roots.

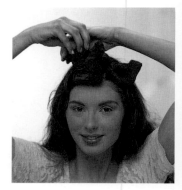

△ **4** To fasten, simply bend each end of the fabric roller towards the centre. This grips the hair and holds it in place.

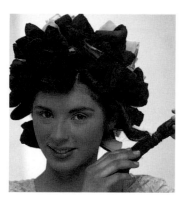

△ **5** Leave the completed set to dry. Then remove the rollers by unbending the ends and unwinding the hair.

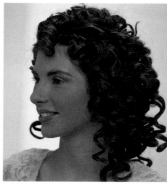

△ **6** When all the rollers have been removed the hair falls into firm corkscrew curls.

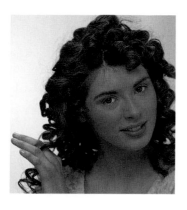

△ **7** Working on one curl at a time, rake and tease out each curl with your fingers for a full, voluminous finish.

TIP

For even more volume, twist each section of hair lengthwise before winding it into the fabric roller.

STYLING CHECKLIST
You will need:
- styling spray
- fabric rollers

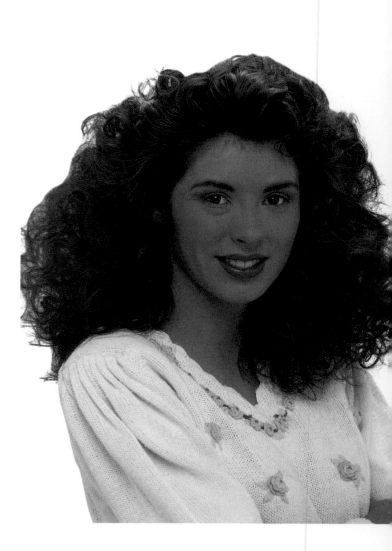

Tong and twist

Tongs can be used to smooth the hair and add just the right amount of movement.

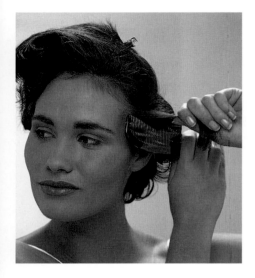

△ **1** Shampoo, condition and dry. Apply a mist of styling lotion. Avoid mousse as it sticks to the tongs and bakes into the hair. Divide off a small section.

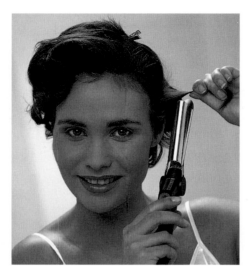

△ **2** Press the depressor to open the tongs.

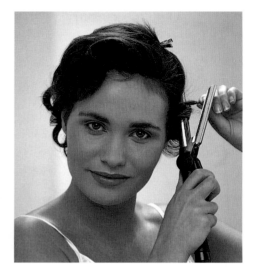

△ **3** Wind the whole section of hair around the barrel of the tongs.

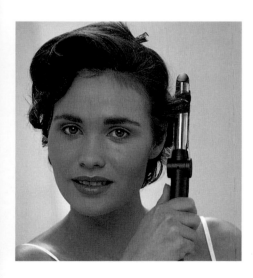

△ **4** Release the depressor to hold the hair in place and wait a few seconds for the curl to form. Remove the tongs and leave to cool as you work on the rest of the hair. Style by raking through with your fingers.

TIP
Never use tongs on bleached hair. The high heat can damage the hair, causing brittleness and breakage.

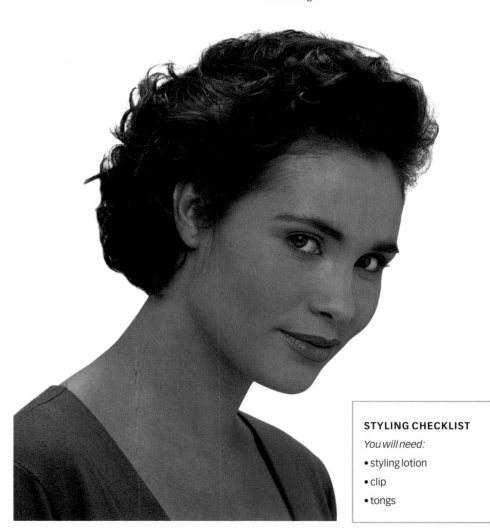

STYLING CHECKLIST
You will need:
- styling lotion
- clip
- tongs

Style and go

Hot brushes with tong attachments enable you to create lots of styles. Here we show you two different techniques, which give two different looks.

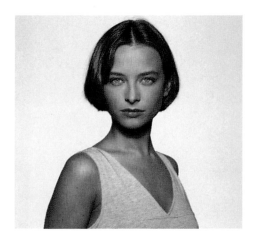

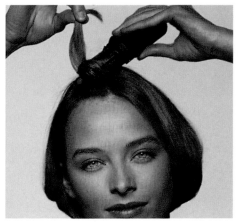

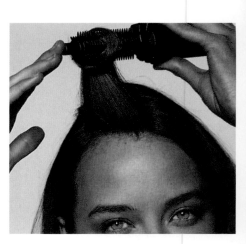

△ **1** Shampoo, condition and dry your hair.

△ **2** Take a section of hair about 5cm/2in square, and apply some styling lotion. Using the brush attachment gently smooth the hair from the roots to the ends. Place the hot brush near the roots, twist the hair around the brush, and hold for a few seconds. Gently unravel the hair and hold without pulling.

△ **3** Place the ends of the hair into the hot brush and wind halfway down the hair length.

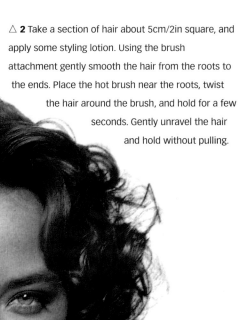

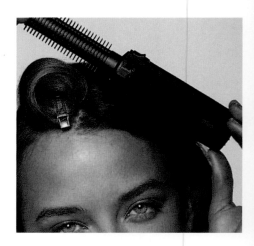

△ **4** Unwind and loop the hair into a barrel curl, securing with a clip. Repeat steps 2 to 4 until you have done the whole head. Remove the clips. Comb.

STYLING CHECKLIST
You will need:
• hot brush with tong attachment
• styling lotion
• clips

TIP
Play with the direction of the waves to see which way they fall best. Draw the fingers upwards from the back of the neck and through the hair for extra lift. Finish with a light mist of hairspray.

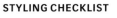

This style uses the tong attachment for a more sculptured, voluminous look.

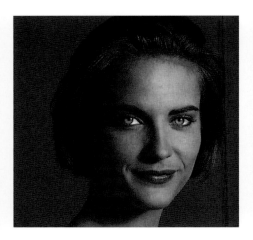

△ **1** Shampoo, condition and dry your hair.

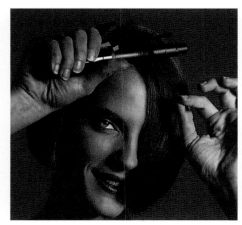

△ **2** Take a section of hair about 1cm/^{1}/$_2$in long and apply some styling lotion. Using the tong attachment on the styler, lift the depressor and keep it open. Slide the tongs on to the hair, just up from the roots. Holding the depressor open, wind the hair around the barrel, towards the face, ensuring the ends are smooth.

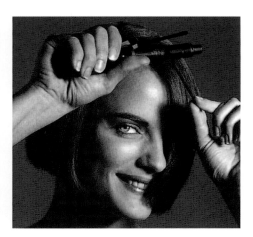

△ **3** Continue wrapping the hair down the length of the barrel, taking care not to buckle the ends of the hair. Hold for a few seconds to allow the curl to form.

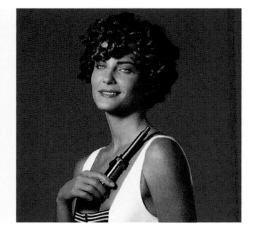

△ **4** Release the depressor and allow the spiral curl to spring out. Repeat steps 2 to 3 until you have curled the whole head, then rake through the hair with your fingers for a softly sculptured look.

TIP

After tonging, don't be tempted to brush your hair or you will lose the curl.

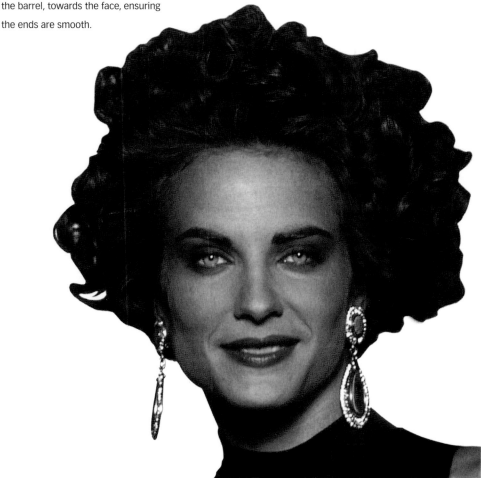

Curl creation

A perm that is past its best can be revived using this diffuser–drying technique.

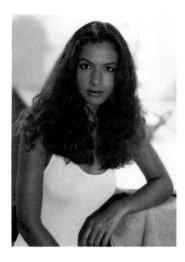

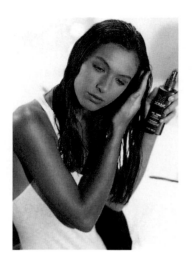

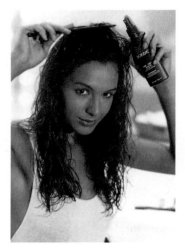

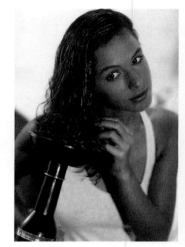

△ **1** The hair has the remains of a perm and is therefore flat at the roots with some curl from the mid-lengths to the ends

△ **2** Wash, condition and towel-dry your hair, then apply curl revitalizer to the damp hair.

△ **3** Use a wide-toothed comb and work from the roots to the ends to ensure the curl revitalizer is distributed evenly.

△ **4** Attach the diffuser to the dryer and dry the hair, allowing the hair to sit on the prongs of the diffuser. This action enables the warm air to circulate around the strands of hair, encouraging the formation of curls. To maximize the amount of curl, use your hands to scrunch up handfuls of hair.

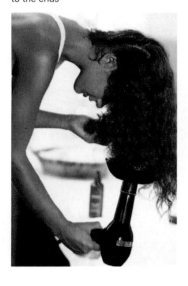

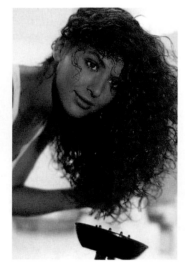

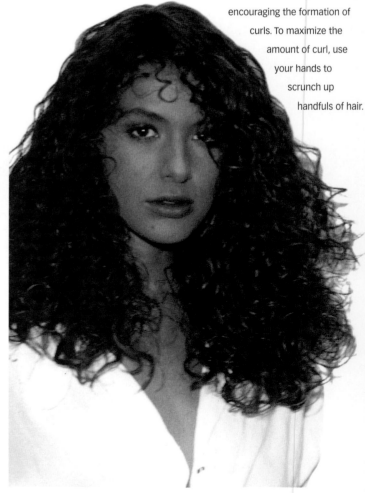

△ **5** Tip your head forwards, allowing the hair to sit in the diffuser cup. Do not pull the hair, simply squeeze curls gently into shape.

△ **6** Repeat steps 4 and 5 until all the hair is dry.

TIP
This technique works equally well on naturally wavy or curly hair, giving separation and definition to curls and waves.

STYLING CHECKLIST
You will need:
- curl revitalizer
- wide-toothed comb
- dryer with pronged diffuser attachment

Smooth and straight

Instant set

Volume can be added to long straight hair by using a dryer with a diffuser attachment that has long straight prongs.

Hair can be given lift, bounce and movement with a quick set using heated rollers.

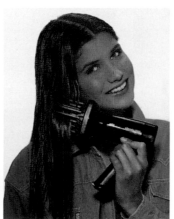

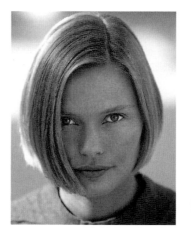

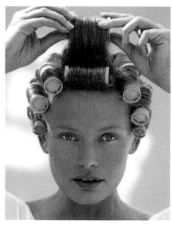

△ **1** Long thick hair often tangles easily and it is difficult to add volume and control.

△ **2** Shampoo and condition your hair, then part it down the centre. Attach a diffuser with long prongs to your dryer and, as the hair dries, comb the prongs down the hair in a stroking movement. This will direct the airflow downwards, smoothing and separating the hair.

△ **1** Shampoo and condition your hair. Apply mousse and blow-dry smooth. Heat the rollers according to the manufacturer's directions.

△ **2** Wind sections of hair (about 5cm/2in wide) on to rollers, taking care not to buckle the hair ends. Use medium and small rollers at the front and sides, larger rollers on the crown.

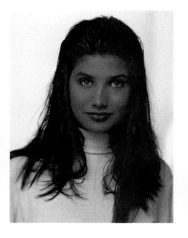

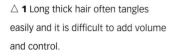

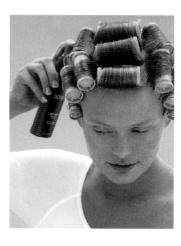

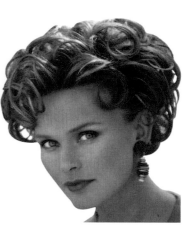

STYLING CHECKLIST

You will need:

• comb

• dryer with diffuser attachment with long straight prongs

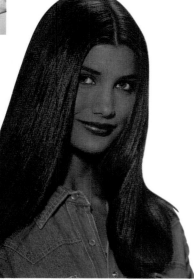

△ **3** To create volume at the top and sides, slide the prongs through the hair to the roots at the crown, then gently rotate the diffuser. Repeat until you have achieved maximum volume.

△ **3** Wind the rollers down towards the root, making sure that the ends are tucked under smoothly. Keep the tension even. Secure each roller with the clip supplied. Mist your set hair with a styling lotion.

△ **4** Allow the rollers to cool and then remove, taking care not to disturb the curls. To finish, loosen the curls by raking your fingers through them.

STYLING CHECKLIST

You will need:

• mousse

• styling lotion

• heated rollers with clips

Double-stranded
braids

These clever braids have a fishbone pattern, which gives an unusual look.

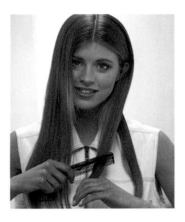

△ **1** Part your hair in the centre and comb it straight.

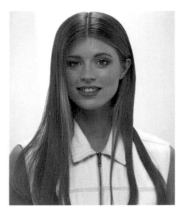

△ **2** Divide the hair on one side of your head into two strands, then take a fine section from the back of the back strand and take it over to join the front strand, as shown.

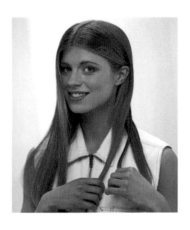

STYLING CHECKLIST
You will need:
- styling comb
- covered bands
- coloured feathers
- two short lengths of fine leather

△ **3** Now take a fine section from the front of the front strand, and cross it over to the back strand. Take a fine section from the back strand again and bring it over to join the front strand. Continue in this way; you will soon see the fishbone effect appear. Secure the ends with covered bands and add feathers, tying in place with fine leather. Repeat on the other side.

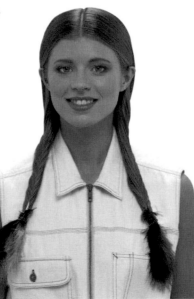

Dragged
side-braids

Curly hair can be controlled, yet still allowed to flow free, by braiding at the sides and allowing the hair at the back to fall in a mass of curls.

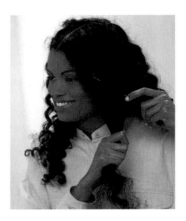

△ **1** Part your hair in the centre and divide off a large section at the side, combing it as flat as possible to the head.

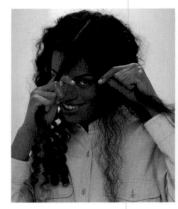

△ **2** Divide the section into three equal strands and hold them apart.

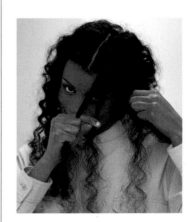

△ **3** Begin to make a dragged braid by pulling the strands of hair towards your face and then braiding in the normal way, that is, taking the right strand over the centre strand, the left strand over the centre, and the right over the centre again, keeping the braid in the position shown.

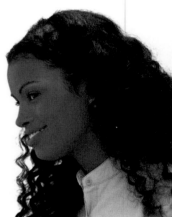

△ **4** Continue braiding to the bottom and secure the end with a covered band. Tuck the braid behind your ear and grip it in place, then make a second braid on the other side.

TIP
Encourage curls to form by spraying the hair with water and then scrunching with your hands.

STYLING CHECKLIST
You will need:
- styling comb
- 4 covered bands
- hair grips

Ponytail styler

A simple ponytail can be transformed easily and quickly using this clever styler.

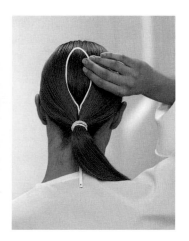

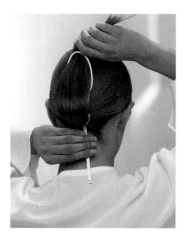

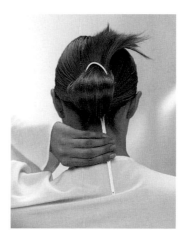

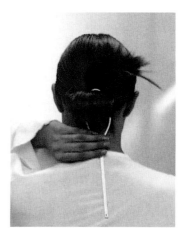

△ **1** Clasp the hair into a ponytail and secure it with a covered band. Insert the styler as shown.

△ **2** Thread the ponytail into the styler and pull it through.

△ **3** Begin to pull the styler down…

△ **4** …continue pulling…

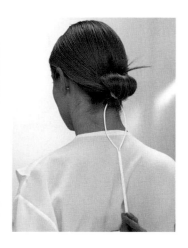

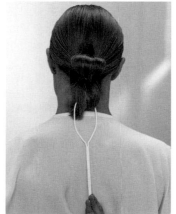

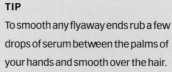

TIP
To smooth any flyaway ends rub a few drops of serum between the palms of your hands and smooth over the hair.

STYLING CHECKLIST
You will need:
- covered band
- ponytail styler

△ **5** …so the ponytail pulls through…

△ **6** …and emerges underneath.

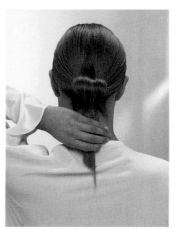

◁ **7** Smooth the hair with your hand and insert the styler again, repeating steps 2 to 6 once more to give a neat chignon loop.

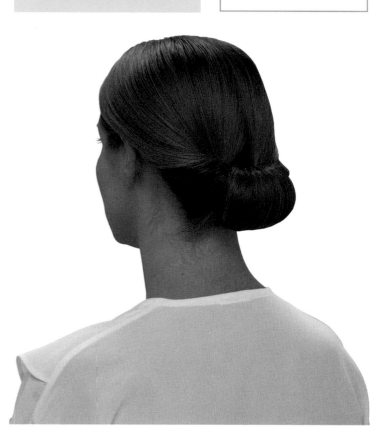

TIP
The same technique can be used on wet hair as long as you apply gel first, combing it through evenly before styling.

Curly styler

The ponytail styler can also be used to tame a mass of curls, creating a ponytail with a simple double twist.

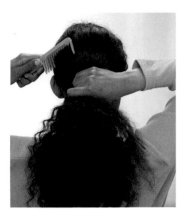

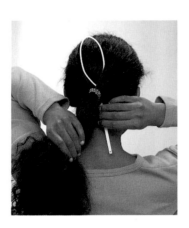

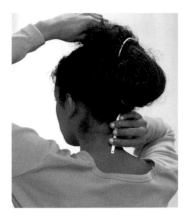

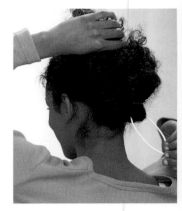

△ **1** Use a comb with widely spaced teeth to smooth the hair back and into a ponytail. Secure with a covered band.

△ **2** Insert the styler as shown.

△ **3** Thread the ponytail into the styler and pull it through.

△ **4** Begin to pull the styler down…

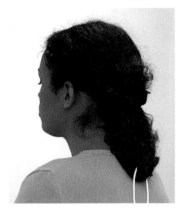

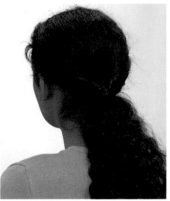

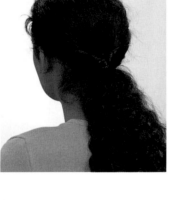

TIP
When inserting the styler through a pony tail, carefully move it from side to side in order to create enough room to pull the looped end of the styler through more easily.

△ **5** …continue pulling…

△ **6** …so that the ponytail pulls through.

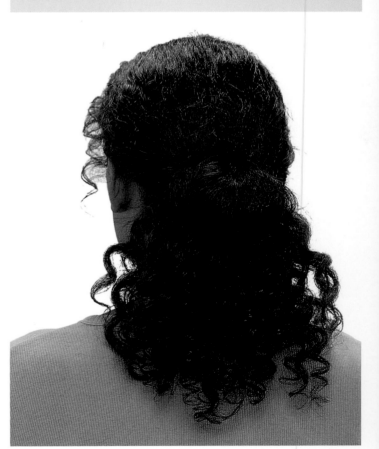

△ **7** Repeat steps 3 to 6.

△ **8** Apply a little mousse to your hands and use it to re-form the curls, scrunching to achieve a good shape.

Crown braids

By braiding the crown hair and allowing the remaining hair to frame the face you can achieve an interesting contrast of textures.

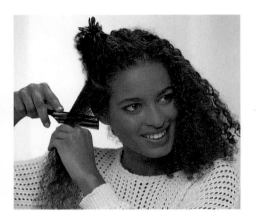

△ **1** Clip up the top hair on one side of your head, leaving the back hair free. Take a small section of hair at ear level and comb it straight.

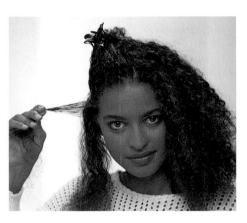

△ **2** Start braiding quite tightly, doing one cross (right strand over centre, left over centre), and then gradually bringing more hair into the outside strands.

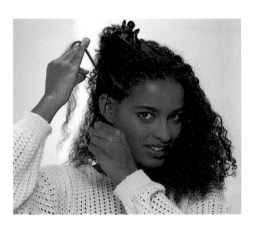

△ **3** Continue in this way, taking the braid towards the back of the head. Secure the braids with small covered bands.

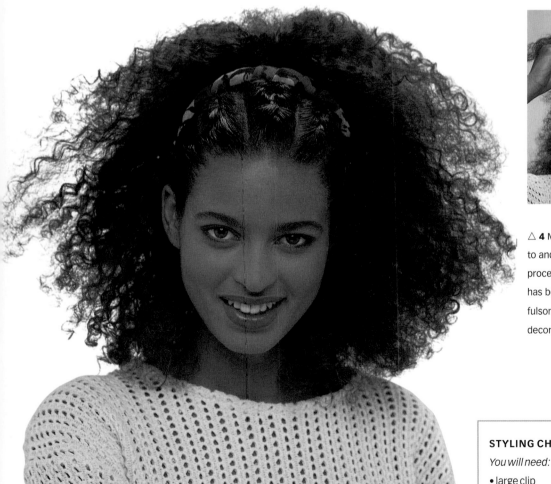

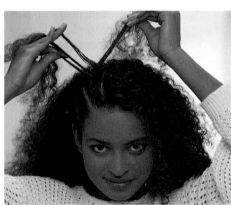

△ **4** Make another parting about 2.5cm/1in parallel to and above the previous braid, and repeat the process. Continue in this way until all the front hair has been braided. Scrunch the remaining hair into fulsome curls to increase the volume. Finally, add a decorative headband.

STYLING CHECKLIST

You will need:
- large clip
- small covered bands
- headband

TIP

The volume of the curls can be increased by tipping your head forwards, then applying styling spray and scrunching the hair lying underneath.

Twist and coil

This style starts with a simple ponytail, is easy to do, and looks stunning.

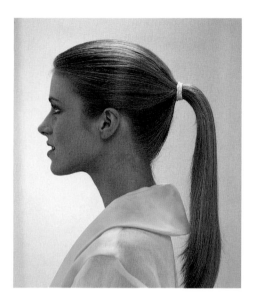

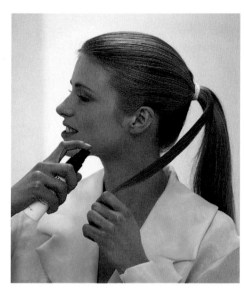

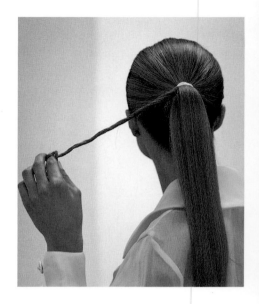

△ **1** Smooth the hair back and secure in a ponytail using a covered band.

△ **2** Divide off a small section of hair and mist with shine spray for added gloss.

△ **3** Holding the ends of a section, twist the hair until it rolls back on itself to form a coil.

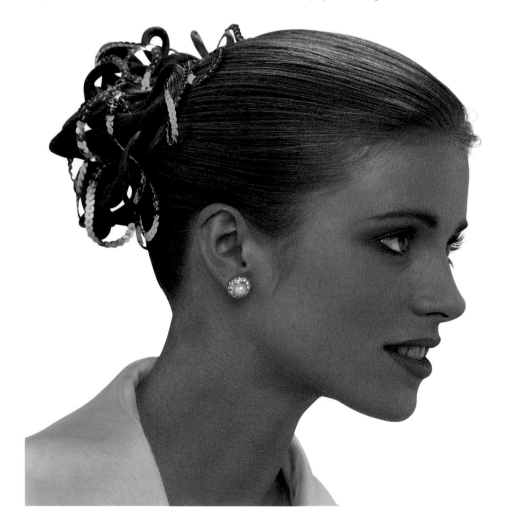

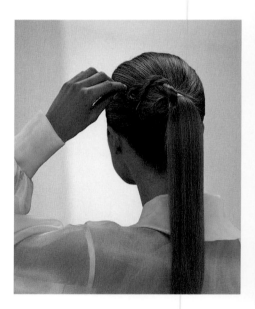

△ **4** Position the coil in a loop as shown and secure in place using hair pins. Continue until all the hair has been coiled. Decorate by intertwining with a strip of sequins.

STYLING CHECKLIST

You will need:
- covered band
- shine spray
- hair pins
- 1m/1 yd strip sequins

Cameo braid

A classic bun is given extra panache with an encircling braid.

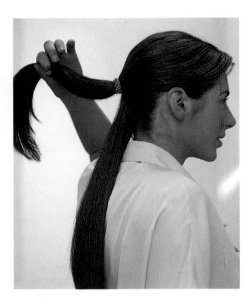

△ **1** Smooth the hair into a ponytail, leaving one section free.

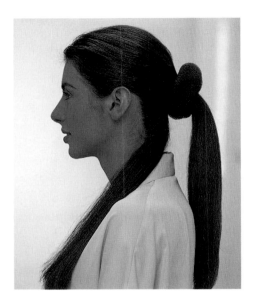

△ **2** Place a bun ring over the ponytail.

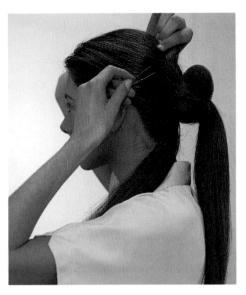

△ **3** Take approximately one third of the hair from the ponytail and wrap it around the bun ring, securing with pins. Repeat with the other two-thirds of hair.

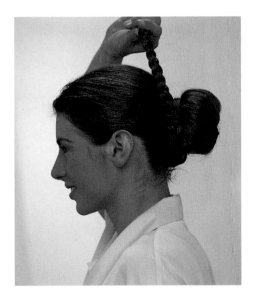

△ **4** Braid the section of hair that was left out of the ponytail, right strand over centre strand, left over centre and so on, and wrap the braid around the base of the bun, then secure with pins.

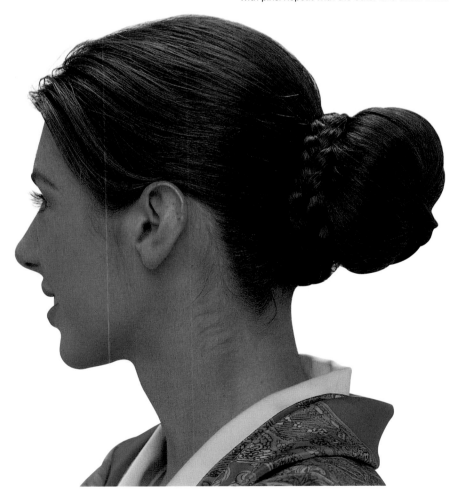

STYLING CHECKLIST

You will need:
- covered band
- bun ring
- hair pins

Band braid

A plain ponytail can be transformed by simply covering the band with a tiny braid.

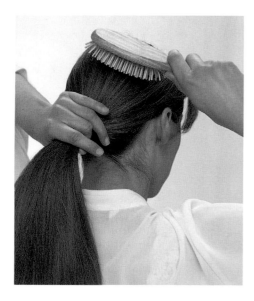

△ **1** Brush the hair back into a smooth, low ponytail, leaving a small section free for braiding. Secure in place with a covered band. Smooth the reserved section with a little styling wax.

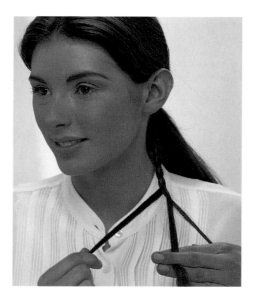

△ **2** Divide this section into three equal strands. Now, braid the hair in the normal way.

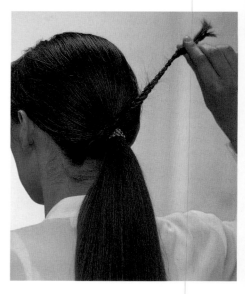

△ **3** Take the braid and wrap it tightly around the covered band.

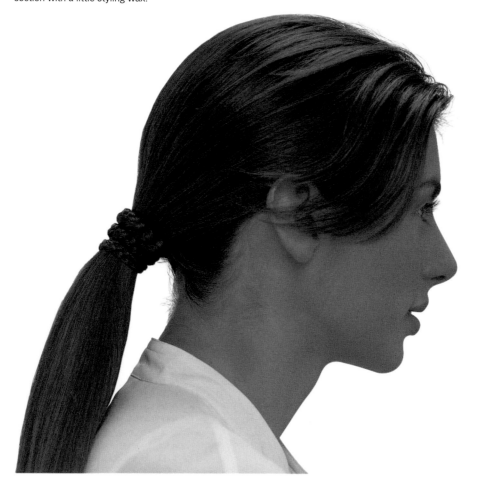

△ **4** Wind it as many times as it goes. Finally, secure with a grip.

STYLING CHECKLIST

You will need:

- brush
- covered band
- wax
- hair pin

Clip up

Long, curly hair can sometimes be unruly. Here's an easy way to tame tresses but still keep the beauty of the length.

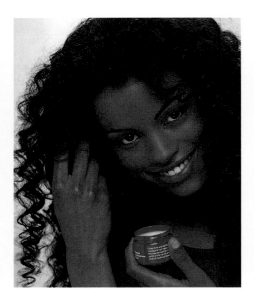

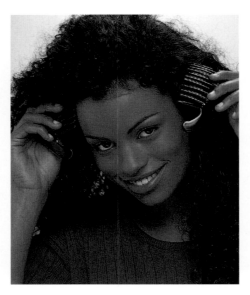

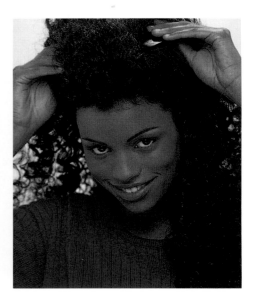

△ **1** Rub a little wax between the palms of your hands, then work into the curls with the fingertips. This helps give the curl separation and shine.

△ **2** Take two interlocking large curved combs and use them to push the crown hair up towards **the centre.**

△ **3** Push the teeth of the combs together to fasten on top of the head.

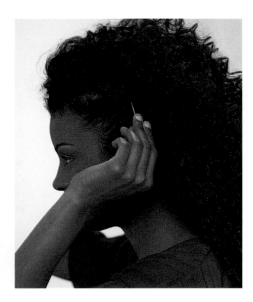

△ **4** Repeat with two more combs at ear level to secure the back hair.

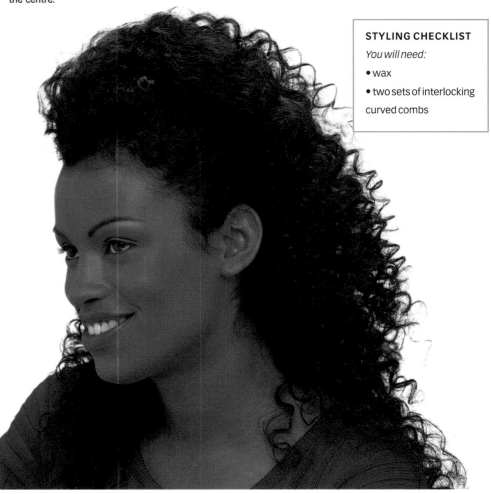

STYLING CHECKLIST
You will need:
- wax
- two sets of interlocking curved combs

TIP
It's easier to disentangle curly hair if you use a comb with widely spaced teeth.

Draped chignon

This elegant style is perfect for that special evening out.

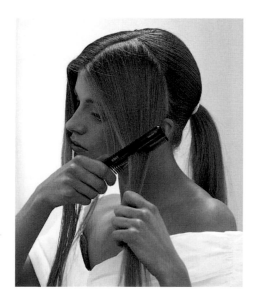

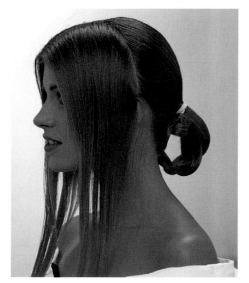

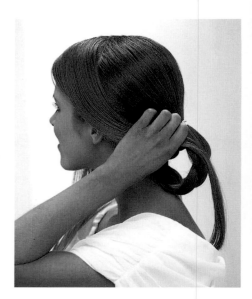

△ **1** Part the hair in the centre from the forehead to the middle of the crown. Comb the side hair and scoop the back hair into a low ponytail using a covered band.

△ **2** Loosely braid the ponytail – take the right strand over the centre strand, the left over the centre, the right over the centre, and so on, continuing to the end. Secure the end with a small band, then tuck the end under and around in a loop and secure with grips.

△ **3** Pick up the hair on the left side and comb it in a curve back to the ponytail loop.

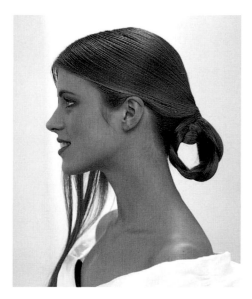

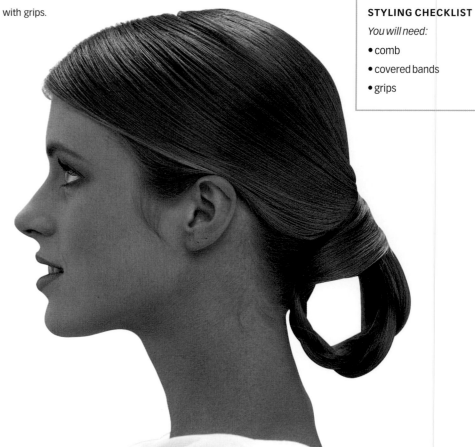

△ **4** Swirl this hair over and under the loop and secure with grips. Repeat steps 3 and 4 on the right side.

STYLING CHECKLIST
You will need:
- comb
- covered bands
- grips

TIP
Even long hair should be trimmed regularly, at least every two months, to keep it in good condition.

City slicker

Transform your hair in minutes using gel to slick it into shape and add sheen.

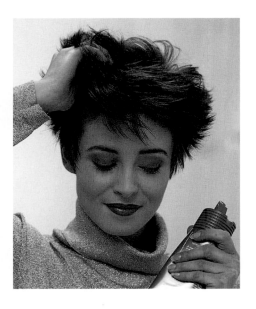

△ **1** Take a generous amount of gel and apply it to the hair from the roots to the ends.

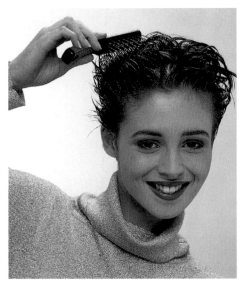

△ **2** Use a vent brush, a comb or your fingers to distribute the gel evenly through the hair.

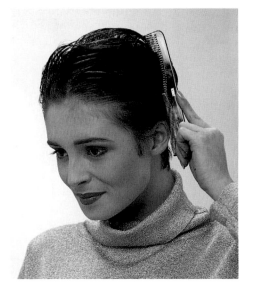

△ **3** Comb the hair into shape using a styling comb to encourage movement.

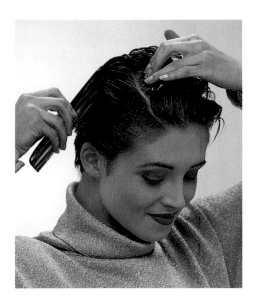

△ **4** Shape to form a wave and sleek down the sides and back.

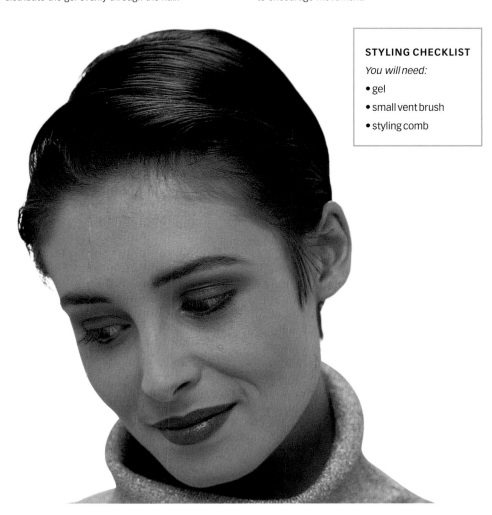

STYLING CHECKLIST
You will need:
- gel
- small vent brush
- styling comb

TIP
Make sure you distribute the gel evenly all over your hair before styling.

Simple pleat

Curly hair that is neatly pleated gives a sophisticated style. The front is left full to soften the effect.

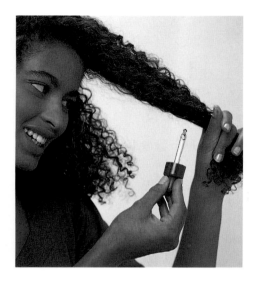

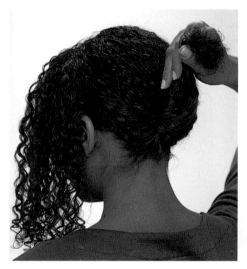

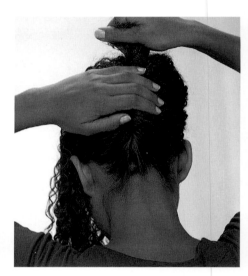

△ **1** Divide off a section of hair at the front and leave it free. Smooth with a little serum. Take the remaining hair into one hand, as if you were going to make it into a ponytail.

△ **2** Twist the hair tightly from left to right.

△ **3** When the twist is taut, turn the hair upwards as shown to form a pleat. Use your other hand to help smooth the pleat and at the same time neaten the top by tucking in the ends.

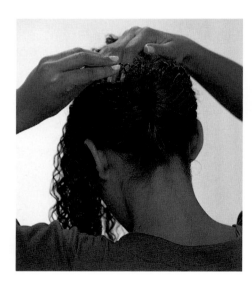

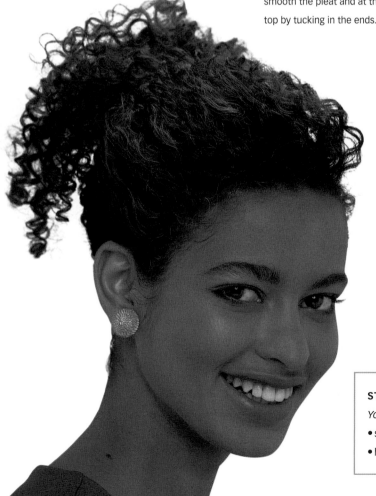

△ **4** Secure the pleat with hair pins. Take the reserved front section, bring it back and secure it at the top of the pleat, allowing the ends to fall free.

STYLING CHECKLIST
You will need:
- serum
- hair pins

Looped curls

Two ponytails form the basis of this elegant style.

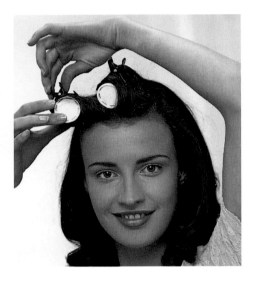

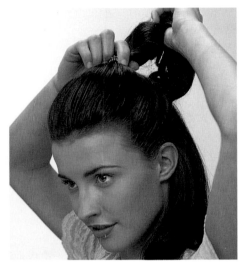

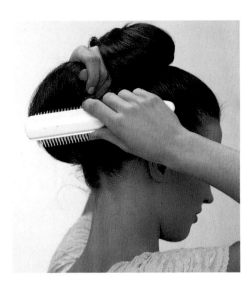

△ **1** Apply setting lotion to the ends of the hair only. This will give just the right amount of body and bounce to help form the curls. Set the hair on heated rollers. When the rollers are quite cool – about 10 minutes after completing the set – take them out and allow the hair to fall free.

△ **2** Divide off the crown hair and secure it with hair pins in a high ponytail. Apply a few drops of serum to add gloss, and brush the hair through.

△ **3** Place the remaining hair in a lower ponytail.

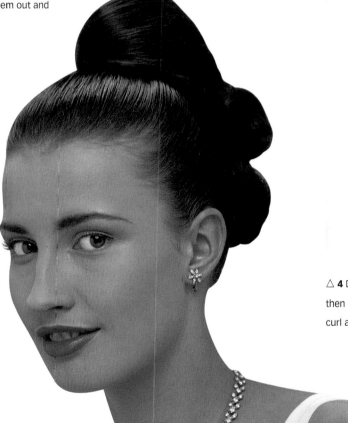

△ **4** Divide each ponytail in sections 2.5cm/1in wide, then comb and smooth each section into a looped curl and pin in place. Set with hairspray.

STYLING CHECKLIST

You will need:

• setting lotion
• heated rollers
• serum
• covered bands, hair pins

French pleat

Mid–length to long hair can be transformed into a classic, elegant French pleat (roll) in a matter of minutes.

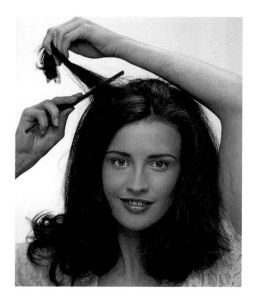

△ **1** Backcomb the hair all over.

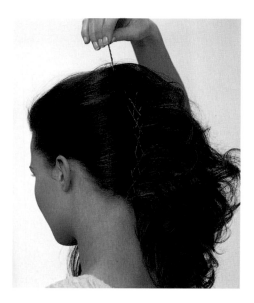

△ **2** Smooth your hair across to the centre back and form the centre of the pleat by criss-crossing hair-grips in a row from the crown downwards, as shown.

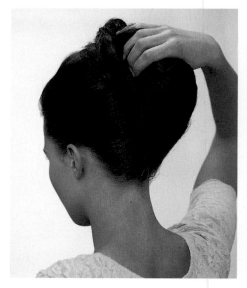

△ **3** Gently smooth the hair around from the other side, leaving the front section free, and tuck the ends under.

STYLING CHECKLIST
You will need:
• comb
• hairgrips
• pins
• hairspray

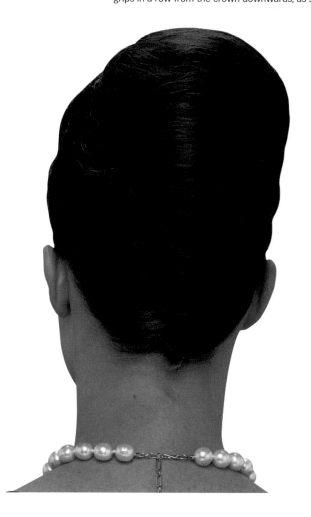

△ **4** Secure with pins, then lightly comb the front section up and around to merge with the top of the pleat. Mist with hairspray to hold.

Short and spiky

Short hair can be quickly styled using gel and wax to create a cheeky, fun look.

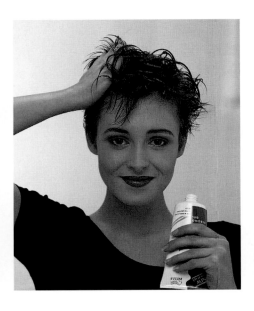

△ **1** Work a generous amount of gel through your hair from the roots to the ends.

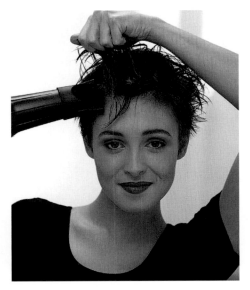

△ **2** Dry your hair using a directional nozzle on your dryer; as you dry, lift sections of the hair to create height at the roots.

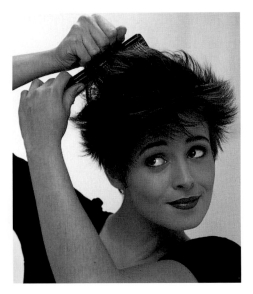

△ **3** When the hair is dry, backcomb the crown to give additional height.

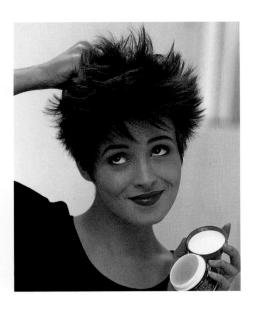

△ **4** To finish, rub a little wax between the palms of your hands, then apply it to the hair to give definition.

TIP
Gel can be reactivated by misting the hair with water and shaping it into style again.

STYLING CHECKLIST
You will need:
- gel
- blow-dryer
- comb
- wax

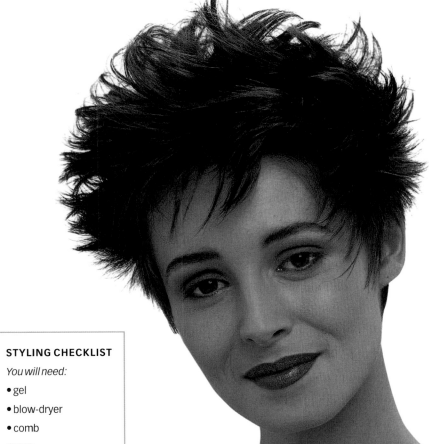

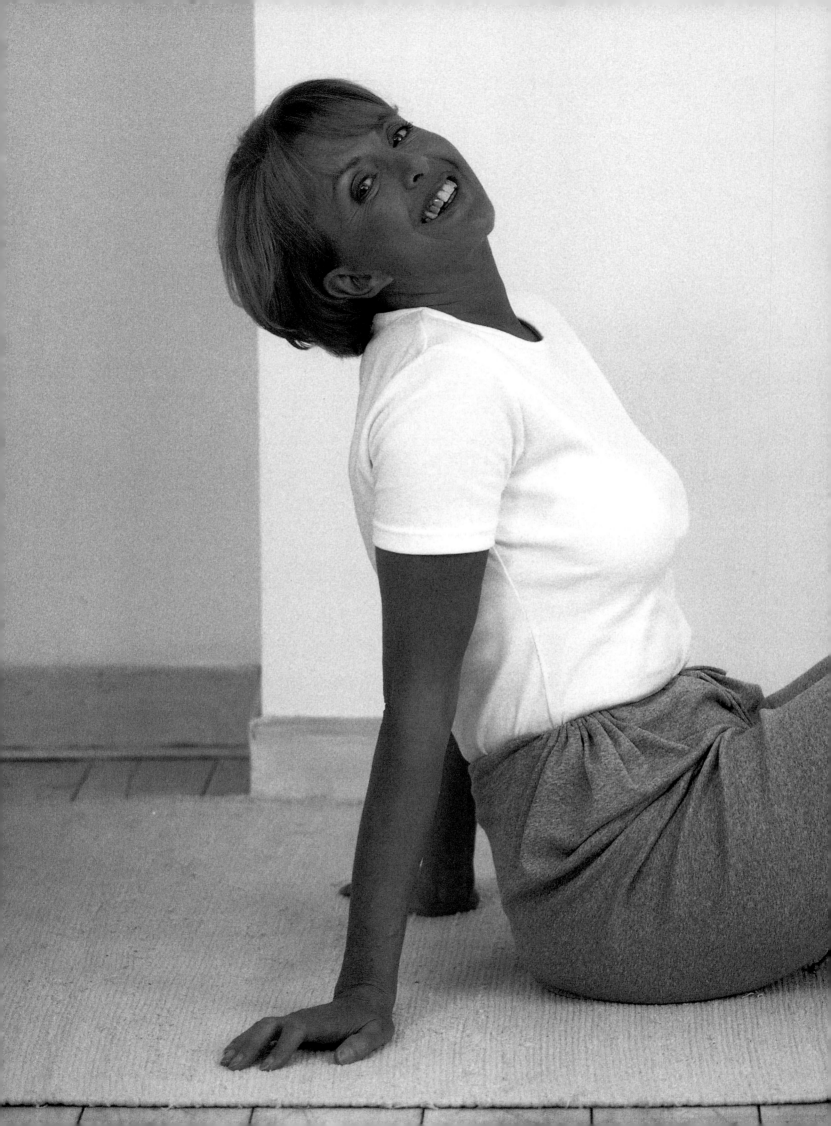

EXERCISE AND HEALTHY EATING

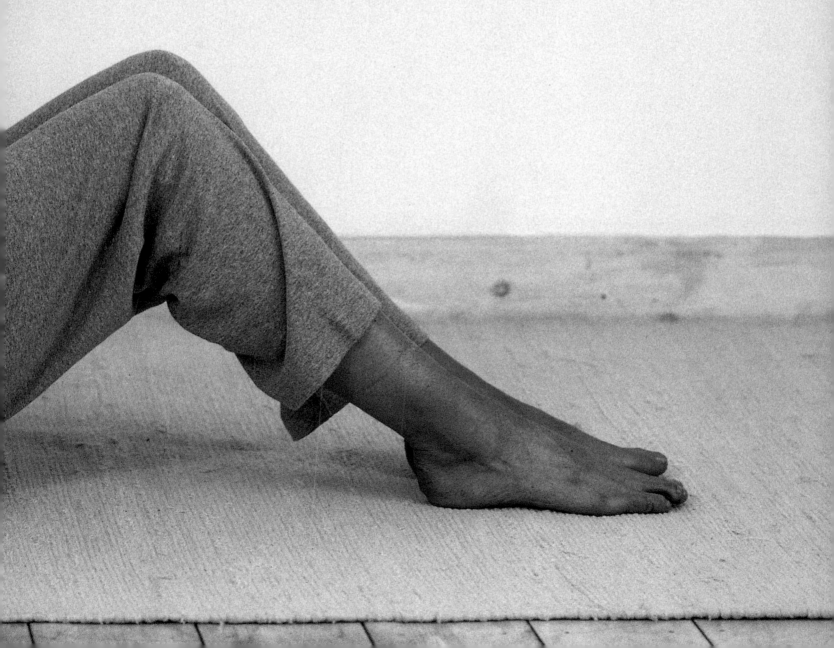

Health and fitness

Fitness is the key to a healthy mind and body. It is based on stamina, strength and suppleness – with better shape and self-esteem as the bonuses. Being fit improves your physical prowess and grace, and also makes you feel better overall. Most of us know that if we were fitter, we would have more confidence and greater zest for life. But although we are more health-conscious about our diet nowadays, regular exercise is still not a part of most people's daily lives. Surveys always draw the same conclusions as to the reasons for this: lack of time, energy, interest and confidence. Becoming fit is neither as difficult nor as time-consuming as it may appear to be: you can get fit – and get a better body into the bargain – more easily and enjoyably than you may think.

how fit do you need to be?

There is no such thing as standard fitness – it depends on your personal make-up and why you want to be fit: being robust enough to run a marathon, for example, is different from honing stamina, strength and suppleness to gain improved physical shape and health. For exercise to be of any help, it should boost your metabolism and improve your cardiovascular (heart and circulation) and respiratory (breathing) systems.

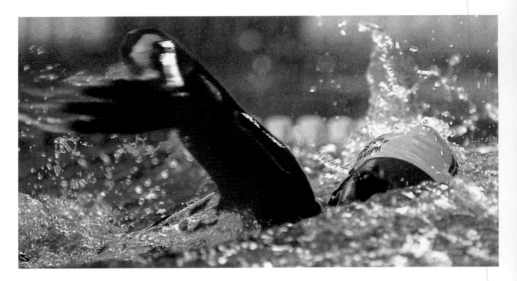

making goals and recording results

Finding a goal that will inspire you is one of the secrets of success. To achieve that goal, you must have a motive that is important enough to give you an iron will, such as improving your figure for a special event (for example, your wedding and honeymoon), buying yourself a longed-for figure-hugging dress, or simply boosting your fitness levels generally. Set the deadline and stick to it. Depending on what you want to achieve, a three-week plan is ideal because it is not too long and if you persevere (take it week by week or day by

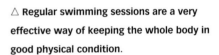

△ **Regular swimming sessions are a very effective way of keeping the whole body in good physical condition.**

day – whichever you find easiest), you will soon see results. However, be realistic: if your goals are too high you are more likely to fail; if they are too low, you will not have enough of a challenge.

Goals will inspire you, but speedy results are the key to keeping up regular exercise – it is perfectly natural that you will want to see rewards for all your hard work – although it is advisable to build up a pattern gradually. The minimum amount of exercise you need to do to improve your personal fitness is 20 minutes three times a week – the "3 x 20" maxim. This means three bouts of exercise vigorous enough to make you fairly breathless (but not gasping for breath). So if you do the general fitness exercises outlined in this book 3 times a week for 20 minutes you will get fitter. If you want to see fast results, though, you need to add extra activities – such as a couple of games of tennis, swimming, or brisk walking – to your exercise quota, so that you are actually exercising six days a week.

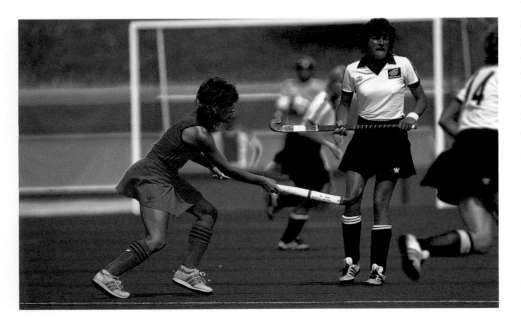

◁ **Hockey is a demanding sport that strengthens the legs, is beneficial to the heart and lungs, and significantly improves co-ordination.**

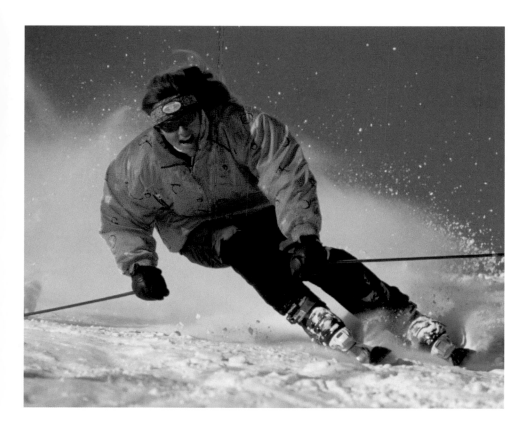

heart rate into a certain range. These are the ideal exercise heart-rate ranges for the different ages:

Age	Pulse Range
20+	130–160
30+	124–152
40+	117–144

To find out your active pulse rate per minute, rest two fingers lightly on your pulse immediately after exercising, count the beats for 10 seconds and multiply by 6.

why bother with keeping fit?

Why are you reading this book? Are you fed up with lacking confidence? Are you tired of running out of puff, being out of shape or always feeling under the weather? Do you regularly suffer from colds, or experience bad pre-menstrual syndrome (PMS), stress or sleepless nights? These are just some of the signs of being unfit. So exercise is worth it, because when you are fitter, recurring problems such as these may ease or even completely disappear.

▽ **A good many water sports demand strength, stamina and a fine sense of balance. Windsurfing is no exception to the rule.**

CAUTIONS

Before taking up any form of rigorous exercise or training, you should consult your doctor – especially if any of the following conditions apply to you:
• diabetes or epilepsy
• over 35 years of age with a long history of inactivity
• cardiovascular or respiratory problems
• chronic joint or back problems.
• obesity
• pregnancy
• heavy drinking or smoking.

amount of exercise gradually. This will avoid any feelings of faintness that may be caused by the pooling of blood below the waist that occurs in the course of vigorous exercise.

monitoring your pulse rate

Checking your pulse rate at regular intervals is crucial because it allows you to monitor whether you are exercising adequately. The maximum heart rate for an adult is approximately 220 beats per minute minus your age in years. The ideal heart rate during exercise is betweem 65 and 80 per cent of this figure. The aim of exercise is to get your

warming up and cooling down

Warm-up activities are important because they ensure that your body is ready for exercise: they ease your muscles into action so that they react more readily to activity, and they also prepare you for a rise in heart rate and body temperature. Warm-ups should be done slowly and rhythmically for 5–10 minutes (depending on age and personal fitness).

In addition, it is very important to set time aside to cool down after exercising: keep walking or moving around slowly for at least 5 minutes. This cool-down period is vital because it allows you to decrease the

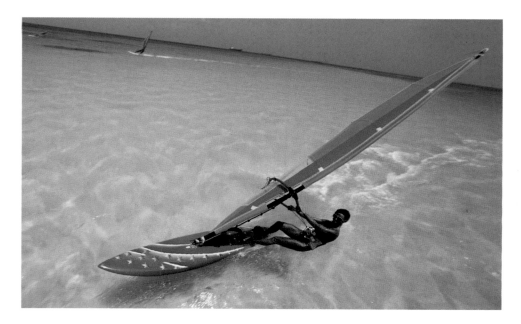

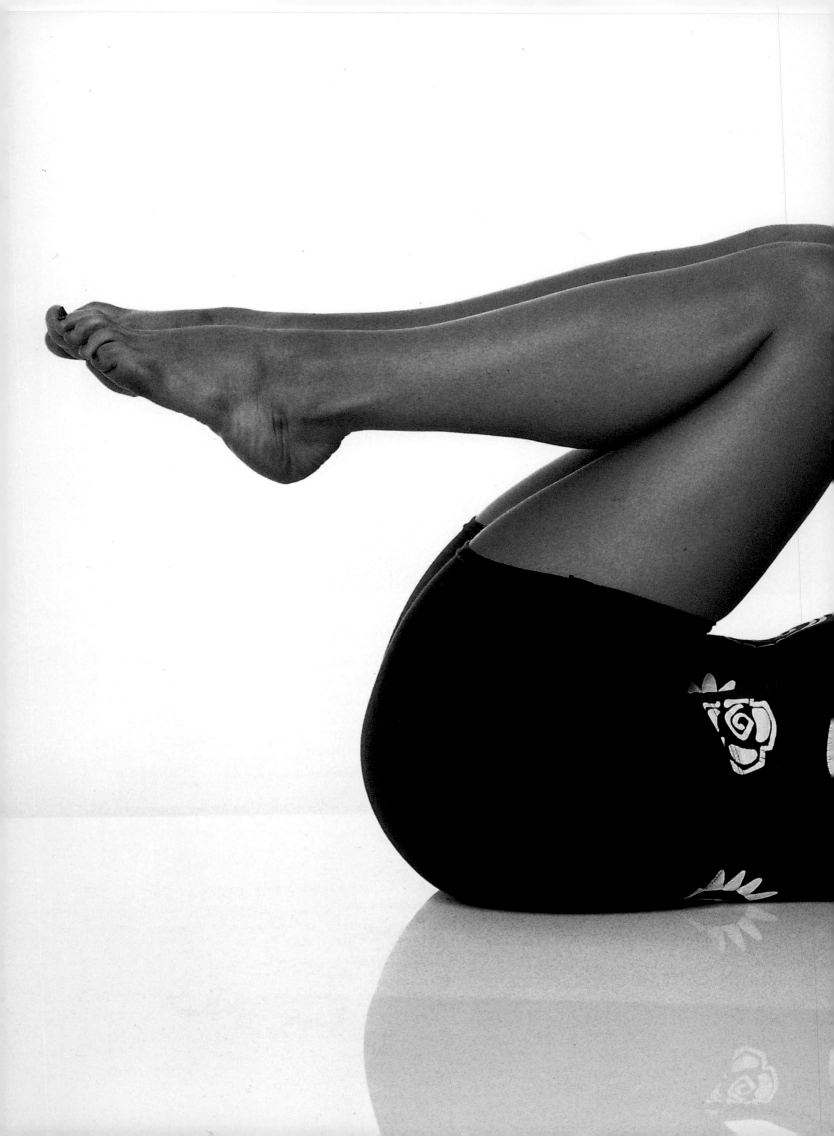

Keeping fit

Are you unfit and out of shape? You might blame your lifestyle because today everything is geared to make life as easy as possible, and you might find it hard to make time to take exercise. However, keeping fit does not need to be hard work and time-consuming. If you want a firmer, healthier body, simply follow the exercise sequences in this chapter.

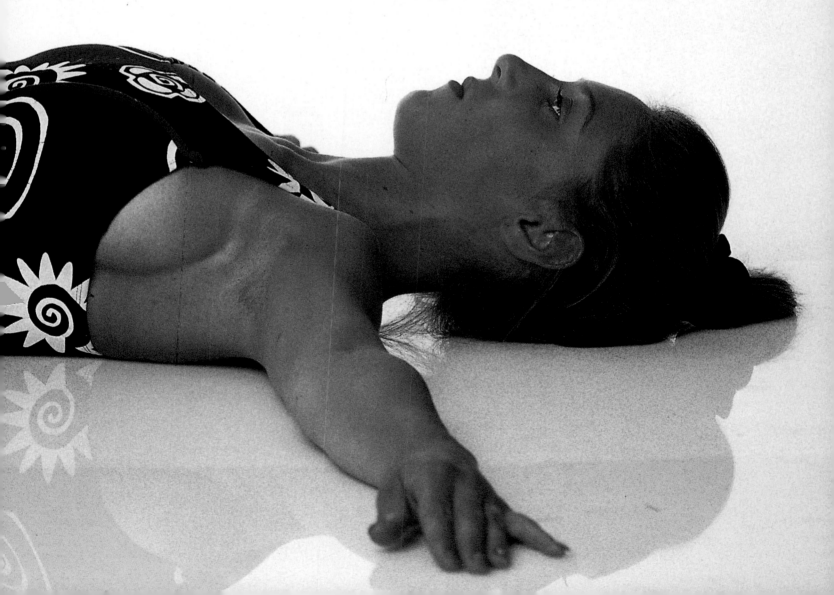

Exercises for general fitness

This exercise routine helps to improve overall fitness and should take you roughly 30 minutes to complete. Aim to do the routine three times a week and try to fit in extra aerobic exercises – such as swimming, walking or cycling – on the other days (aerobic exercises include activities that can be done rhythmically and continuously and that boost the efficient uptake of oxygen).

SOME POINTS TO REMEMBER BEFORE YOU EXERCISE

- If you are not in the habit of exercising regularly, it is advisable to check with your doctor that this exercise routine is suitable for you.
- If you feel any pain or feel dizzy – or experience anything other than the normal sensation of muscle fatigue – stop exercising.
- Always work out at your own pace; don't feel you have to work faster than feels comfortable or do more than you feel capable of.
- It is advisable to avoid exercise if you are ill, or have a virus or a raised temperature.

warm-up exercises

Before you start the general exercises, it is extremely important that you set aside the time to warm up your muscles. A warm-up routine can take as little as 2 or 3 minutes and the aim is to stretch and loosen your muscles. If they are feeling tight or stiff, it can be risky to start exercising vigorously immediately because this can result in strains and even injuries. You can follow the special warm-up exercises outlined on these pages, or carry out your own routine of stretches for a couple of minutes. If you do your own routine, remember to include exercises to warm up your whole body.

Think of warm-up exercises as a way of easing your body slowly and gently into increased activity. Focus on making the movements relaxed, slow and rhythmical, not sharp and jerky. Each of the exercises focuses on warming and stretching a particular area of the body. It is crucial that you take the time to repeat the sequences and make sure that you follow each movement exactly. Concentrate particularly on stretching and extending the neck, spine and legs, which are more susceptible to injury than other parts.

Warm-up exercise A

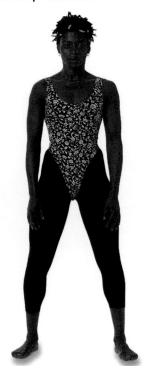 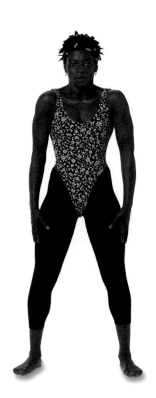 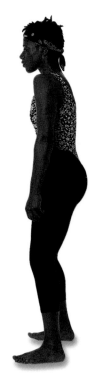 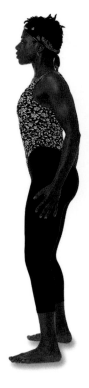

△ **1** Stand upright with your feet apart and in line with your shoulders, with your arms hanging loosely at your sides and your shoulders down.

△ **2** Bring your shoulders forwards.

△ **3** Then raise them as high as you can.

△ **4** Now move your shoulders back as far as possible. Finally, bring them back to the starting position.

Warm-up exercise B

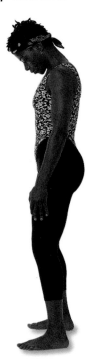

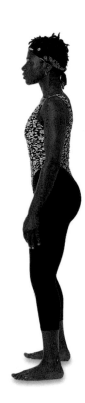

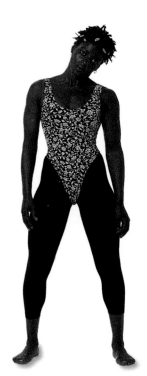

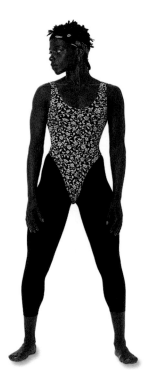

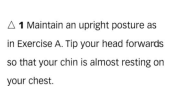

△ **1** Maintain an upright posture as in Exercise A. Tip your head forwards so that your chin is almost resting on your chest.

△ **2** Raise your head, stretching and lengthening your neck as you return to the upright position. Repeat 4 times.

△ **3** Tip your head to the left, keeping the shoulders down, then return to the centre, stretching to lengthen your neck. Repeat with your head to the right. Repeat 4 times on each side.

△ **4** Keep your head up and look over your left shoulder. Then face forwards and stretch to lengthen your neck. Repeat 4 times. Now do 4 times turning to the right. Repeat this sequence twice.

Warm-up exercise C

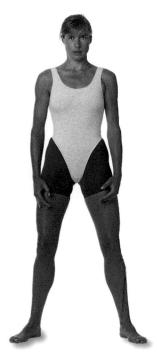

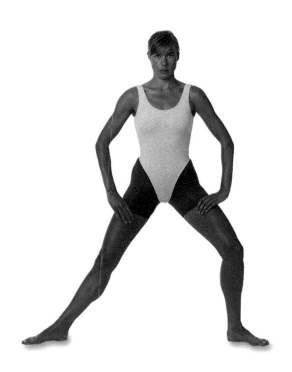

△ **1** Stand with your feet fairly wide apart; lean forwards slightly from your hips keeping your chest lifted and back straight.

△ **2** Rotate and bend your left leg out from the hip so your knee is over your left foot and pointing in the same direction. Keep your right leg straight. You will feel a stretch in the inner thigh; if not, move your feet wider. Repeat 5 times, hold for 5 seconds; swap legs and repeat.

REPETITION GUIDE FOR GENERAL FITNESS EXERCISES

Toning Exercises	Repeats/Time Allowance
Warm-ups	5 minutes
Press-ups	10 repeats
Lying Flies	10 repeats
Squats	10 repeats
Reverse Curls	10 repeats
Sit-ups	10 repeats
Cool-downs	3–5 minutes
Aerobic Exercise	20–30 minutes

The recommended 10 repeats are for beginners – you should aim to repeat each exercise (from Warm-ups to Cool-downs) 15 times, or as often as is comfortable. Start by doing this set of exercises twice a week, then work up to three times a week and combine it with some other form of exercise – ideally aerobic – for the time suggested above.

working on the chest, back and legs

Once you have warmed up properly, you are ready to begin these exercises which focus on your chest, back, legs and abdominal muscles. Read the instructions carefully and make sure you understand how to carry out each movement. If you follow this routine at least twice a week, and combine it with another form of exercise, you will soon have a fitter, firmer and healthier body.

chest muscles: press-ups

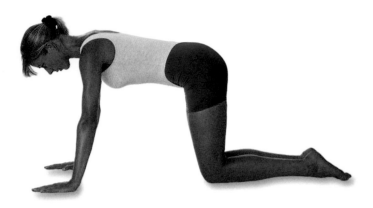

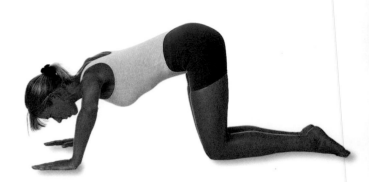

△ **1** Place yourself on all fours with your knees directly under your hips, your hands beneath your shoulders with your fingers pointing forwards, and your palms flat. Make sure your back is straight – that is, parallel with the ceiling – all the time. Achieve this by pulling your stomach in and tucking your pelvis under.

△ **2** Steadily lower yourself – nose first – towards the floor. Then raise yourself back to the starting position, breathing in as you go.

upper back muscles: lying flies

◁ **1** Lie on your front on the floor with your hips down, and keep your body relaxed. Rest your forehead on the floor, your arms out on each side at right angles to your body, elbows bent.

◁ **2** Keeping your elbows bent, steadily lift both arms, making sure they are parallel to the floor. Lower your arms once again. Make sure you don't pull your elbows back; keep them in line with your shoulders and keep your hips and feet in contact with the floor all the time.

leg muscles: squats

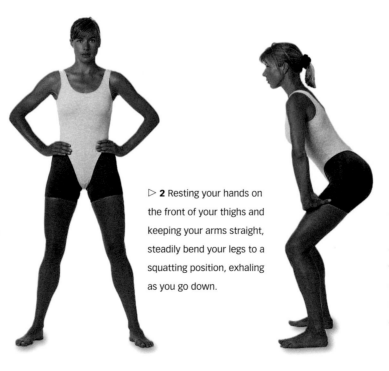

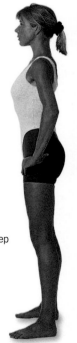

▷ **1** Stand up straight with your feet a little more than shoulder-width apart. If you stand on tiptoe, this exercise tones your calf muscles and your quadriceps, the muscles on the front of your thighs; if you angle your toes slightly outwards while on tiptoe, it benefits your inner thighs.

▷ **2** Resting your hands on the front of your thighs and keeping your arms straight, steadily bend your legs to a squatting position, exhaling as you go down.

▷ **3** Then, inhale as you rise steadily back to the starting position. When you do this exercise, it is important to keep your back straight and your knees flexible. Don't let your knees bend further forward than your toes.

working on the abdominal muscles

When you carry out these exercises, you need to make sure that you keep your lower back pressed into the floor throughout and focus on working slowly, with total control. In the upper abdominals exercise, lift your head and shoulders as one unit, never separately. Roll up from the top of your head; you might find it helpful to imagine you are trying to hold a peach between your chin and your chest, as it is important to try to keep this gap constant throughout. Make sure your face muscles are completely relaxed all the time.

lower abdominals: reverse curls

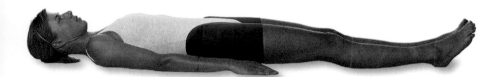

△ **1** Lie flat on your back on the floor, arms by your sides, palms flat on the floor beside you. Keep your shoulder blades down and relax your neck.

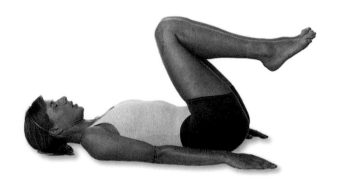

△ **2** While keeping your arms and hands flat on the floor, bring your knees in towards your chest one at a time, and once there, keep both knees together in the bent position.

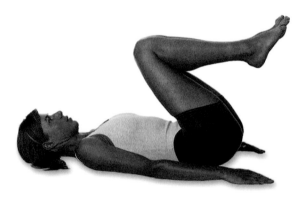

△ **3** Breathe in and, keeping your spine firmly pressed into the floor, pull in your abdominal muscles while at the same time curling up your coccyx (tail-bone) to bring your knees closer to your chest. Keep your feet relaxed throughout. Lower your body to the starting position, exhaling as you go down.

upper abdominals: sit-ups

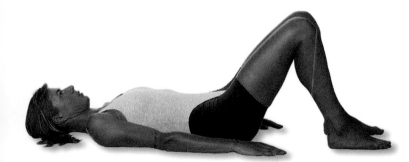

△ **1** Lying flat on the floor with your arms by your side, palms flat on the floor, bend your knees and keep your feet flat on the floor a little distance apart in line with your hips.

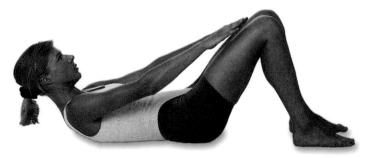

△ **2** Lift your head and shoulders – inhaling as you move up – and push your fingertips towards your knees keeping your arms straight. Lower your body back to the starting position, exhaling as you go down; repeat the movement.

Choosing the right sport

Team sports and work-outs at the gym are fun; they also add to your exercise quota for the week, helping you reach your self-improvement goals that much faster. The benefits of taking part in specific sports and of working out are given here.

make exercise easy to do

Your body cannot "store" fitness, so once you have started, you have to keep exercising regularly. Make your routine flexible: if you think it is going to be hard to maintain, don't choose an activity that requires good weather or a long detour from your office or home.

sports and work-outs

Badminton: Aerobic; improves joint flexibility, stamina, leg and shoulder tone and strength; 30–40 minutes' continuous play burns up around 200–800 calories.
Golf: Anaerobic; improves arm, shoulder and leg tone, and strength (you walk 6.5–8km/4–5 miles when you do a round of golf and burn off around 100–200 calories).
Jogging: Aerobic; improves stamina and leg strength and tone; an hour's jogging burns up 200–350 calories. Before taking up jogging take the usual precautions: check with your doctor and, as with all aerobic exercise, increase the pace gradually.

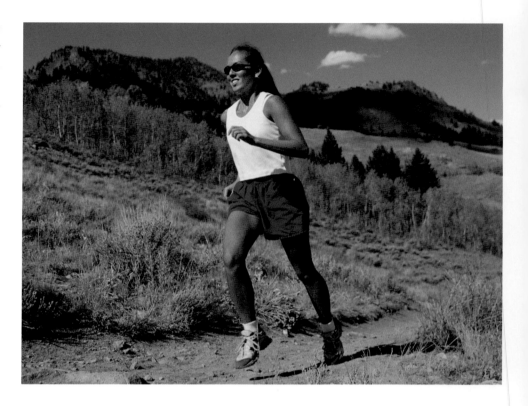

Tennis: Aerobic; boosts stamina and suppleness; strengthens and tones your shoulders, forearms, calves and thighs; if you play very energetically (with plenty of running around the court) at least twice a week for an hour, you will burn up around 300–400 calories per session.

△ When you go jogging always wear a good-quality pair of trainers and support bandages if your joints are weak.

Brisk walking: Aerobic; strengthens and tones your legs. (You should lose up to 100 calories per hour.)
Cycling: Aerobic; builds stamina; tones legs. (An hour's cycling could lose you 250–400 calories, depending on the terrain.)
Skipping: Aerobic; boosts stamina, strength and leg tone. Start with 3 skipping sets of 30 seconds with a 5-minute break after each;

DIETING COMBINED WITH EXERCISE
You will lose weight if you limit your food intake, but not as quickly or as evenly as you would if you combined a balanced weight-loss diet with regular exercise. This is because exercise increases your metabolism, and, if you want to lose weight more quickly, you need to exercise in conjunction with dieting.

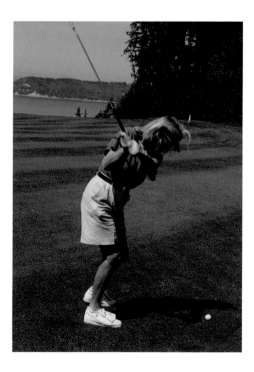

▷ Golf is a sport that particularly benefits shoulders, arms and legs. Playing a round of golf involves a good deal of walking.

THE RIGHT FOOTWEAR
What you wear on your feet is crucial to your performance and to the benefits you will get from exercise. Good sports shops will give advice on the right trainers to wear for different activities, but cross-trainers – designed to be worn for most sports – are probably your best investment because they are good all-rounders.

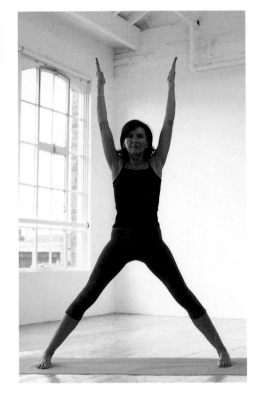

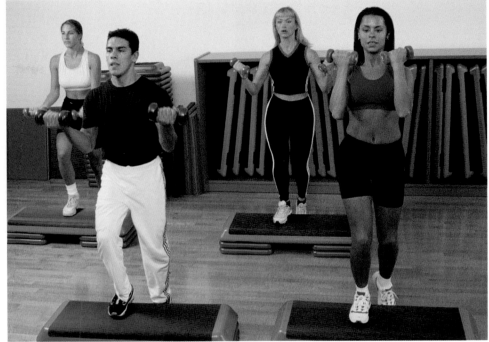

△ **A step class is a fantastic calorie-burning exercise and if you use weights as well it can provide all over body toning.**

◁ **With minimal equipment and easy to fit into a daily routine, yoga is excellent for building up strength and tone thoughout the body.**

then build up to skipping for 2 minutes with a 10-minute break and also increase the repetitions. (Expect to lose up to 500 calories per hour.)

Rebounding: Aerobic; bounding on a mini trampoline is a fun way to get fit at home. (In an hour expect to lose 300 calories.)

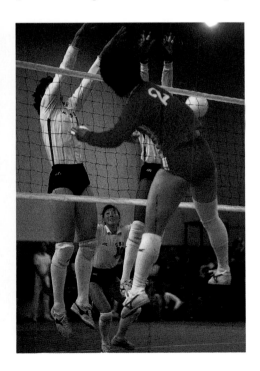

Swimming: Aerobic; swimming is one of the fastest (and best) ways to boost overall fitness, muscle tone, joint flexibility and relaxation. Do 4 lengths of a 25m/25yd pool, rest for a minute and build endurance by reducing rest time and increasing your swim time; within a fortnight you will be noticeably fitter and firmer; an hour's breaststroke burns 500–800 calories.

Football: Aerobic; improves stamina; strengthens and tones your legs; an hour's play burns up around 250–1000 calories.

Boxing: Aerobic; tones and strengthens your chest, shoulders and arms; an hour's boxing burns up around 400–600 calories.

Volleyball: Aerobic; improves stamina; tones and strengthens the whole body, especially your legs and arms; mobilizes joints; an hour's play burns up 200–600 calories.

Squash: As above; an hour's play burns up 400–1000 calories.

◁ **Taking part in a team sport once a week is a good idea: not only will it make you fitter, slimmer and happier, but the competitive spirit will also strengthen your resolve.**

Aerobics: Specific aerobics classes combine exercise with constant movement for up to an hour; fast fat-burners are an ideal activity to do regularly if you are after speedy results. In an hour-long class you would lose 250–500 calories, depending on intensity.

Circuit, cross, resistance or weight training: Aerobic; increase stamina, strength and suppleness; an hour of circuit training burns up 350–550 calories.

Step classes: Aerobic; improves stamina; tones and strengthens your lower torso (bottom, thighs and calves); an hour-long class burns up 500–800 calories.

Yoga: Improves posture; tones; strengthens and relaxes the body; loosens joints; an hour of yoga burns up about 200 calories.

Body shape

The shape of your body is unique, and it is important to remember that this is because the basic skeletal and muscular form that you have inherited is unchangeable. Features such as your height, foot size, shoulder width and the length and shape of your legs, nose, fingers and toes combine to produce a whole. Each person is an individual, with characteristics and features particular to their genetic make-up.

body types

Although we come in a variety of shapes and sizes, the human body is cast from three basic moulds. Often, features from two or three of these body types are jumbled with our individual characteristics, but it is the more dominant features that slot us into one of the following groups: ectomorphs, mesomorphs and endomorphs.

Ectomorphs are usually small- and slender-framed with long limbs and narrow shoulders, hips and joints. They usually have little muscle or body fat. Mesomorphs have medium to large – but compact – frames with broader shoulders and pelvic girdle, and well-developed muscles. Endomorphs are naturally curvaceous, with more body fat than muscle, wider hips, shorter limbs and a lower centre of gravity than the other two body types.

self-image

If you are a little overweight, it can be annoying to hear someone who you think is slim moaning about being overweight. Remember though that this stems from self-image. Very few of us actually see ourselves as we really are. We tend to misjudge our bodies with sweeping claims to fatness, even when we have only a spot of excess flab around our midriff to show for it. And although it sounds amazing, the way we behave in everyday life (and think others see us) often tallies with our self-image. It's a vicious circle: we think we don't measure up to the standard beauty ideal so our self-

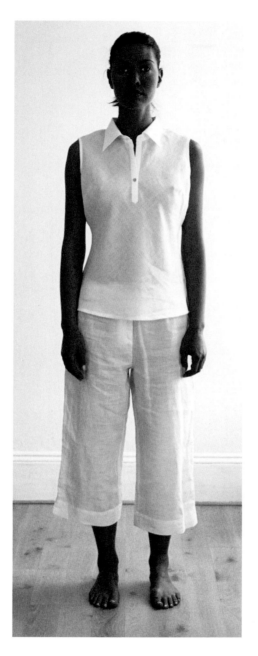

esteem dips again, often so low that we feel we will never have a better body. This in turn causes self-confidence to plummet further, we feel even worse, and so the vicious circle continues.

Taking control of your self-image brings enormous bonuses. And the faster you can do this, the greater the rewards, as speedy results boost your confidence more quickly. But before you undertake a scheme to get into better shape, you must work on your positive thinking: realize your potential by deciding on (and accepting) your body

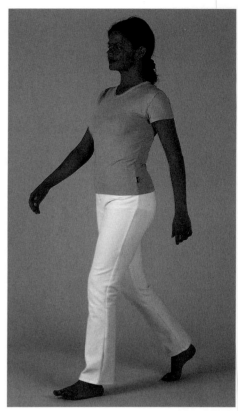

△ Alexander Technique focuses on improving posture and ease of movement during simple activities such as walking, bending and lifting. It explores how the mind and body work together to perform everyday tasks.

◁ We all have things about our bodies we would like to change. Standing up straight and feeling confident about how we look is vital for a positive self-image.

model, then use this as your goal. Forget conventional beauty ideals – you don't have to have mile-long legs to have a good figure, and what you already have – your basic shape – is great. It just needs perfecting, and that is something that everyone can do.

good posture

The difference that good posture makes to the look of our bodies is enormous, mainly because when we are standing properly our abdominal muscles are in their correct supporting role and the whole body is

▷ Improving self-image can be as simple as making positive affirmations while in a calm, meditative state. We all have qualities in which we can take pride and pleasure, and it is important to focus on these positive attributes.

aligned so that it looks leaner and taller. Good posture is also beneficial for our mental and physical health; some alternative therapies (such as the Alexander Technique) are based on the principle of correct posture because it can be very helpful for easing back pain, stress and even headaches.

STRAIGHTENING THE SPINE

This is a very simple exercise to carry out to improve your posture.

Kneel on the floor, take a deep breath in, and then on the out breath drop and relax your shoulders. Imagine your head is attached to a cord tied to the ceiling. Every time you breathe out imagine the cord pulling your head up, and your spine lengthening and straightening.

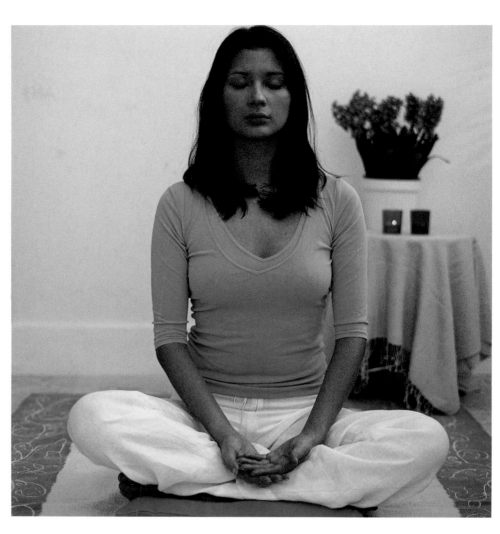

neck care for improving posture

▽ A poor posture profile, such as a curved back, slumped shoulders and a head that juts forward, is commonplace. Stretching exercises can help reverse this trend before the poor posture becomes habitual.

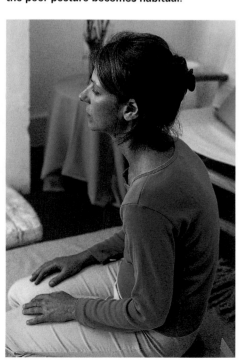

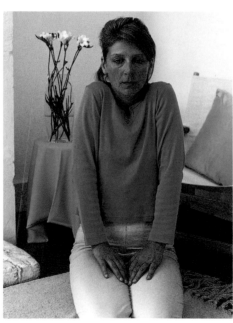

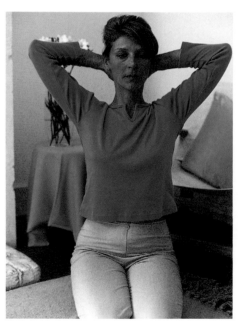

△ **1** Take a deep breath in and slowly begin to lift your shoulders up and back as far as they will comfortably go. On the out breath, slowly release, beginning the upward movement again on the next breath. As your shoulder blades come down, imagine them meeting in the middle of your back. Shoulder shrugs help to release tension in the large muscles of the upper back that pull on the neck.

△ **2** Centre your head and tuck in your chin. Put your hands behind your head, push your head against them and hold for 3–5 seconds. Repeat 10–20 times. Then place one hand on the side of your head. With your chin in, push your head against your hand and hold for 3–5 seconds. Repeat 10–20 times. Swap hands and repeat on the other side. These movements help to strengthen the neck muscles.

Tackling problem areas

Very few people are able to say honestly that they are totally happy with their body. Everyone has at least one gripe – if it is not big feet, it is thin hair or knobbly knees. All these perceived "flaws" can be improved or disguised, but as anyone who has ever tried (and failed) to move the fat that sits on strategic points such as hips, thighs, stomachs and buttocks knows, it is much easier to hide the flaws than to tackle them. Trouble spots such as these are notoriously stubborn to shift, but it is possible to alter your outline with a combination of diet and exercise.

common problems

Any of the following can be discouraging, but remember – each problem has a solution.

Slack stomachs: Our stomachs become flabby when the abdominal muscles slacken; this usually happens through lack of exercise. Your abdomen extends from just under the bustline to the groin, and it is packed with muscles that criss-cross to form a wall to hold the abdominal contents in place – a bit like a corset. Exercise is not the only way to keep your stomach flat though: weight is also an important factor and the long-term answer is both diet and exercise.

Thunder thighs: Like bottoms and busts, thighs are a great source of discontent, whether it is because they are too flabby, muscular or skinny. You inherit the basic shape of your thighs, but that does not necessarily mean that you were born with the excess fat that may be covering them. Thigh size and tone can certainly be altered with the right diet, correct body care and regular exercise. Sports such as cycling, skiing, tennis, squash and riding (a great inner-muscle firmer) will tone your thighs, as will weight-training for specific areas of the body.

Large bottoms: There are three large muscles in our buttocks: gluteus maximus, medius and minimus. These create the shape, but not the size, of our rear ends. It is the tone of these muscles and the fatty tissue around them that gives us the bottoms we have. The good news is that buttock muscles respond well to exercise, which means that any effort you put into bottom-toning exercises will be rewarded quite quickly. Locomotive exercises – such as fast walking, running upstairs and jogging – are especially good bottom trimmers. Other exercises are given in the Exercises for Specific Problems.

Slack upper arms: Arms do not really change shape a great deal during our lives, unless we lose or gain a lot of weight. Muscle tone is the main problem, but, as in the case of thighs, exercise and specific weight-training will tone up and reshape flabby arms. It is very often the case that any changes in body shape that happen through exercise and diet are noticeable most quickly on your upper arms.

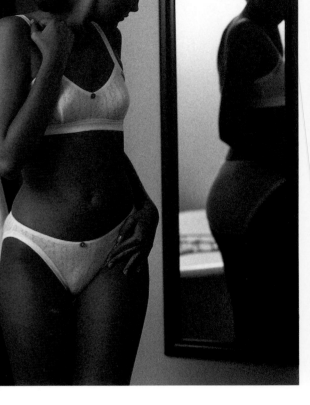

△ The best way to assess your figure is to stand in front of a full-length mirror. Be honest with yourself, and look for areas that need improving.

Droopy breasts: Breast shape and size only really change when our weight swings dramatically, during pregnancy, breast-feeding, menstruation, or if taking oral contraceptives. Gravity is the bust's worst enemy, especially if the breasts are not given proper support, because it literally drags the breasts down and slackens their tone. Although the breasts are supported by suspensory ligaments, they do not contain any muscle (the milk glands are buffered by protective fatty tissue) so you cannot noticeably reverse lost tone. However, if you exercise the pectoral muscles beneath your armpits you will give your breasts a firmer base and more uplift.

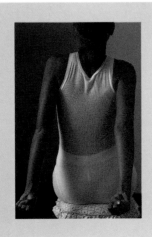

FLABBY ARM FIXER

To firm up flabby arms, add this exercise to your daily exercise routine, or spend five minutes doing it twice a day. Sit on a chair holding your hands in loose fists and, with your arms extended behind, make downwards punching movements backwards and forwards.

TWO QUICK THIGH-TONERS

If you do not have time to do a full exercise routine, grab 10 minutes in the morning and evening to warm up and do these two exercises.

outer thighs

Sit on the floor with your legs straight out in front and hold your arms out to the sides as shown. Roll sideways on to your bottom – go right over on to your outer thigh and then roll right over on to the other thigh. Do this 20 times.

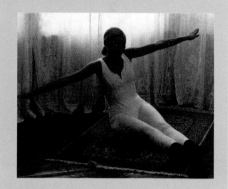

inner thighs

Stand upright and consciously tighten – and hold – your buttock muscles for a slow count of five. Repeat with your thigh muscles and then your calf muscles. You can do this while you are waiting for your bath to run, standing at the bus stop, and so on.

Thick ankles: Trim and slender ankles are seen to be a great asset. But if you are not blessed with these, or if your ankles tend to become stiff and puffy from fluid retention, you need to brush up on some ankle-improving exercises.

Assess the flexibility of your ankles by sitting on a chair or stool with your feet on the floor and, while keeping your heel down pull the rest of your foot up as far as it will go: if the distance between your foot and the floor measures 12–15cm/5–6in your joint flexibility is good; if it is between 10–12cm/4–5in it is fair; and if it is less than that, your joint flexibility is poor.

improving your true form

Obviously there are certain things about your body shape that you will never be able to change. However, it is important to focus on your good points and remember that there is a great deal you can do to improve on your natural shape and form.

Confront your body: Go on, be brave. Strip to your underwear, stand in front of a mirror and have a good look at your body. Take your time and be tough but realistic. You may have disliked your thighs since you were 16 – and they will probably never be those of a supermodel – but if you look hard enough you might just find that they are not as bad as you have always thought, and that improving them is not going to be that hard after all.

Write it all down: Note down all the things that annoy you (and that you can do something about) as well as those that you like or do not mind. Then go through your list of dislikes, ticking the things that you really want to do something about. Also,

make a mental note to start appreciating your good points: the more you focus on them the less you will notice the not-so-good zones.

Make an action checklist: Add a set of action points under the problem zones you have listed. If you want to firm up your arms for that sleeveless sundress you have been unable to wear for a decade of summers, make notes like this:

Flabby Upper Arms

Do Basic Exercises

Check diet

Exfoliate/moisturize.

Finally, add your goal(s) and your deadline to the top of the list and put it somewhere where you are going to see it frequently.

▽ **Making an action checklist will help you focus on your goals.**

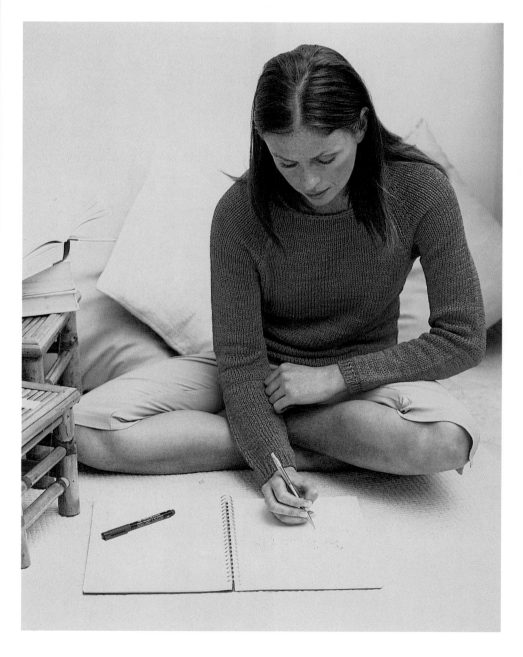

Exercises for specific problem areas

Add these basic exercises to your general fitness routine to give special problem areas extra work, or do them on their own as an isolated routine. If you do them on their own, use the abdominal muscle exercises from the general fitness plan for your stomach – and remember to warm up first and cool down afterwards.

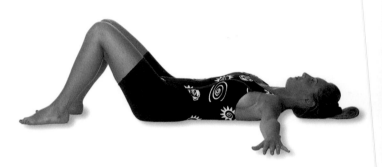

thigh muscles

exercise A

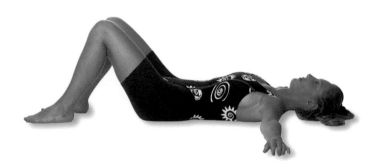

△ **1** Lie on your back on the floor with your arms resting straight out at right angles to your body and your feet apart in line with your hips.

△ **2** Hold a cushion between your knees and, keeping your back pressed into the floor, press your knees together 10 times quickly and 10 times slowly, keeping the cushion in place throughout.

△ **3** Now repeat the sequence from step 2 again, but this time holding a tennis or golf ball between your knees.

exercise B

▽ **1** Lie on your back on the floor with your legs straight and your lower back pressed to the floor. Put your arms along your sides, palms to the floor.

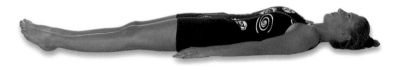

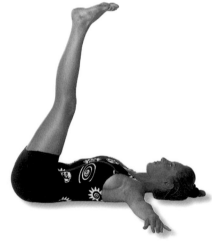

◁ **3** Keeping your legs together, steadily straighten them so that they are pointing up towards the ceiling. Keep your feet relaxed, do not point them.

▷ **2** Stretch your arms out to the side at right angles to your body. Bend your legs and bring your knees in towards your chest.

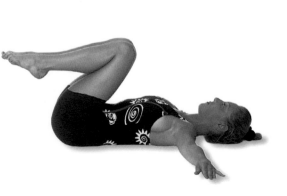

◁ **4** Slowly open your legs out sideways – as wide as you can – then close them again. Repeat the exercise 4 times. When you feel completely comfortable with this exercise, you can try doing it with small weights tied to your ankles.

exercise C

▷ **1** Stand alongside a chair or table (lightly holding the edge to maintain your balance), with your shoulders down and relaxed. Have your knees slightly bent and your feet facing forwards.

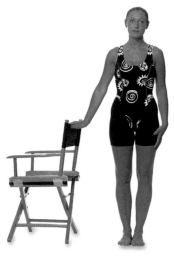

▷ **2** Lift your left hip slightly and slowly move your leg out and up (no higher than 45 degrees), keeping your foot and knee facing forwards. Make sure you do not let your body tilt – keep it as straight as possible. Carefully lower your leg. Repeat the whole exercise 10 times, then turn and repeat with the other leg.

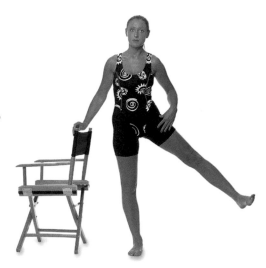

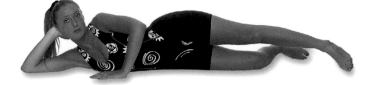

exercise D

△ **1** Lie on your right side on the floor with your legs out straight. Support your head with your right hand.

△ **2** Bend your lower leg behind you to maintain balance and tilt your hips slightly towards the floor; your head, hips, knees and feet should all be facing forwards. Balance yourself with your left hand on the floor in front of you.

◁ **3** Slowly lift your upper leg, then bring it down until it touches the lower one; raise it again and repeat this movement 6 times. Turn over and repeat steps 1–3 on the other side.

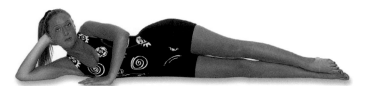

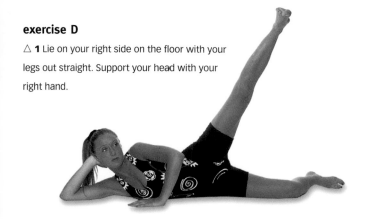

ankles and calf muscles

exercise A

▽ **1** Sit up straight on a chair, with your knees together and heels on the floor and slightly apart, in line with your hips. Bring your big toes up (as high off the floor as possible) and roll your feet in towards each other.

exercise B

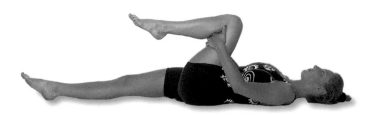

△ **1** Lie flat on your back on the floor with your legs straight.

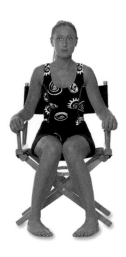

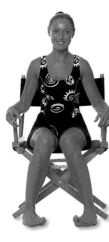

▷ **2** Now tilt and move both feet down and outwards from the ankle, keeping your big toes raised as much as possible as you roll your feet on to their outer edges. Repeat this 10 times.

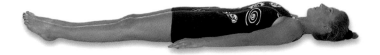

△ **2** Bring one leg up and hold it beneath the back of your thigh so that it is pulled towards your chest. Rotate your foot 10 times clockwise and 10 times anti-clockwise. Repeat with the other leg. Increase the number of repeats to 20 for each foot, working alternately in groups of 7.

buttock muscles

exercise A

▷ **1** Stand upright and lightly hold the back of a chair or the edge of a table with both hands to maintain your balance. Put your weight on your right leg and turn your left leg out from the hip.

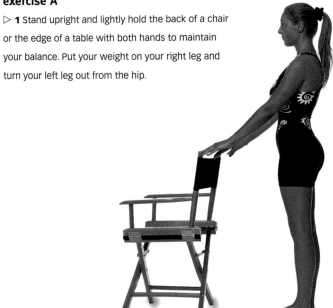

▷ **2** Keeping your foot flexed, take your left leg back as far as you can without bending it at the knee, forcing the movement or over-arching your back. Repeat with the other leg. Repeat 5 times for each leg and gradually build up to 20 repetitions.

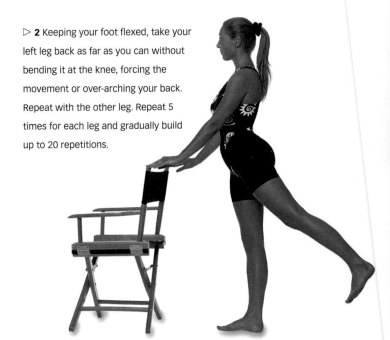

exercise B

▽ **1** Lie on your back with your knees bent and your feet slightly apart, in line with your hips. Place your arms by your sides, palms flat on the floor.

▽ **2** Place your weight on your shoulders and upper back (not your neck), raise your bottom to a comfortable height and tighten your buttock muscles, keeping your feet flat on the floor and your arms by your sides. Hold for several seconds. Lower your bottom to the floor. Repeat 5 times, building up to 20 repetitions.

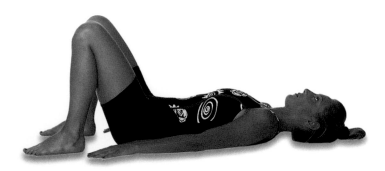

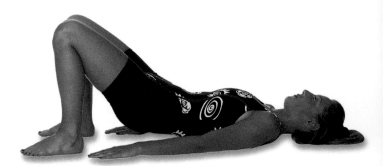

exercise C

▽ **1** Kneel on all fours with your knees slightly apart, in line with your hips, but keeping them tucked right under your hips. Place your hands in front of you, shoulder-width apart and facing forwards. Bend your elbows so that you are leaning on your forearms.

▽ **2** Keeping your foot flexed, push your left leg out straight behind you, keeping your back and hips parallel. Bring your leg and foot down to the floor, keeping your foot flexed and your leg straight. Repeat 12 times. Return to the original position, then repeat the exercise with your other leg. Build up to 20 repetitions.

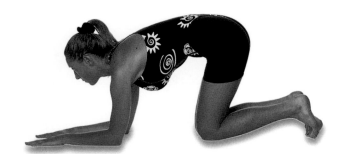

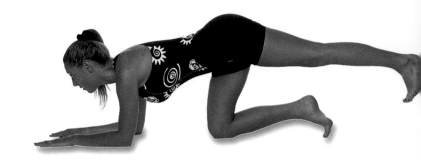

upper arm muscles

▷ **1** Stand upright with your feet shoulder-width apart and your arms hanging loosely by your sides.

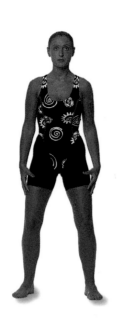

▷ **2** Lift your arms, flex your hands and make 5 small circles forwards and then backwards with both arms moving simultaneously. Aim to build up to 20 circles, and when you are used to the exercise, hold a can of beans in each hand and repeat. You can vary the exercise by bringing your arms around to the front and tracing the circles there as well. As you improve with practice, move your feet closer together.

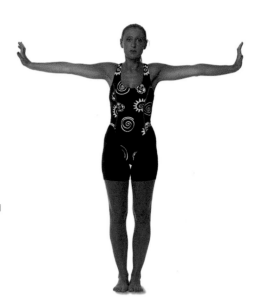

bust (pectoral) muscles

exercise A

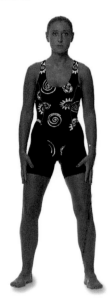

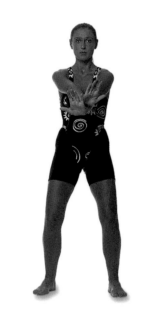

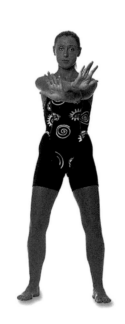

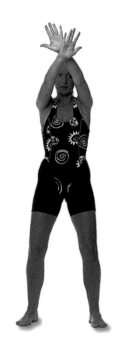

△ **1** Stand upright with your feet apart in line with your shoulders. Keep your shoulders up, back straight, bottom and stomach tucked in, legs slightly bent and arms loosely by your sides.

△ **2** Make a scissor movement across the front of your body (at waist-level) by crossing one hand over the other while holding your arms straight out in front.

△ **3** Raise your arms to chest level and repeat the action.

△ **4** Then repeat the action holding your arms at head level. Keep the scissor movements controlled as you swing; do 20 repetitions at each level.

exercise B

▽ **1** Kneel on all fours as if you were about to do press-ups, with your legs raised at the back and your feet crossed. Your arms should be straight.

▽ **2** Bend your arms as you lower your body to the floor. Do this 10 times to begin with, and build up to 30 repetitions. Remember to keep your back straight.

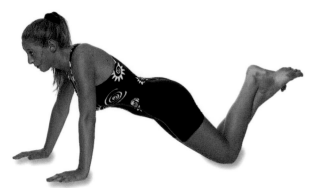

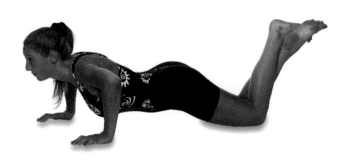

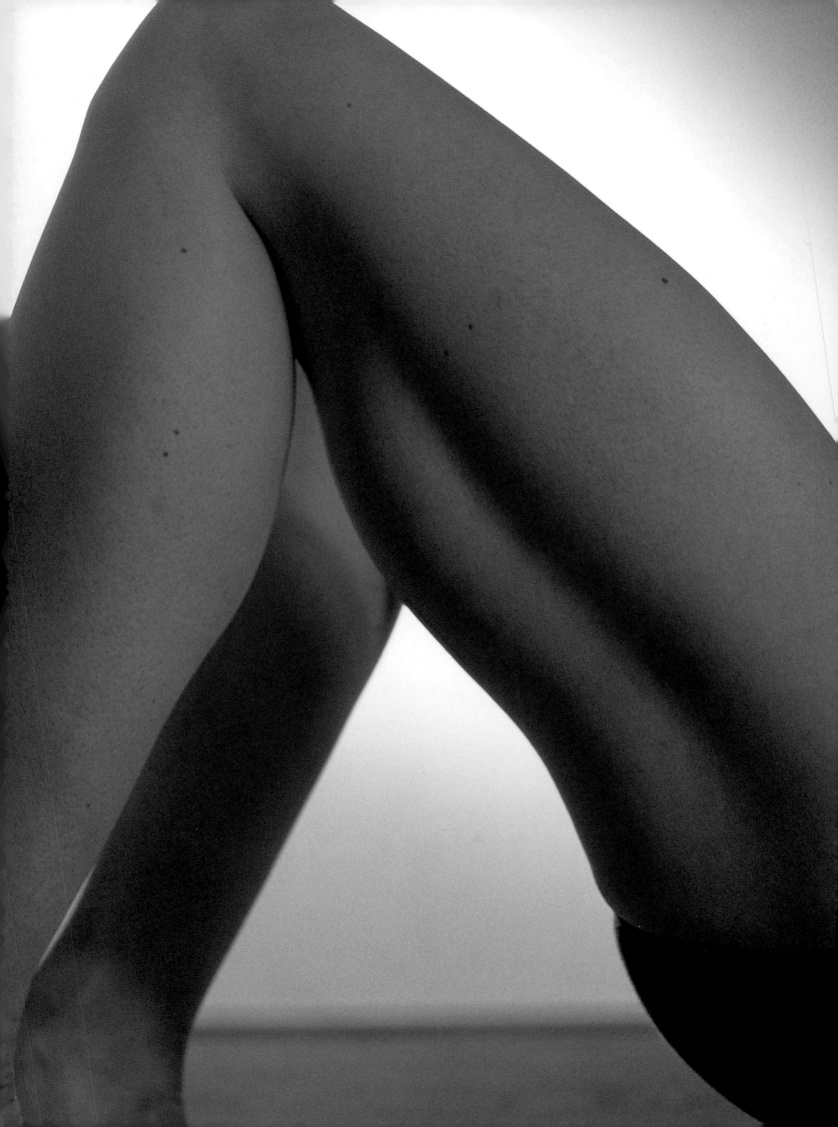

Introducing Pilates

This section explores the benefits of Pilates and what you can expect to achieve. If you have tried other exercise programmes and wondered why your success was limited, find out why Pilates is different and why its practice will become an essential and enjoyable part of your life.

The benefits of Pilates

This chapter explains the key elements of Pilates and takes you through a range of exercises. The programme aims to be user-friendly: it is designed for beginners but advanced variations of many exercises are included so that you can progress.

The "first position" in each exercise is the most basic. If you are new to Pilates, start with this one, or you will not master the control and focus needed to perform the exercise correctly. Your main concern is doing the movement correctly, not how many repetitions you can do. The "second position" should be attempted only when you understand the first position. For some people this may take two or more months. Others may take as little as three weeks. Just progress at your own rate. The "third position" is a more intense variation still.

a holistic approach

It is important to look at exercise in a holistic way and to integrate it into your daily life with minimal disturbance. The programme does not set out to turn you into an Olympic athlete. It might, however,

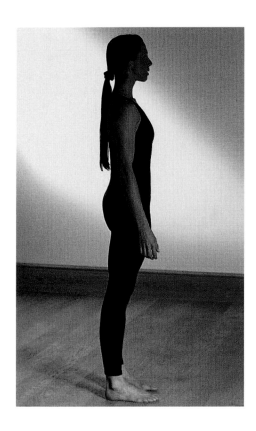

△ Pilates helps to re-define posture, creating a relaxed, confident stance. It is worth remembering that the correct posture can give an illusion of a 2kg/6lb weight loss.

give you that push you need to start exercising by explaining just why it is important, not just for aesthetic purposes but to help you avoid pain and injury, to make you feel good about your body and to increase your self-esteem.

We hope that the programme is clear, logical and simple to remember, so that it will be easy to make it a regular part of your daily routine – just like brushing your teeth – because exercise really should be a matter of course. It's just common sense.

everyone can benefit

Pilates can benefit everyone, whatever your age or fitness level. Although you will get stronger all over, one of the main benefits of Pilates is to increase core strength. This is a phrase that is used a great deal in Pilates, and it refers to the important abdominal and

back muscles at your centre that support your whole body whether moving or at rest. As these muscles are strengthened, your posture will improve.

If you are new to Pilates, you will find these exercises different from others you may have tried. Pilates involves a series of movements that flow into one another without pauses, and concentrates on the body as a whole, stretching some muscles, strengthening others and, by helping you to function more effectively, reducing the risk of injury in everything you do.

In Pilates only a few repetitions are needed per exercise in comparison with other methods. If you are performing the movements correctly, up to 10 repetitions will be more than adequate. This means that you can give each repetition your full effort and concentration: you will maximize the potential of the exercise without growing tired or bored with continual repetitions.

the importance of focus

Another distinguishing feature of Pilates is that to practise it you must be totally focused and concentrated. This concentration creates a mind–body connection. A Pilates sequence can help to still the insistent clamour of your daily life, acting like meditation to calm your mind and help you see things more clearly. This focus and attention to alignment and detail makes Pilates unique and very satisfying.

correct, controlled movements

You should check throughout the exercises that your spine is in neutral (unless otherwise stated), that the abdominals are contracted, that you are not holding your breath at any time, that the muscles not involved in the movement are relaxed (it is common to hold tension in the jaw and shoulders) and that the movements are controlled. All these factors are the key elements that make Pilates so effective, and they are fully explained on the following pages.

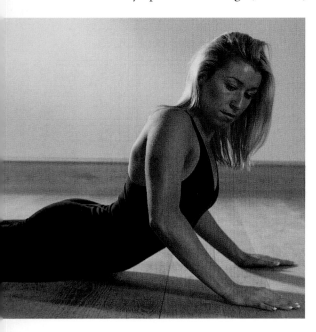

△ Pilates combines stretches and strengthening exercises, making it one of the safest and most effective forms of exercise.

▷ Pilates creates a strong, lean, balanced body. This reduces the risk of injury and helps to eliminate nagging aches and pains.

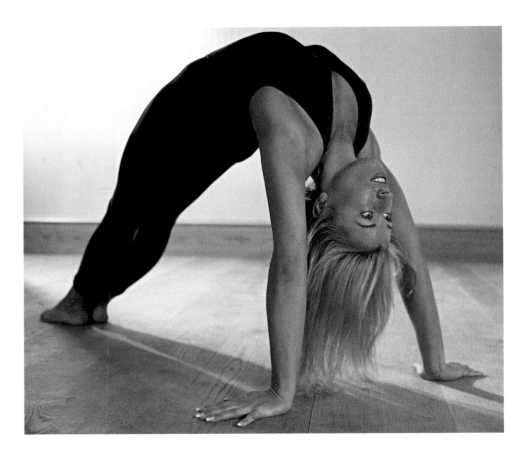

stabilizing muscles

Muscle imbalances occur through repetitive strain or faulty mechanics, and result in an uneven pull of the muscles around a joint. This imbalance may cause injury to that joint. The pain that results inhibits the postural or stabilizing muscles around the joint and, as a result, these muscles weaken, making the injured joint more unstable and more susceptible to further injury and pain. And so the cycle repeats itself. Even when the area is no longer painful, these muscles do not automatically strengthen again. This is why injuries tend to recur. To recover fully, the muscles in that area need to be specifically strengthened and their co-ordination retrained.

Trunk or core stability requires strength, endurance and co-ordination of the stabilizing abdominal, pelvic floor and lower back muscles. Stability is vital to support and protect the lower back from injury, to help with general postural alignment and to allow the release of the hips for greater freedom of movement. So, better core stability can reduce the chance of injury. Improving it is often the way to get rid of back problems that you may have suffered from for years. Core stability exercises are a crucial part of Pilates, which focuses on improving the strength and control of stabilizing muscles.

the endorphin effect

You may hear regular exercisers talking about the high they get from activity: this is the production of endorphins, chemicals in the brain that are stimulated by exercise and have similar effects to opiates. Tests have shown that people who suffer from illness and depression are significantly helped by taking exercise.

As well as describing each exercise in detail, this chapter gives advice on putting together a sequence to help you achieve the benefits you are seeking, and on incorporating Pilates into a fitness regime of exercise and healthy eating. Start investing in the present and future health of your body.

▽ Within weeks of beginning regular Pilates practice, you will see a clear improvement. Pilates creates long, lean muscles with no risk of developing a bulky, overdeveloped physique.

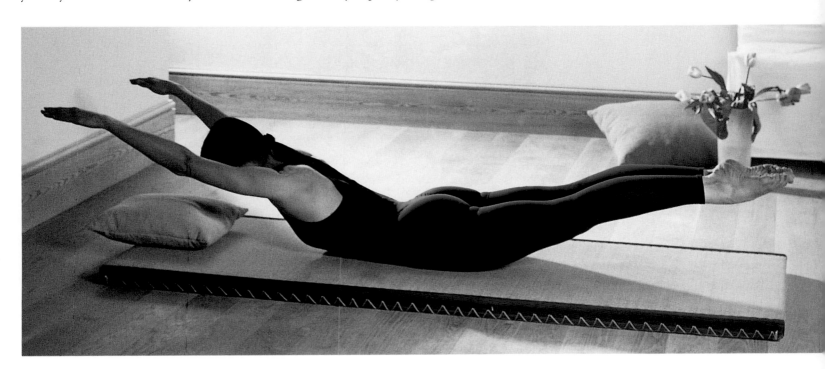

The key elements of Pilates

Some concepts are referred to repeatedly in Pilates: these are the "key elements" that make it more than just a sequence of movements. Keep them in mind throughout your sessions, relating them to each exercise, and as you become more familiar with the technique they will start to make more sense to you. They will help you to get the most benefit from each movement, and also keep the exercises safe and comfortable. Some of these key elements will come more naturally to you than others, but do not feel discouraged. They will eventually become automatic and you will find yourself applying the same principles to other forms of activity, because they are based on attention to detail and alignment, safety and common sense.

breathing

You breathe unconsciously, however, when you are completely relaxed and calm your breathing pattern is very different from when you are tense, anxious or negative.

At times of tension and stress, breathing is usually irregular and shallow, and does not completely meet your need for oxygen. If you learn to control your breathing while practising Pilates as well as during daily activity, it will help you to maintain your energy and stay relaxed.

Holding your breath causes tension in your muscles, which decreases when you exhale. For this reason, athletes learn to exhale when executing certain movements such as a tennis serve, a basketball dunk or a golf swing: they are programmed to exhale on the maximum effort. In sports that require a maximum effort during a longer period of time, such as power-lifting, elite athletes will hold their breath. This gives their muscles added stability but has several potentially negative effects on their blood pressure. Remember that these athletes are aiming at a particular goal: they want to win medals at all costs, sometimes even by endangering their health. You should never

hold your breath when exercising. In Pilates, it is sometimes difficult to gauge which of the movements is the one that takes maximum effort. Most of the movements maintain tension in the torso at all times, but your breathing should always be regular and relaxed.

When starting out on this or any other exercise programme, strive to master the general movement first, then focus on the breathing patterns. It is often the case that correct breathing patterns start to come naturally as the body tries to help itself, but you can practise breathing control exercises when you are not moving to help you learn the correct technique. During the exercises try not to let the ribs flare up (push upwards and outwards away from your spine), which sometimes goes hand in hand with arching the spine. Aim to keep the ribs the same distance from your hips, just sliding them out to the sides and then back again as you breathe. This is described as breathing laterally.

breathing exercise

Here is a simple breath-control strategy that you can practise at any time. Regulating your breathing will enhance your body awareness and control and make you feel calm and centred.

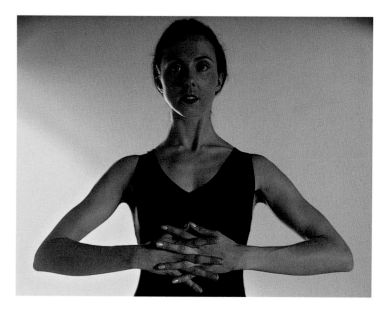

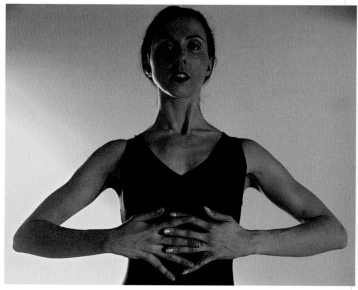

△ **1** Place your hands with your palms under your chest, on your ribs, and your fingers loosely interlocked. Inhale slowly and continuously through your nose, to a count of four. Do not strain, keep yourself relaxed.

△ **2** As you inhale concentrate on allowing your ribs to expand laterally: your fingers should gently part. Don't let your ribs jut forward. Exhale slowly, expelling all the breath from your lungs, then repeat.

concentration

Your muscles respond better to a training stimulus if the brain is concentrated on the effort. Remember that it is the brain that sends out the signal to the muscle to contract. So, it is imperative that you concentrate on the work you expect the muscle to perform.

It is very easy to get distracted while exercising if you do not set the right mood, avoiding intrusive sounds or disturbances that will take your mind off what you are doing. It is also necessary to prepare yourself mentally to focus on your body and the work that it will be doing.

control

All movements should be performed slowly and with absolute control. The faster you do anything, the less actual muscle mass you will use to do the exercise; instead, you will be using momentum. Most Pilates movements are not static; they should be continuous but at the same time controlled and precise.

flow

Pilates movements cannot be likened to repetitions of a conventional exercise. They are continuous. Try to "link" one movement with the next, maintaining a steady flow of energy throughout the session. You will not be stopping and starting as in conventional exercise, but flowing like a steadily turning wheel.

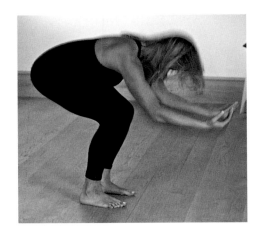

△ **Maintain a steady flow of energy, keeping movements graceful and fluid.**

relaxation

Pilates is a gradual re-education of the body, and in order to benefit from it you must try not to create unnecessary tension. This would eventually create an imbalance in the body, which is the very thing you are trying to remedy. Watch especially for tension in the neck and jaw, but you may hold it anywhere – even in the feet. During a session, give yourself little mental checks from head to toe and you will start to see where you tend to hold tension. Awareness is half the battle.

adherence

No exercise programme works unless you do it! Adopt this programme as part of your life and make it as much a part of your daily routine as brushing your teeth. Physical activity is as much a way of taking care of your body as personal hygiene.

▽ **The anterior and posterior views of the human muscular system show the main muscles of the front and back of the body. Although this is a simple diagram only, it will help you to gain a clear understanding of the location of the muscles used throughout your Pilates practice. Be aware, though, that Pilates uses many other supporting muscle groups during different phases of a movement.**

THE MUSCULAR SYSTEM

deltoid

pectorals

biceps

abdominals

hip flexors

adductors

quadriceps

triceps

lower trapezius

latissimus dorsi

erector spinae

gluteals

abductors

hamstrings

gastrocnemius

ANTERIOR VIEW   POSTERIOR VIEW

Core strength

The principal aim of the exercises is to create core strength, which will be the powerhouse for the rest of your body. When you reach a level of understanding of core strength Pilates starts to feel like an altogether different form of exercise: you begin to get a feel for your body working as a whole in a very focused, concentrated way.

The abdominals and back form the centre of the body, from which all movements in Pilates are initiated. If you look at a ferris wheel in a funfair, there is movement around the wheel but the powerhouse is the centre because everything is controlled from there. This is how you should view your body. Your centre should be your first priority, because without sufficient strength in this area you are vulnerable to injury. So, what are these muscles and how do you locate them?

THE KEY ABDOMINAL MUSCLES

▷ **The illustration displays the key abdominal muscles used in Pilates. These are the muscles used when we refer to "working from a strong centre" or developing "core strength".**

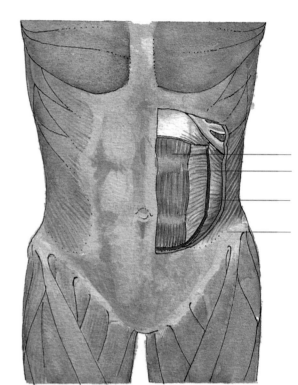

rectus abdominis

transverse abdominis

internal abdominal obliques

external abdominal obliques

muscles that stabilize the torso

Rectus abdominis: This is a wide and long muscle that runs all the way down from the sternum (breast bone) to the pubic bone. The rectus abdominis helps to maintain correct posture and allows forward flexion.

Obliques: These are located at the waist, and there are actually two sets: the internal and external obliques. They allow you to rotate at the waist as well as flexing laterally (to illustrate this, imagine that you are picking up a suitcase by your side).

Transverse abdominis: This muscle is located behind the rectus abdominis, like a "girdle" wrapped around your stomach. It is used when you draw your navel towards your spine, and is the muscle that contracts when you cough.

building core strength

By stabilizing the torso you are creating a "co-contraction" between the abdominal muscles and the back muscles. This means that all these muscles are working together to create a stable entity. In most people they are weak, and in the back they can be tense and tight. In this situation the spine may be pulled out of alignment, causing improper posture and risk of injury. When the back muscles and the abdominals are strong and flexible it becomes easier to maintain correct posture. Pilates strengthens and stretches these core muscles, helping to correct imbalances and reducing the chances of suffering back pain.

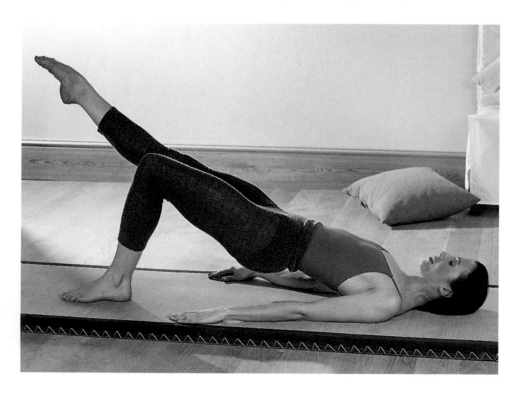

◁ **Pilates exercises are designed to build up your core strength.**

locating the transverse abdominis

Sit or stand upright, inhale and pull your stomach towards your back, imagining that you are wearing very tight jeans and trying to pull your tummy away from the waistband. This is what you will be doing during all the Pilates exercises.

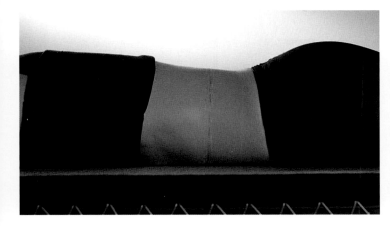

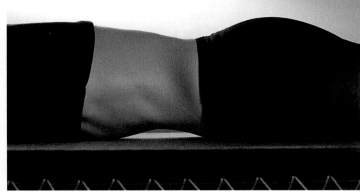

△**1** Lie on your tummy with your head relaxed and supported on your folded hands or on a small cushion under your forehead. Keep your head in alignment with your back and the back of your neck long, without shortening the front. Try to keep your hip bones on the floor and relax your shoulders.

△ **2** Inhale, then as you exhale pull your navel towards your spine, trying to create an arch under your abdominals. You may not be able to lift very far up at first: this is not important as long as you understand the concept. Gently lift your shoulders back and draw your shoulder blades down your spine.

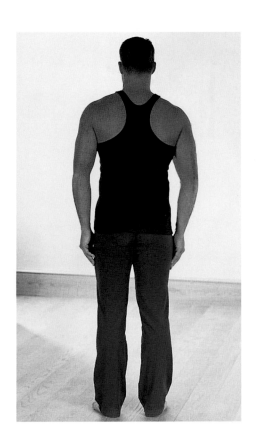

△ **If sliding your shoulder blades down your spine is a baffling request, practise this subtle movement by standing up with your arms by your sides. Keeping your back straight, push your fingertips towards the floor. Do not force your arms down or lock them into position. Try to keep the shoulder blades close to the back of the ribcage. This is very useful for limiting tension around the shoulders, which tends to make you pull your shoulders up to your ears.**

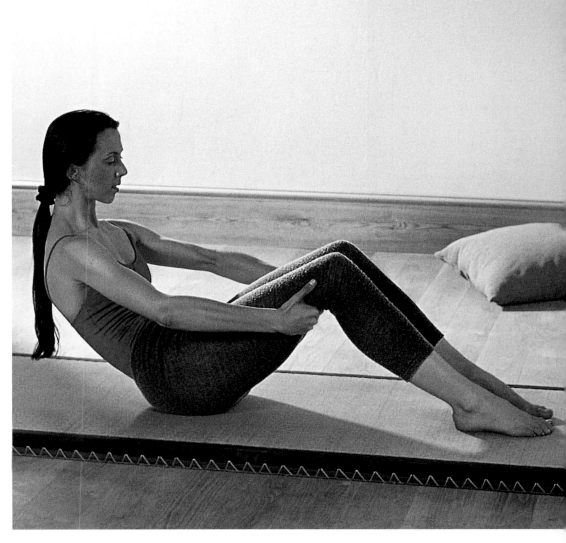

△ **Every movement should be controlled via your abdominals. Keep bringing your attention and focus back to pulling your navel towards your spine.**

Neutral spine

A healthy spine has natural curves that should be preserved and respected but not exaggerated. The term "neutral spine" refers to the natural alignment of the spine. If you have any serious pain in your back, check with a physician before embarking on any exercise programme. The main curves are:

- **The cervical spine**: the area behind the head, along the back of the neck, is concave; it should curve gently inwards.
- **The thoracic vertebrae**: the largest area of the back curves very slightly outwards.
- **The lumbar spine**: the lower back should curve slightly inwards; it should not be flat or over-curved.
- **The sacral spine**: the sacral curve is at the bottom of your spine and curves gently outwards.

It is important to allow the spine to rest in its natural position to prevent stresses and imbalances. During Pilates movements you should ensure (unless otherwise directed) that your back is not flat or pushed into the

THE AREAS OF THE SPINE

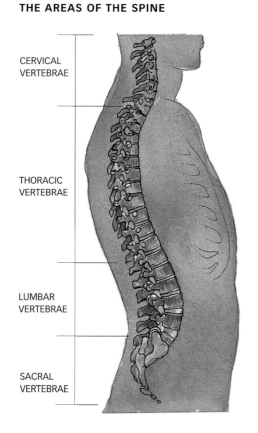

CERVICAL
VERTEBRAE

THORACIC
VERTEBRAE

LUMBAR
VERTEBRAE

SACRAL
VERTEBRAE

Finding neutral spine

The importance of neutral spine cannot be emphasized enough, as it allows your spine to elongate and relax. Before starting an exercise it can be helpful to roll gently between the two extreme positions and then try to fall comfortably between the two.

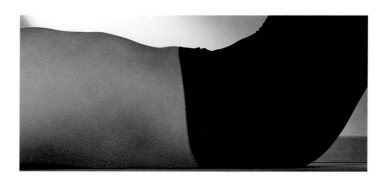

◁ **1** Tilt your pelvis, flattening your back into the floor.

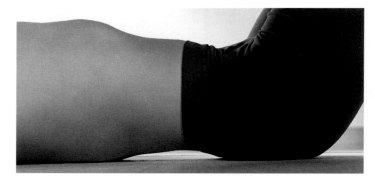

◁ **2** Tilt your pelvis in the opposite direction, creating an arch under your lower back. Make this movement slow and take care not to hold for too long or you may cause tension in your lower spine.

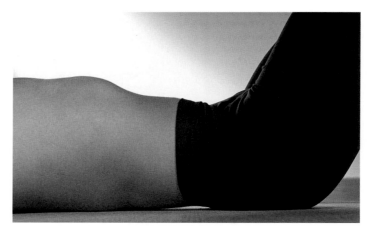

◁ **3** Find a position between these two extremes in which your back feels natural and comfortable: this is neutral spine. Unless otherwise stated, you should always work from this position during your Pilates routine.

floor, although this can be tempting in order to achieve a flatter tummy. What you tend to do in this position is grip at the hip flexors (the muscles located at the top of the thighs) thus creating tension in a place that is commonly tight anyway. You must also try to avoid over-curving your spine, as this pushes the abdominals forwards and tightens the muscles around the spine. "Neutral spine" lies in between these two extremes and echoes the natural and safe position that your spine prefers.

◁ **The diagram shows the four natural spinal curves. These curves help to cushion some of the shock from our daily activities – even walking creates some mild stress. One of the key elements of Pilates is the close attention given to the alignment of the spine during all movements.**

Planning a Pilates programme

To be effective any exercise needs to be organized into a programme that is easy to remember and that you will want to do regularly. At the end of this exercise section there is guidance on devising a successful Pilates programme that will help you achieve your goals. Keep your programme balanced and combine it with cardiovascular work and good nutrition to give you a total fitness plan.

With Pilates, it can be difficult to identify the muscles that are being challenged as most movements involve a combination of several muscle groups all working together. A Pilates exercise may be overtly working the arms or the legs and may also be demanding constant stabilization from the torso. So you will find that even though a movement is targeting a certain muscle group, you will often feel it in other parts of your body as well.

In general, Pilates movements can be divided into three main categories:

- **Strengthening exercises** that concentrate on making certain muscle groups stronger and more toned.
- **Flexibility exercises** that improve the range of motion around a joint.
- **Mobility exercises** that train the body to move more easily.

exercise categories

The following list groups the exercises according to both the action that is being reinforced and the dominant muscles that are being used. Once you have worked through the exercises on the following pages, you can use it to plan a programme.

exercises that strengthen the upper body

- Push-ups (deltoids, pectorals, biceps, abdominals and stabilizing back muscles)★
- Triceps push-ups (triceps, deltoids, abdominals and pectoral muscles)
- Leg pull prone (abdominals, stabilizing back muscles)★
- Triceps dips (triceps, abdominals)

exercises that strengthen the lower body

- Cleaning the floor (quadriceps, supporting muscles of the feet and ankles, abdominals)
- Open V (adductors, abdominals, hip flexors and stabilizing back muscles)
- Outer thigh blaster (abductors, abdominals, adductors and hamstrings)
- One-leg kick (hamstrings, abdominals, lower gluteals and erector spinae)★
- Inner thigh lift (adductors and abdominals)

exercises that strengthen the abdominals and back

- One-leg stretch (abdominals and stabilizing back muscles)★
- Side kick (hamstrings, hip flexors, abdominals, abductors and stabilizing back muscles)★
- Leg pull prone (abdominals and stabilizing back muscles)★
- Roll-up (abdominals and hip flexors)★
- Side bend (obliques, abdominals, stabilizing back muscles; stretches the latissimus dorsi)★
- Side squeeze (internal and external obliques, abdominals, shoulder stabilizers and abductors)
- Hundred (abdominals and stabilizing mid-back muscles)★
- Swimming (abdominals, gluteals and erector spinae)★

exercises that promote flexibility

- Gluteals stretch (gluteals)
- Chest stretch (pectorals)
- Side stretch (latissimus dorsi)
- Hip flexor stretch (hip flexors)
- Spine twist (obliques, adductors and hamstrings; promotes thoracic mobility)★
- Abdominal stretch (abdominals)
- Spine stretch (erector spinae, hamstrings, adductors)★
- Deep chest and shoulder stretch (pectorals and latissimus dorsi)

- Lower back stretch (erector spinae and gluteals)
- Spine press (erector spinae)

exercises that promote mobility

- Rolling back (spine)★
- Spine twist★ and Spine press (spine)
- Spine stretch (spine)★
- Rolling back (spine)★

core exercises

These are marked with a star and you will get the best results if you choose a few "core" exercises – movements that are considered pure Pilates exercises – and concentrate on these for a period of time, say four to six weeks, giving your muscles a chance to adapt to the work. Start with these, and once you have mastered them (not necessarily advancing to a higher level, just feeling comfortable and confident about the movement) add on a few more.

▽ Shoulder circles are a useful warm up exercise and a good way to relieve tension in the shoulders and upper back. Make the movement slow and controlled, keeping the spine in neutral.

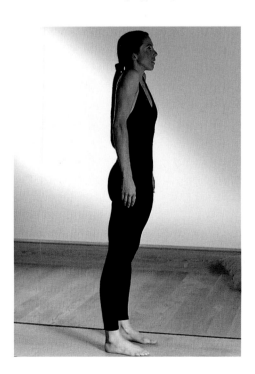

Rolling back

As you work on these exercises that concentrate on the abdominals and back, feel the abdominals getting stronger and flatter as you progress. Your back will be free from the burden of aches and stiffness. Make sure you work on a mat that gives plenty of support, and once you have practised rolling down the spine with your hands on the floor, try progressing on to rolling back: you may not roll back up on your first attempt, but keep practising. When pulling in abdominals, imagine you are squeezing a sponge held between your navel and your spine. Squeeze the sponge as hard as you can. Take care not to roll back on to your neck. Pay careful attention to the alignment of your body as you work.

Purpose: To mobilize and massage the back and strengthen the abdominals
Target muscles: Erector spinae, abdominals
Repetitions: Repeat 6 times

Checkpoints
- Keep your feet flat on the floor
- Lengthen up through the spine at the end of the movement
- Tilt the pelvis

first position

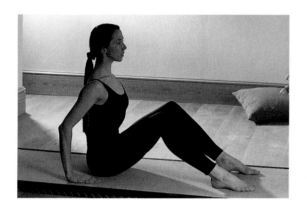

△ **1** Sit with your spine in neutral and your knees bent with both feet flat on the floor. Place your hands near your hips with your fingers facing your feet. Inhaling wide and full through the ribs, draw your navel towards your spine. Lower your chin towards your chest then, using your hands for support, start to roll down to the floor. Try to place each vertebra on the floor, one by one. To do this, tilt your pelvis and curve your spine into a C-shape.

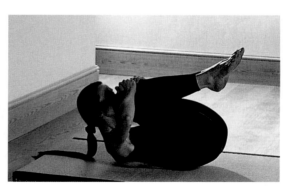

△ **2** Once you have rolled down as far as you find comfortable, exhale and, using your core strength, return to the starting position. Pull up through the crown of your head to create a long spine, then repeat. Use your arms only as support and avoid transferring all your weight on to your triceps.

second position

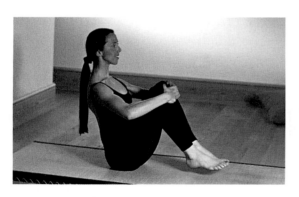

△ **1** Sit upright with your spine in neutral. Lengthen up through the spine and imagine your head floating up to the ceiling. Place your feet flat on the floor and your hands just below your knees. Don't overgrip; keep your elbows bent and your chest open. Take care not to tense or grip around your neck.

△ **2** Inhale as you tilt the pelvis and curve the spine into a C-shape to roll back, tucking in your chin and keeping your thighs close to your chest. As you exhale, use your abdominals to pull you back up to the starting position. Try not to use momentum, but make the movement flow at a consistent speed. Between each roll lengthen up through the spine.

Checkpoints
- Keep the chin tucked into the chest
- Do not grip the neck
- Use your abdominals to get you back to the starting position again

The roll-up

In spite of the name of this exercise, you begin by rolling down. It is an excellent way to strengthen the abdominals but is very challenging, so ensure you are comfortable and confident with the first position before moving on. Although you are curving your spine do not collapse into the movement. Roll down only a little way at first to get the feel of the movement, then roll lower as you become stronger. At all times, do a mental check that you are not tensing other parts of your body, such as your neck or face. As you come back to an upright position imagine that you are sitting against a cold steel door.

Purpose: To strengthen the abdominals

Target muscles: Abdominals, hip flexors

Repetitions: Repeat 10 times

first position

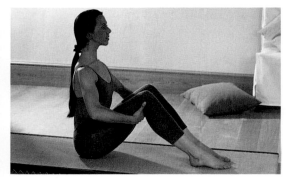

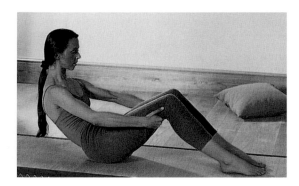

△ **1** Sit upright with your feet flat on the floor and your knees bent. Hold the back of your thighs, with your elbows bent and your arms open; don't overgrip. Your spine should be in neutral. Lengthen up through the spine but do not grip the neck. Slide the shoulder blades down the spine.

△ **2** Inhale and tilt your pelvis to create a C-shaped spine. Keeping your feet flat on the floor, roll down bone by bone, creating space between the vertebrae. Your hands are there to support you if you lose control but try to rely on abdominal strength to stabilize the movement. As you curl down, imagine your spine is a bicycle chain that you are placing down link by link. When you have lowered down as far as you can, exhale and contract the abdominals to roll back up to the starting position. Sit upright, keeping the spine in neutral.

Checkpoints
- Do not overgrip the legs, use them only as support
- Lengthen up through the spine in the starting position
- Feel the abdominals pull you up

second position

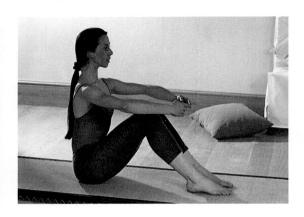

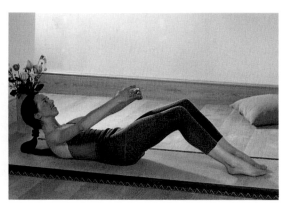

△ **1** This time, hold your arms directly in front of you, level with your shoulders. Your elbows should be bent, arms rounded. Let your shoulder blades glide down your spine and feel the crown of your head "float" up towards the ceiling. Inhale and tilt your pelvis to begin the downward roll as before.

△ **2** When you first progress to this position try a few small roll-downs to get the feel of the movement before going down further. Feel the support of the abdominals throughout the downward and upward roll. Keep your feet flat on the floor all the time.

Checkpoints
- Use the abdominals, not momentum, to pull you up
- Lower bone by bone
- Do not collapse into the movement
- Keep the feet on the floor

The hundred

This static contraction builds core strength and is one of the most commonly taught Pilates exercises. Challenge yourself to reach a hundred. The Hundred really tests your co-ordination. Try not to stagger your breathing as you count your taps: the breath should be flowing and even. Pay special attention to any tensing in the neck and face in this position. To help you do this exercise well, visualize a heavy weight balancing on your abdominals and pulling your navel down towards your spine.

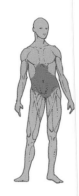

Purpose: To strengthen core muscles, co-ordinate breathing patterns and build endurance.
Target muscles: Transverse abdominis, rectus abdominis, stabilizing mid-back muscles
Repetitions: 20 x 5 beats

first position

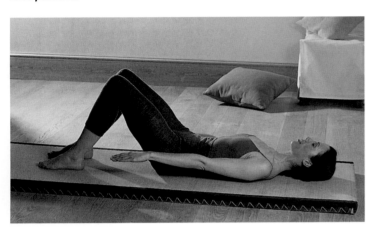

◁ Lie on your back with your knees bent, your feet flat and your head in alignment. The spine should be in neutral and the abdominals hollowed, drawing the navel to the spine. Your arms are by your sides, lifted off the mat. Slide your shoulder blades down your spine. Inhale as you count to five then exhale for five. Gently tap your fingertips on the floor and co-ordinate your breathing with your taps. Breathe steadily and laterally into your ribs.

Checkpoints
• Keep your arms lengthened
• Draw the shoulder blades down the spine
• Keep the abdominals hollowed

second position

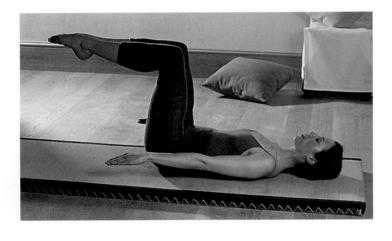

◁ When you feel confident about the first position, lift your feet off the floor. Your knees should be directly above your hips and your feet level with your knees. Do not allow your knees to fall away as this will cause your spine to curve. If this is too much of a challenge you can raise just one leg, but do not twist your hips. Repeat the breathing pattern as before. Keep the abdominals flat throughout and maintain the distance between your hips and ribs.

Checkpoints
• Glide your shoulder blades down your spine
• Keep your knees above your hips
• Toes are pointed
• Feet stay level with knees

third position

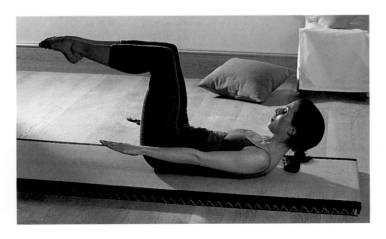

◁ Curl your upper body off the floor, dropping your chin towards your chest so that you are facing your thighs. Do not grip your neck and keep drawing your shoulder blades down your spine. Maintain the breathing pattern for a hundred beats as before. If you want a greater challenge, try straightening the legs. Lower your eyes in this position to check that your abdominals are flat and your ribs are not flaring up.

Checkpoints
• Release tension from the neck
• Do not clench your jaw
• Keep the abdominals flat

The swimming

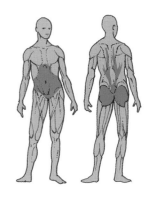

This exercise is a favourite with physiotherapists as it is a very effective way of developing strength in the core muscles. It is a very challenging exercise but is an easy one to cheat on, so read the instructions carefully to make sure that you are performing the exercise correctly. Ensure that you keep your abdominals lifted. Instead of just raising your arms and legs, visualize them lengthening away from your trunk. Do not try to lift them too high from the floor. Make your movements elegant and flowing and avoid throwing your arms and legs or collapsing back on to the floor on the way down. Take care not to lift your hips off the floor or to overbalance on to one side or the other.

Purpose: A strength exercise, challenging co-ordination and core strength
Target muscles: Abdominals, gluteals, erector spinae
Repetitions: Repeat 10 times

first position

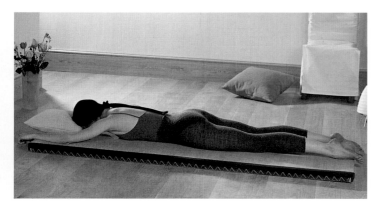

◁ Lie on your front, placing a small pillow under your forehead to keep your head in alignment with your spine, which is in the neutral position. Keep your neck long. Stretch your arms over your head and lengthen them away. Point your toes and lengthen your legs away. Breathe laterally, wide and full. Draw in your abdominals, imagining that there is a drawing pin on the mat that you are lifting away from.

Checkpoints
• Do not tip your head back
• Keep the abdominals lifted
• Breathe laterally

second position

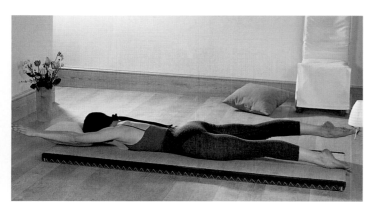

◁ Introduce a challenge to your core strength by lifting one leg. Exhale as you lift and inhale as you lower the leg. Keep both hips in contact with the floor, and do not try to lift the leg too high. Keep lengthening as you lift, maintaining the distance between the ribs and hips. Do not lose the lift in your abdominals. Take care not to twist the raised leg but keep your knee and foot in line with your hips. Repeat with the other leg.

Checkpoints
• Lengthen as you lift the leg
• Do not twist the hips

third position

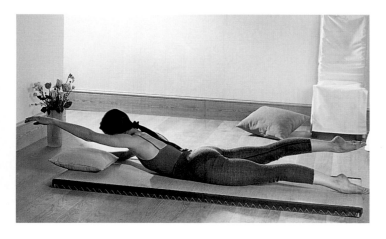

◁ As you exhale, lift your opposite arm and leg together. When you lift your arm raise your head and upper body with the movement, but keep facing the floor so that your head stays in line with your spine. Lengthen through your arms and legs and keep your hips in contact with the floor. Remember the drawing pin under your navel: if you lose the lift in your abdominals, continue to work in the second position for a while longer.

Checkpoints
• Keep your head in line with your spine
• Do not twist the torso
• Lengthen from a strong centre

One-leg stretch

Do not be fooled into thinking that this is a relaxing leg stretch – it is actually a very challenging movement which builds core strength and is also good for improving co-ordination. Keep your hips still throughout as if they were being held in a vice. Take care not to curve your spine, and keep your shoulder blades pulled down your spine and close to the back of your ribs throughout. If you find the hand position difficult, you can lightly hold either side of your knee instead. Make sure that you are just making light contact and do not over-grip as this causes tension in the neck and jaw. Your upper body should be stabilized by your abdominal muscles.

Purpose: To strengthen abdominals and improve co-ordination
Target muscles: Abdominals, stabilizing back muscles
Repetitions: Repeat 10 times on each leg

Checkpoints
• Hollow your tummy throughout
• Keep the hips still

first position

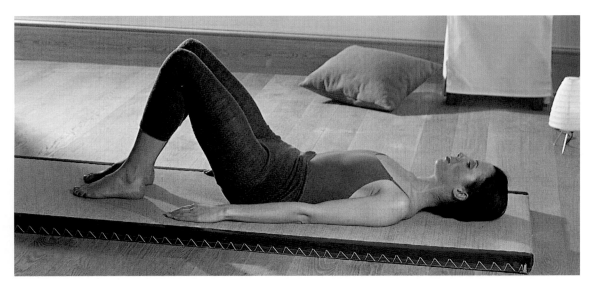

△ **1** Lie on your back with your knees bent and your feet flat on the floor. Your spine should be in neutral and your head in alignment: do not shorten your neck by tipping your head back or dropping your chin to your chest. Draw the navel to the spine.

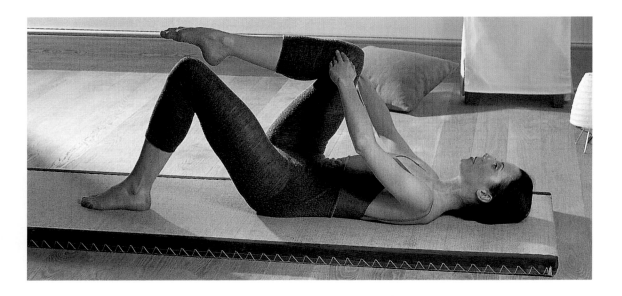

△ **2** Lift one foot off the floor, keeping the knee bent, and pull the leg gently towards you, supporting it at the knee. Try not to over-grip, causing tension in the neck, and keep your foot in line with your knee. Take care not to let the ribs flare up. Repeat with the other leg, inhaling as you lift and exhaling as you lower.

second position

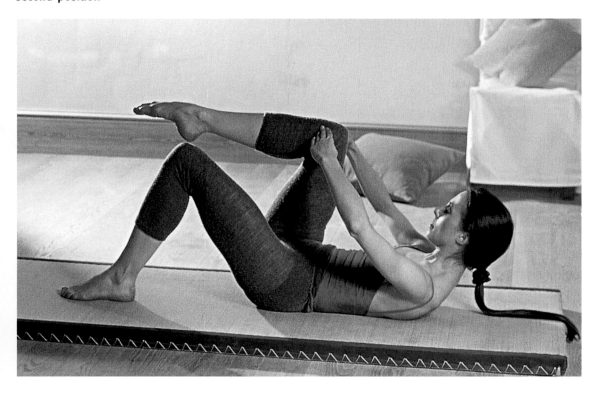

Checkpoints
- Do not tip the head forward or back
- Watch for tension in the neck

△ Once you understand the first position, curl the upper body off the floor and continue the same movement. Let the chin fall towards the chest, and try to limit tension in the neck. Keep the hips very still, controlling any movement from the hips via your abdominals. Breathe laterally. Keep the stomach hollowed throughout the movement, trying to make it as flat as possible.

third position

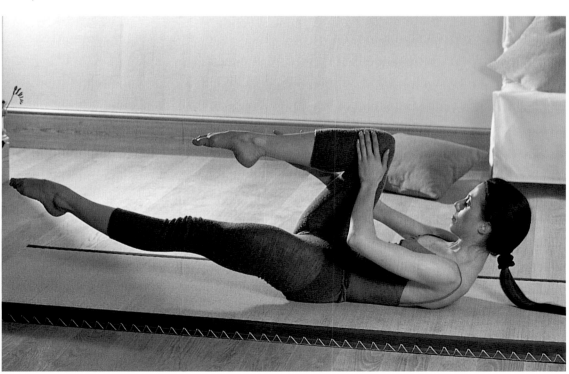

Checkpoints
- Pull the shoulder blades down your spine close to the back of your ribs
- Lengthen the legs away
- The lower your straight leg, the harder your abdominals have to work

△ This position really challenges your co-ordination. As you raise the right leg, place the right hand on the ankle and the left hand on the inside of the knee. Change hands as you change legs. As one leg comes in to the body the other leg lifts and lengthens away on an exhalation. Keep your toes pointed and stretch down through the straight leg. The movement is controlled by the abdominals: keep them hollowed, and maintain the distance between the ribs and hips. Do not twist the hips: imagine they are being held in a vice. Keep the pace slow and consistent.

Leg pull prone

This is actually a yoga position as well as a modified Pilates one. You will gain a lot of torso strength and stability from this exercise, and if you do it properly it will feel as if every muscle in your body is being challenged. Remember to breathe freely throughout the exercise and do not hold your breath when holding the position. It is common to shrink down into your shoulders in this position so try to maintain the length in your neck throughout. Keep checking for tension around the neck, face and shoulders. Focus on your abdominals; they should be stabilizing your whole body. You could try to visualize a drawing pin inserted through your navel and attaching to your back.

Purpose: To strengthen the abdominals and spine and challenge the upper body
Target muscles: Abdominals, stabilizing back muscles
Repetitions: Repeat up to 10 times

first position

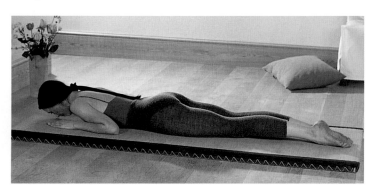

◁ Lie on your front with your head in line with your spine. Bend your arms and keep your upper arms close to your body. Lift the abdominals off the floor, imagining that you are creating an arch under your stomach. Breathe wide and full. Concentrate on this abdominal lift and aim to hold it for one minute before relaxing again.

Checkpoints
• Slide your shoulders down your spine
• Keep the upper arms close to your body

second position

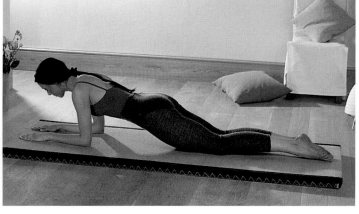

◁ Your elbows should be directly under your shoulders. Do not push your buttocks towards the ceiling or arch your spine. Keep your head in line with the spine and lengthen it away: don't sink into your shoulders or squeeze the shoulder blades together. Make sure that your hips stay square. The abdominals are lifted throughout. If this is too difficult, lower your hips and curl just your upper body off the floor. Try to hold this for one minute.

Checkpoints
• Maintain a straight line from your head to your knees
• Do not let the abdominals sag

third position

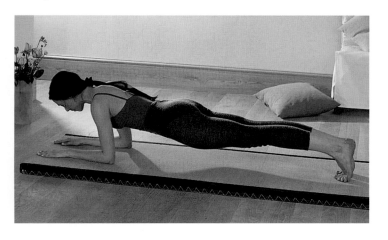

◁ Lift up on to your toes, straightening your legs. This is a real challenge, so be sure to have worked on the first and second positions for quite some time before progressing. Take care not to transfer all the weight into your shoulders or upper body, and keep your hips square. Pull your navel to your spine, maintaining the distance between your ribs and hips, and breathe laterally. Aim to hold for up to one minute.

Checkpoints
• Keep a straight line from your head to your heels
• Do not transfer all your weight into your upper body
• Draw your shoulder blades down your spine

The side kick

This is another good exercise for core strength, concentrating on the lower body. Have patience and work gradually through the progressions to achieve the best results. When performing the side kick take care not to use momentum to lift and lower your leg. It may help to visualize moving your leg through mud as this will slow you down.

Keep your foot or knee in line with your hip. Note the alignment of your hips and keep them stacked on top of one another as it is common for the hips to roll forwards and the posture to collapse. This is stabilized by the abdominals and the obliques (the muscles at the side of the waist). Try to keep a steady connection with their involvement.

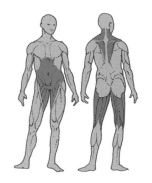

Purpose: To challenge core strength and work the lower body
Target muscles: Hamstrings, hip flexors, abdominals, stabilizing shoulder muscles, abductors
Repetitions: Repeat 10 times each side

Checkpoints
• Do not transfer all your weight on to the arm in front
• Keep your abdominals flat

first position

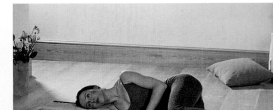

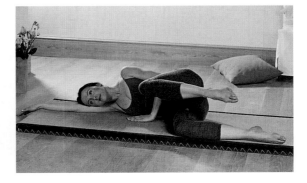

△ **1** Lie on your side, resting your head on your outstretched lower arm. Keep your head in line with your spine, which is in neutral, and your hips stacked vertically; they must not roll in or out. Your knees are bent, one on top of the other. Place your free hand in front for balance but do not lean into the supporting arm or transfer your weight forward.

△ **2** Lift the top knee directly above the other knee. Inhale and, with your toes pointed, move the knee back as you exhale until it travels behind your body. The challenge is to keep your hips stacked and your abdominals hollowed. Your shoulder blades should be pulled down your spine and your ribs should not be pushed up. You should feel this in your side. If you want to increase the challenge straighten the top leg, keeping the toe pointed.

second position

Checkpoints
• Do not let the hips collapse
• Lengthen out through the legs

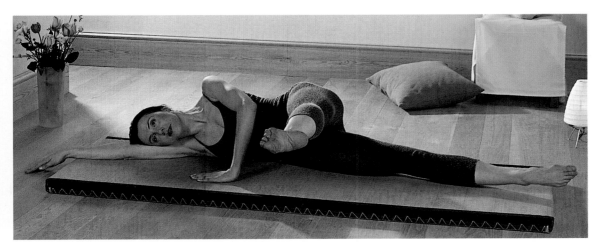

△ Straighten both legs. This is very challenging so be sure to advance only after working with the previous position. Bring the bottom leg forward slightly from your hip; it should not be in line with your spine. Keep the hips vertical and lengthen out through both legs. The control comes from your centre. Exhale as the leg travels backwards.

The side squeeze

This exercise will shape the waist and abdominals, so it is especially good for the area that hangs over your waistband when you wear fitted clothes. As you lift, check for tension in your neck or other parts of your body, and watch that your ribs stay down. Do not let the abdominals sag but hold them taut throughout.

If you wish to add an extra challenge, raise the top knee, keeping it in line with your hips – no higher. Make this a slow, controlled movement. Take care not to overgrip with your hands. Perform the movement with flow, avoiding any jerk when lifting and lowering.

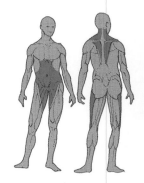

Purpose: To strengthen the waist and mid-section, stabilizing and improving balance
Target muscles: Obliques, shoulder stabilizers, abdominals and abductors
Repetitions: Repeat 10 times on each side

Checkpoints
- Do not allow the abdominals to sag
- Keep your hips stacked
- Maintain the distance between your ribs and hips
- Really feel the muscles in your side working

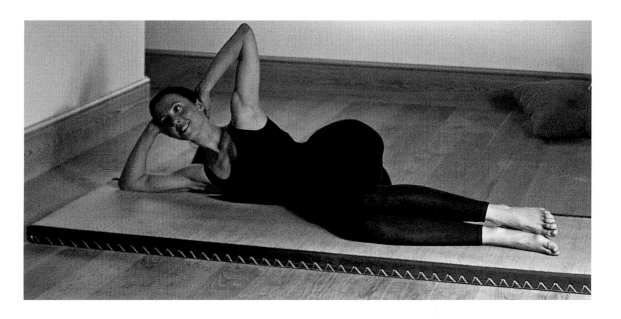

△ **1** Lie on your side with your knees bent and in line with your hips. Your hips are stacked and your abdominals hollowed. Place your hands on your head, directly opposite each other. Do not tip your head back or drop your chin to your chest. Breathe in.

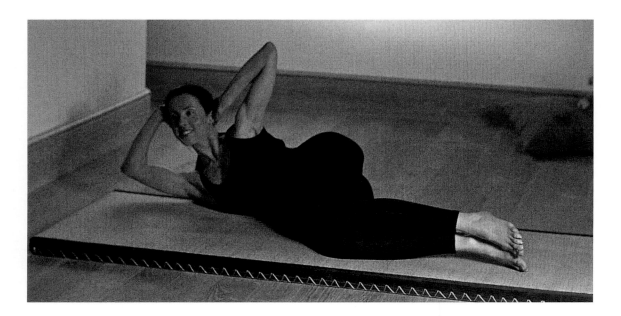

△ **2** Exhale as you lift your upper body off the floor and inhale as you lower. Make the lift slow and controlled. Don't jerk your neck or grip too hard with your hands. Maintain the length through your spine and take care not to let your hips collapse, but keep them stacked. Make sure your knees stay level with your hips. Draw your shoulder blades down your spine.

The side bend

This movement may look simple but it creates a marked improvement around the waistline if you practise it regularly, as well as developing core stability and balance. Feel the movement being controlled by your torso. Take care in this position not to let the hips roll either inwards or outwards. Imagine that you have a red dot on your hips that should always face the ceiling as you lift. Maintain the length in your neck and avoid sinking into your shoulders. You may not be able to lift very far off the floor initially but do not worry as the real benefit comes from maintaining the correct alignment and performing the exercise accurately. You might find that this exercise is less challenging on one side than the other – it is common for one side to be a little stronger than the other.

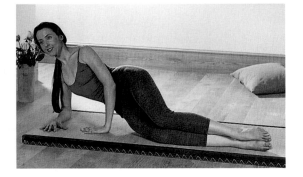

Purpose: To strengthen the abdominals and sides and improve balance

Target muscles: Obliques, abdominals, stabilizing shoulder muscles and latissimus dorsi

Repetitions: Repeat up to 10 times on each side

first position

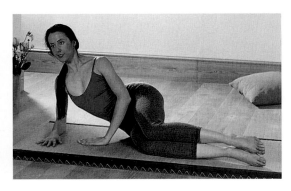

△ **1** Lie on your side with your legs bent, knees level with hips and feet in line with knees. Imagine there is a rod running vertically through your hips. Rest on your elbow, which should be directly under your shoulder, and bring the other arm in front for support. Resist the temptation to push all your weight on to the supporting hand or the resting elbow.

△ **2** Inhale, breathing into your sides, and as you exhale lift your hips off the floor. Use the muscles in the side closest to the floor to initiate the movement and control it via a strong centre. Hollow the abdominals, drawing navel to spine, slide your shoulder blades down your spine and ensure that your ribs are not pushing up.

Checkpoints
- Initiate the movement via a strong centre
- Do not transfer all your weight on to your arms
- Keep the neck soft

second position

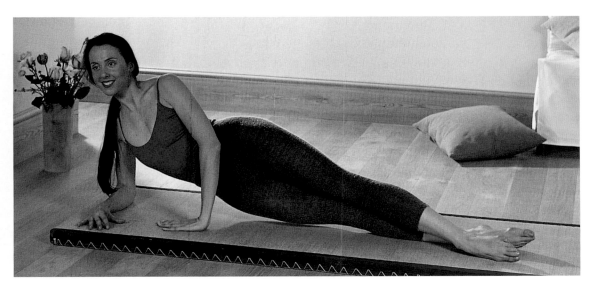

△ Progress only after reaching a level of ease in the first position. If you feel ready, straighten your legs and lengthen them away. Cross one foot over the other, with the toes pointed, to support you as you lift your hips. Keep your head in line with your spine and lengthen up through the top of your head.

Checkpoints
- Make sure the hips do not collapse
- Keep the abdominals hollowed
- Lift straight up, not veering to either side
- Keep the movement flowing

Push-ups

These push-ups are great for shaping the upper body: the shoulders and biceps. If they are performed properly, your abdominals will get a workout too. Once you progress beyond the first position, if your previous exercise was a standing one you can preserve the flow of movement and loosen up the spine by using a transitional move to get to the floor. Follow the instructions for the mobilizing exercise called "Rolling Down the Spine" and, once your hands are hovering at floor level, bend at the knees, place your hands on the floor and move into the start position for push-ups.

In every position, pull the abdominals in tight, never allowing them to sag, and keep your spine in neutral. Check for tension in your neck. Build up gradually to the full push-up.

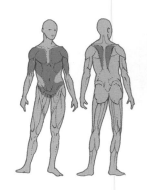

Purpose: To strengthen the upper body

Target muscles: Deltoids, pectorals, biceps, stabilizing back muscles and abdominals

Repetitions: Repeat up to 10 times

Checkpoints
- Keep your head in line
- Do not let the abdominals sag

first position

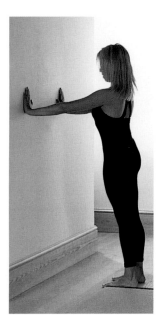

◁ **1** Stand facing a wall and place your hands on it. Your hands should be level with and just wider than your chest and flat against the wall, with the fingers pointing upwards. Your feet stay flat on the floor. Keep your spine in neutral and lengthen up your body, feeling your head "float" towards the ceiling.

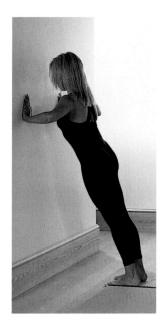

◁ **2** Bend at the elbows to bring your chest towards the wall. Keep your head in line with your body, slide your shoulder blades down your spine, and check that you are not pushing up your ribs. Push away from the wall to come back to your starting position. Keep the movement slow and controlled.

second position

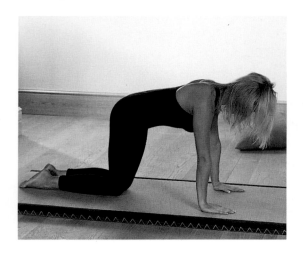

△ **1** Position yourself on all fours, knees directly under your hips and hands directly under your shoulders, with the fingertips facing forwards. Keep your spine in neutral and don't let your head sink into your neck.

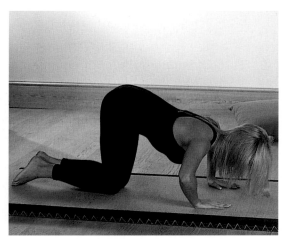

△ **2** Keeping your head in line with your spine, exhale as you lower your chest to the floor between your hands by bending your elbows. Do not allow the abdominals to sag. As you push up, straighten the arms without locking the elbows.

Checkpoints
- Do not lock the elbows
- Lower only as far as you can control
- Keep your chest at hand-level and your head in front of your hands

third position

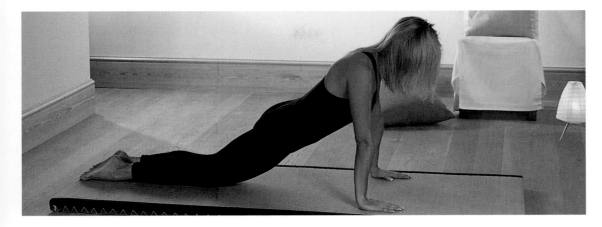

Checkpoints
- Keep a straight line from your head to your knees
- Do not let your buttocks stick up
- Do not arch or curve your back

△ **1** Drop your hips so that there is a straight line from your head to your knees. Your fingertips should be facing forwards and your hands directly under the shoulders. Keep the abdominals strong and your hips square.

▷ **2** Exhale as you lower and inhale as you lift. Keep your head in line with your spine and in front of your hands. Don't let your ribs flare up. Keep your weight evenly distributed between your knees and your hands.

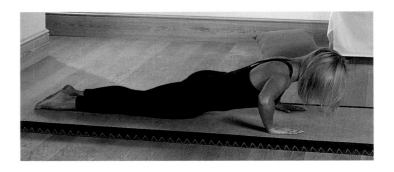

fourth position

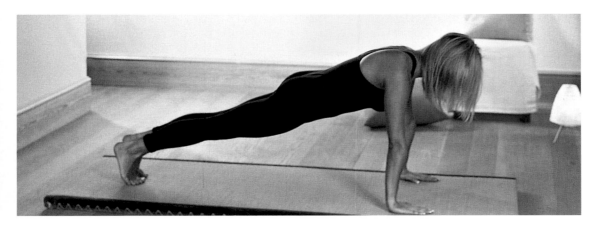

Checkpoints
- Keep your shoulder blades down the spine
- Make it a controlled, flowing movement
- Breathe laterally

△ **1** Form a straight line from your head to your feet, supporting yourself on your toes and hands. The fingertips should face forwards and your head should be in alignment with your spine.

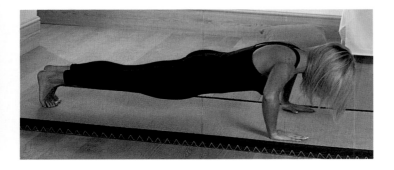

◁ **2** Lower your chest to the floor between your hands, then push up, keeping your elbows soft. Keep the movement controlled and continuous. Lower only as far as you can control.

Tricep push-ups

A common complaint is the lack of muscle tone at the back of the upper arm; this is excellent for challenging this area. It works by adapting the classic push-up to work on the triceps. The movements may look the same but there are subtle – and very important – differences. The elbows stay close to the body this time. To help you keep your elbows by your sides, visualize doing the movement in a narrow space between two walls. Try to maintain a constant, slow speed throughout the exercise, although this can be very difficult to maintain on the last few repetitions.

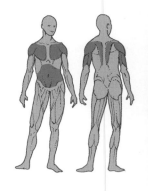

first position

▷ **1** Stand facing a wall. Place your hands flat against the wall, fingers pointing upwards. Your hands should be level with and just wider than your chest. Your feet stay flat on the floor. Keep your spine in neutral and slide your shoulder blades down.

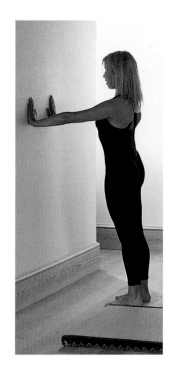

▷ **2** Bend at the elbows to bring your chest towards the wall as you exhale. Unlike in the classic push-up, your elbows should remain close to the body and pointing down at all times. Keep your head in line with your body and check that you are not pushing up your ribs. Push away from the wall to come back to your starting position.

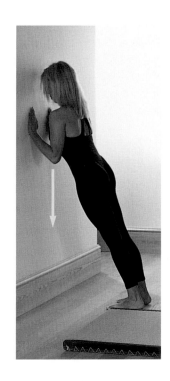

Purpose: To strengthen the upper body and the abdominals

Target muscles: Triceps, pectorals, deltoids and abdominals

Repetitions: Repeat up to 10 times

Checkpoints
- Do not let your elbows "wing" out to the sides
- Watch for your shoulders moving up towards your ears
- Lengthen up through the top of your head

second position

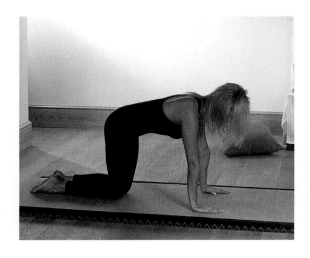

△ **1** Position yourself on all fours, with your hands directly under your shoulders, fingertips facing forwards. Keep your spine in neutral and maintain a straight line from your head to your hips. Don't let the abdomen sag.

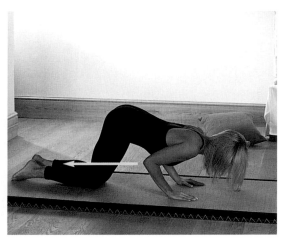

△ **2** Exhale as you lower your chest to the floor. This time, bend at the elbow and ensure that your elbows point towards your feet, with your upper arms staying close to your sides. As you push up, straighten the arms without locking the elbows.

Checkpoints
- Keep your chest level with your hands
- Keep your head in front of your hands
- Keep your feet flat on the floor

third position

▷ **1** Drop your hips so that there is a straight line from your knees to your head. Glide your shoulder blades down your spine. Your fingertips should face forwards.

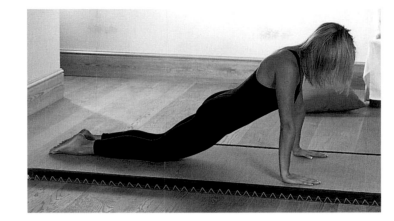

▷ **2** Exhale as you lower and inhale as you lift. Keep your head in line with your spine. Ensure that your head stays the same distance from your hands and that the elbows are pointing in the direction of your feet. Try to perform the exercise with flowing, continuous movements.

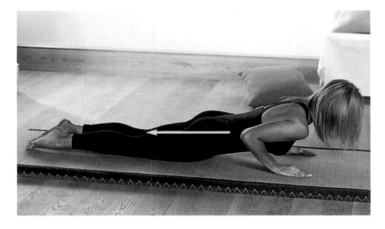

Checkpoints
- Do not let your buttocks stick up
- Feel the movement in the back of your upper arms
- Do not rely on momentum

fourth position

Checkpoints
- You should really feel this in the triceps
- Keep your body in alignment
- Hollow the abdominals
- Maintain a straight line from your head to your feet

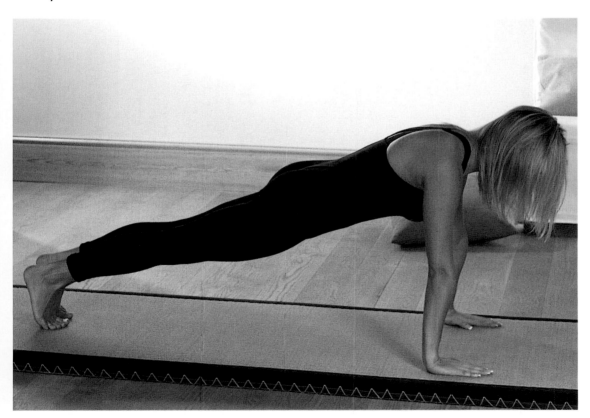

△ Make sure you have been practising the modified positions for some time before progressing to this position. This time your whole body should be in one straight line. Don't let your head sink into your shoulders. Lower the chest to the floor, keeping your elbows pointing towards your feet and using the same breathing pattern as for the previous positions.

Tricep dips

This exercise is indispensable for firming up the muscles at the back of the arms. The tricep runs from the shoulder to the elbow and can be hard to work, but if neglected, this is the part of your arm that wobbles when you wave. Find a chair that offers support at the correct height and check that it will not slip away from you. Work through the full range of the movement by straightening the arms, but take care not to "lock out" the elbows. Lengthen up through the top of your head.

Purpose: To tone the triceps

Target muscles: Triceps, abdominals

Repetitions: Start gently but work up to 20 times

Checkpoints
- Keep your back close to the chair
- Do not lock your elbows
- Keep your head in line

first position

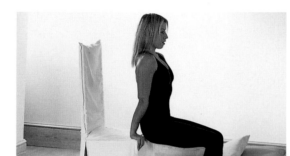

△1 Place yourself in front of the chair with bent knees and feet flat on the floor. Support yourself on your hands with your fingers pointing down. Lengthen up through your spine, which is in neutral. This is your starting position. Make sure that your abdominals are hollowed throughout the exercise.

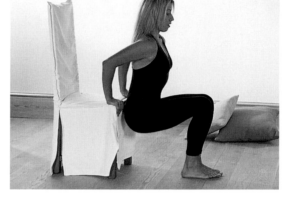

△ 2 Bend your elbows and lower your body as you inhale. Glide your shoulder blades gently down your spine and watch that your ribs do not push up. As you return to the starting position on an exhalation, take care not to "lock out" your arms, just straighten them. Keep your back close to the chair and make sure your elbows travel backwards rather than out to the sides. Execute the movement with control.

second position

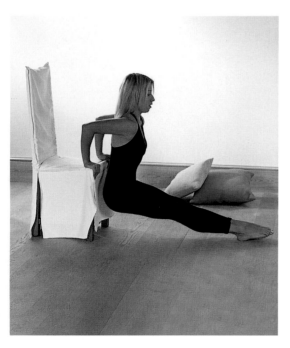

◁ Start in the same basic position as above, but this time put your legs straight out in front of you with your toes pointed. Keep your back close to the chair, your elbows pointing straight behind you and fingers pointing down. In this advanced position it is very tempting to let the elbows travel out to the sides, particularly if you are tired or not paying full attention. Ensure that your head does not sink into your shoulders. Your breathing should be wide and full allowing your ribs to expand fully, but keeping your abdominals hollowed out throughout the exercise. Aim to keep the movement flowing and continuous, and don't let the pace speed up or slow down. In this way you will work the triceps and abdominals harder and get the most benefit from the exercise.

Checkpoints
- Do not use momentum
- Keep the abdominals hollowed
- Maintain an even flow

Exercises for thighs

The following exercises pay attention to the inner thighs and hips. Although you will be predominantly toning the lower body, you should still focus on hollowing out the abdominals. Ankle weights can be added to both of these exercises. Alignment is very important for these exercises, so follow the directions carefully, letting the movements flow rather than "throwing" the leg.

The outer thigh blaster

If practised regularly, this exercise will really firm up the outsides of the hips and thighs and strengthen the lower body. Do not let the abdominals sag, and slide your shoulder blades gently down your spine. Maintain a constant distance between your ribs and your hips and keep the hips square, moving only your leg. Watch for tension elsewhere in the body as you do the exercise.

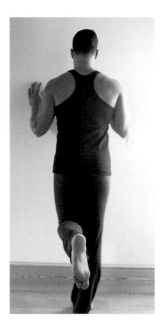

◁ **1** Stand facing the wall with your hands at chest level and flat against the wall. Bend one leg at the knee so that your foot is level with your knee and both knees are in line. Your spine should be in neutral and your foot flexed. Check that there is a straight line from your head to your feet, resisting the temptation to lean into the wall or bend at the hip.

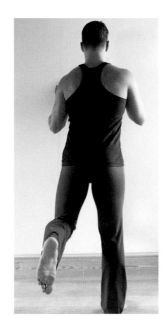

◁ **2** From this starting position, take your knee out to the side. It is important to keep your foot flexed and your knees aligned. Exhale as your leg travels away from your body, inhale as you bring it back. You should not swing the leg. Don't "sink" into the supporting leg, but keep lengthening up through the spine.

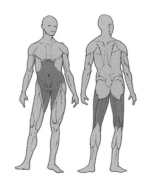

Purpose: To tone the hips and lower body

Target muscles: Abductors, abdominals, adductors and hamstrings

Repetitions: Repeat 10 times with each leg

Checkpoints

• Keep your lifted foot in line with your knee

• Keep the rest of your body still; move only the working leg

The inner thigh lift

This is a popular exercise that is often done badly. However, when it is performed correctly it works wonders with that much complained about area, the inner thigh. To progress the exercise you could use ankle weights, but you should really get a feel for the inner thigh initiating the movement before moving on.

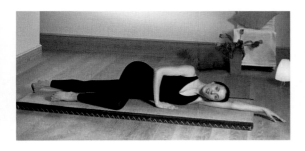

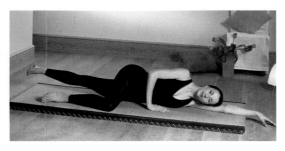

△**1** Lie on your side, supporting your head on your outstretched arm. Your hips should be stacked and your other hand can rest in front of you on the floor for support. Bend the top leg and rest your knee on the floor. Straighten the lower leg and lengthen it away on the floor with the foot flexed. Do not curve your back or allow your ribs to jut forwards. Glide your shoulder blades down your spine.

△ **2** Inhale, and as you exhale, lift the bottom leg as high as you can, keeping the abdominals hollowed all the time, then lower it. Make the movement flow, trying to avoid any jerky movements or, worst of all, swinging your leg. You should feel the muscle of the inner thigh doing the work. Take care not to twist the knee. Keep your foot in line with your leg; there is a tendency to lead with the toes in this position.

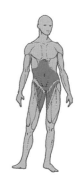

Purpose: To tone the inner thigh

Target muscles: Adductors and abdominals

Repetitions: Repeat 10 times with each leg

Checkpoints

• Do not roll hips

• Do not curve the spine

The open V

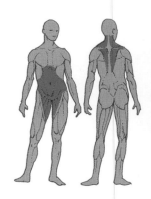

This is not one of the most graceful-looking movements, but it works wonders for the thighs, especially the inner thighs, and also benefits the abdominals. It is very important to pay special attention to keeping your knees (and feet in the second and third positions) directly above your hips at all times. If your feet fall towards the floor, your lower back may curve upwards which could cause stress. Check that you are not holding any tension in the shoulders or neck. To create an extra challenge try placing a cushion between your knees. Of course, you won't be able to open your legs so far.

Purpose: To firm up the inner thighs

Target muscles: Adductors, hip flexors, abdominals and stabilizing back muscles

Repetitions: Repeat 10 times

Checkpoints
- Check that your feet do not drop down
- Keep your feet flexed
- Do not curve your spine

first position

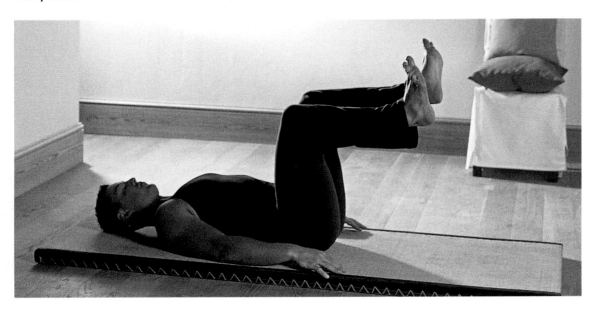

△ **1** Lie on your back, with your knees bent and directly above your hips, and your feet level with your knees. Your feet should be flexed. Your arms are on the floor, lengthening away, your shoulder blades slide down your spine, and your head is in alignment with your spine. Start with your knees apart.

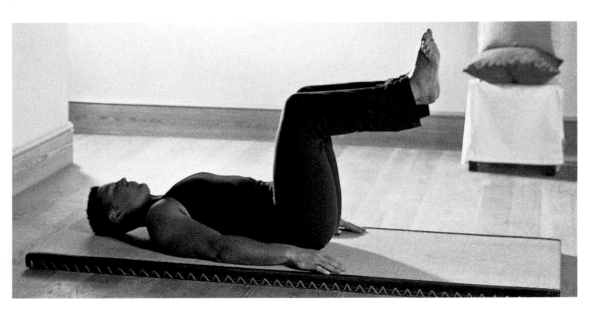

△ **2** Keeping your feet in line with your knees, bring your knees together and squeeze to feel your inner thighs working. Hold for a few seconds, then return to the starting position. Keep your abdominals hollowed throughout and your spine in neutral.

second position

Checkpoints
- Do not allow the legs to drop away from your body
- Do not let the legs open too far
- Squeeze the knees together

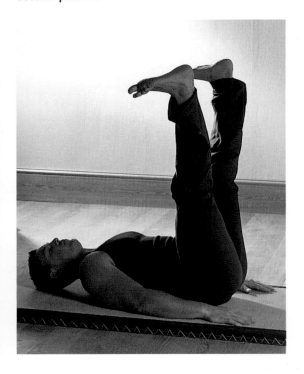 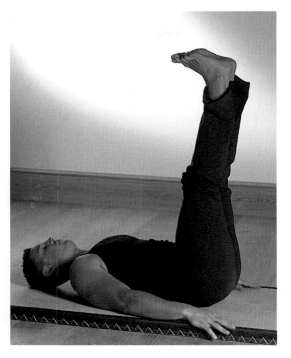

△ **1** The basic movement is the same as before, but is done with straight legs. Lengthen up through your heels and keep your feet flexed. Start with your legs apart.

△ **2** Bring your legs together and squeeze to work your inner thighs. Keep the hips still via the abdominals, which are hollowed throughout. Keep your arms strong, and really feel your inner thighs working.

third position

Checkpoints
- Watch for tension in the neck
- Lengthen the arms away
- Lengthen up through the heels
- Slide your shoulder blades down your spine

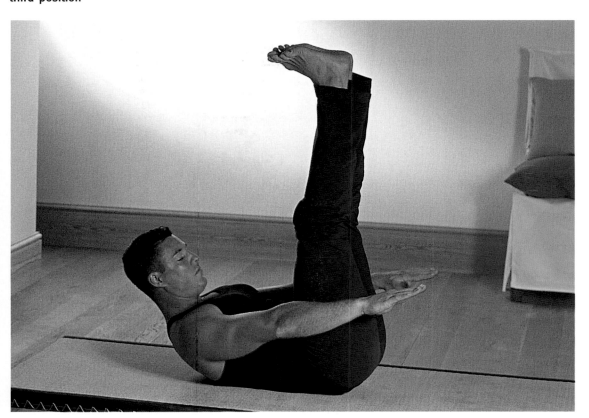

△ Curl your upper body off the floor, watching for tension in the neck and shoulders. Don't let your head sink into your shoulders, but glide your shoulder blades down your spine. Watch that your ribs do not flare up. Keep hollowing the abdominals; you can glance down and check that they are held flat. Squeeze the legs together as before.

Cleaning the floor

This movement will improve your balance and strengthen your lower body and all the small muscles in your feet and ankles – it is great for weak ankles. Initially, you may find the balance quite challenging. If so, it may help to look at a fixed point on the wall. It is common to find that your balance is better on one side than the other as most people favour one side. One of the objectives of this exercise is to balance any subtle differences in strength. Concentrate on maintaining the alignment between your foot and knees. If it helps, imagine that your supporting leg is held in a narrow gap between two walls.

Purpose: To strengthen the lower body, feet and ankles
Target muscles: Quadriceps, supporting muscles around feet and ankles, abdominals
Repetitions: Repeat up to 10 times with each leg

Checkpoints
- Watch for your knees rolling inwards or outwards
- Keep your supporting foot flat on the floor
- Lengthen up through the spine
- Make the movement smooth and continuous

first position

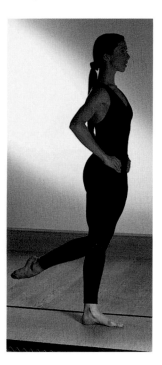

◁ **1** Stand up tall and imagine the crown of your head floating up to the ceiling. Feel your spine lengthening. It should stay in neutral throughout. Keep your abdominals as flat as possible. Place your hands on your hips and keep your head in line with your spine. Keeping your knees in line with one another, let one foot hover above the floor as you balance evenly on the other.

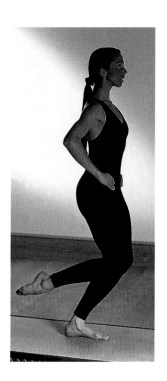

◁ **2** Bend the supporting leg and lower your body as far as you can control. Do not collapse into the movement. The supporting foot may feel a little wobbly at first. Check that the knee of the supporting leg stays in alignment with the foot. Inhale as you come back up to standing. Keep your upper body strong and watch that your ribs do not travel away from your hips.

second position

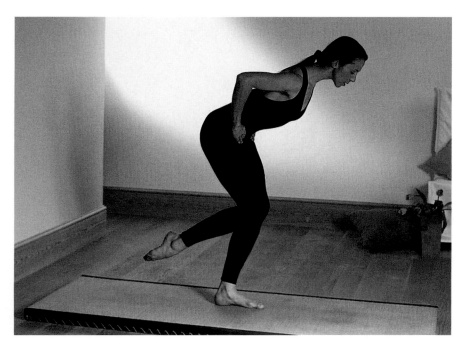

◁ Bend your knee and lower as far as you can into the position as before. This time, you are going to hold this position and then very carefully lower your chest towards the floor. Bend only a little initially. To get back to the starting position, straighten your torso first then come back up to standing. Keep your head in line.

Checkpoints
- Do not try to lower too far
- Do not collapse into the movement
- Keep lifting the abdominals

One-leg kick

This core exercise really challenges your co-ordination as you cannot see the movement – you just feel it. It is fantastic for toning up the lower body while challenging core strength. A good way to visualize the movement is to imagine that you are squeezing a pillow between your hamstrings and your calf. Try to resist just placing the leg: really feel the hamstrings working. This is a deceptively hard movement so do not worry if it takes practice. You may find it easier to get a feel for the movement first, then add the correct breathing pattern and work on lengthening down through the other leg.

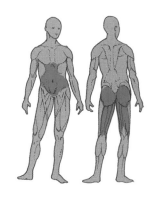

Purpose: To tone the lower body and develop core stability and strength
Target muscles: Hamstrings, erector spinae (when upper body is lifted), abdominals, gluteals
Repetitions: Repeat 10 times with each leg

first position

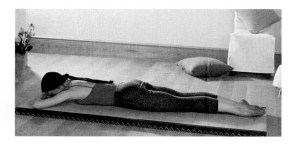

△ **1** Lie on your front, supporting your forehead on your folded hands to keep your head in alignment. Draw your navel to your spine, trying to form an arch under your abdominals.

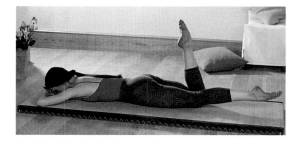

△ **2** Relax the neck. Avoid clenching the jaw. Relax your shoulders and slide the shoulder blades down your spine. Bend one leg at the knee. This is your starting position.

Checkpoints
• Keep the movement swift and continuous
• `Limit any movement by keeping the abdominals hollowed throughout
• Slide the shoulder blades down your spine

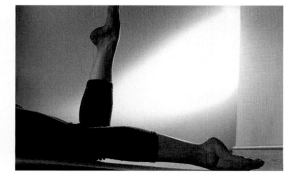

△ **3** Inhale, and as you exhale, point your toes and make a stabbing movement with your foot towards your buttocks. Keep your knees together and lengthen through the legs.

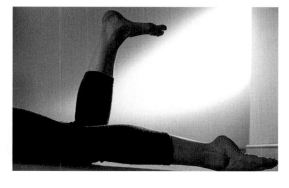

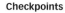

△ **4** Ease out of this position then repeat, this time with your foot flexed. Then extend your leg back to its original position. Meanwhile, the supporting leg on the floor should be lengthening away at all times.

second position

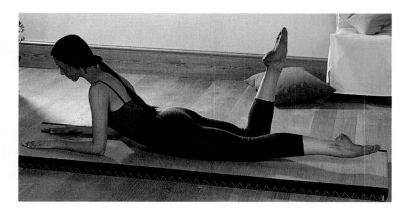

◁ Perform the same movements, but this time curl your upper body off the floor and rest on your elbows. Slide the shoulder blades down. Keep your neck long throughout and watch that your ribs do not travel away from your hips. Lengthen through the spine. If you feel a pinch in your spine in this position, stay with the first position for a while.

Checkpoints
• Keep your neck in line throughout the exercise
• Breathe wide and full
• Do not push all your weight on to your arms

Spine stretch

If your back feels tight or if you just want a healthy and mobile spine then this is the stretch for you. You will feel longer, stretched and more flexible. This is a flowing movement, not a static stretch. To keep your spine lengthening up and to stop you collapsing into the stretch, imagine that you have a beach ball in front of you, and lift up and over the ball. As you come upright again, imagine that your back is rolling up a pole, vertebra by vertebra, and take care to keep this alignment from your head to your hips; do not lean forwards, or away from the imaginary pole.

Purpose: To stretch the spine

Target muscles: Erector spinae, hamstrings, adductors and abdominals

Repetitions: Repeat 10 times

Checkpoints

- Do not collapse into the stretch
- Keep the movement flowing and continuous
- Let your head float up to the ceiling

first position

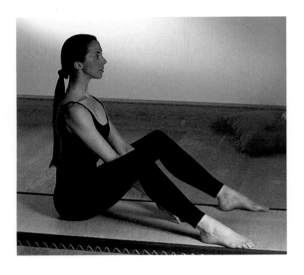

△ **1** Sit upright with your knees bent and your feet flat on the floor. Create as much length through your spine as possible. Keep the shoulders relaxed.

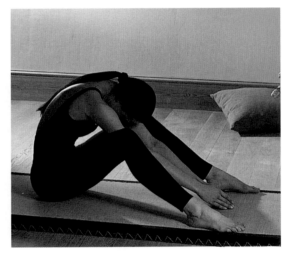

△ **2** Let your chin gently drop to your chest, then roll down bone by bone through your spine. As you do so, gently reach forwards with your hands. Keep your abdominals hollowed throughout. Roll back up to the starting position and lengthen up through your spine. Do not collapse into the stretch, but lift up through the abdominals and spine. Exhale as you lower into the stretch.

second position

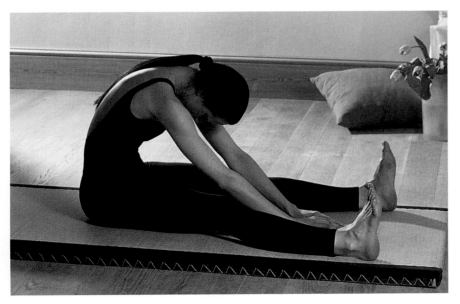

◁ The movement is the same as before, but this time straighten the legs and flex your feet, lengthening the heels away. Bend the knees slightly if you find this uncomfortable. The legs should be parted as far as is comfortable. As you roll up create as much length as possible between the vertebrae. Keep your buttocks on the floor.

Checkpoints

- Do not have the legs too far apart
- Visualize reaching up and over a beach ball
- Roll up vertebra by vertebra

Spine twist

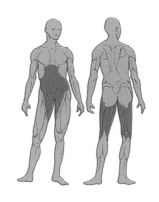

A deceptively challenging movement, this twist will stretch the waist and lower back while strengthening the abdominals. To gain the maximum benefit, it is important to keep your bottom on the floor throughout this movement. Let your head float up to the ceiling and pull your navel towards your spine. Try to keep the movement smooth and continuous. On your first attempts at this exercise you may be surprised at how hard it is to sit correctly aligned. We all develop certain postural habits and this exercise challenges them so it will feel intense at first. It gets easier with practice.

Purpose: To stretch the sides, strengthen the abdominals and promote thoracic mobility
Target muscles: Obliques, abdominals, adductors and hamstrings
Repetitions: Repeat 10 times on each side

first position

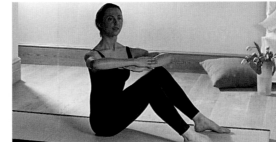

△ **1** Sit upright, lengthening up through the spine, with your knees bent and feet flat on the floor, legs slightly apart. Cross your arms loosely across your chest. Maintain a straight line from your head to your bottom.

△ **2** Breathing laterally, inhale and, as you exhale, turn the upper body to one side, keeping your buttocks firmly on the floor. Repeat on the other side. Remember that this is a flowing movement, not a static position.

Checkpoints
- Keep the movement flowing
- Hollow the abdominals
- Lengthen up through the spine

second position

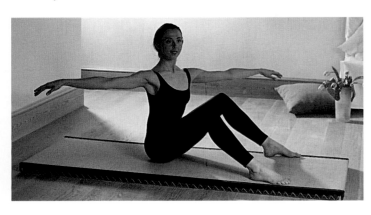

◁ The basic movement is the same but is performed with straight arms, lengthening out through the arms from the shoulders. Take care not to drop them. Now you are stretching in two directions: lengthening out through your arms and up through your spine. Slide your shoulder blades gently down your back and keep your feet flat on the floor.

Checkpoints
- Do not collapse into the movement
- Keep the whole of your buttocks on the floor
- Do not curve the spine

third position

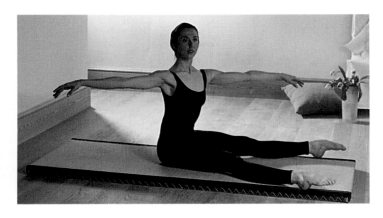

◁ The movement is the same but this time straighten the legs and point your toes. You are now stretching in three directions: up through your spine, out through your arms and through your legs. Be sure to keep your buttocks on the floor. You may be tempted to lean into one side as you turn.

Checkpoints
- Lengthen all the way to the toes
- Feel the abdominals working

Lower back stretch

This is a good warm-up stretch. Taking deep breaths can help you to relax into the stretch and you may find your muscles becoming more pliable, allowing you to ease yourself further into the movement. The stretch is great for easing mild tension in the lower back, which is a common complaint. Some people find it beneficial to rock slightly from side to side while in this stretch as this can gently mobilize the lower back. To do this, keep your upper body on the floor and make the movement very subtle. Although a small number of repetitions are recommended, these are only a guideline until you are confident about your instincts. Hold the stretch for longer or repeat if you need to.

Purpose: To stretch the lower back

Target muscles: Erector spinae and gluteals

Repetitions: Stretch twice; hold for 30 seconds each

Checkpoints
- Check for tension in the neck and shoulders
- Relax into the stretch
- Do not overgrip with your hands

first position

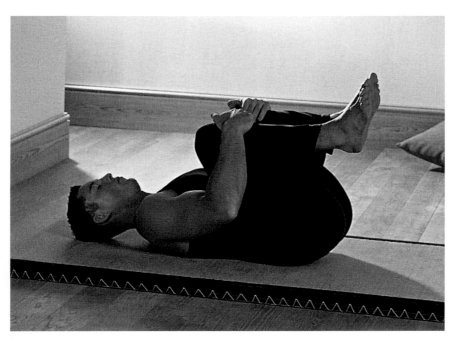

◁ Lie on your back and bring both knees up towards your chest. Support your legs with your hands, just below your knees. Relax your shoulders and feel the stretch in your lower back. Remember to keep your abdominals hollowed. Inhale to prepare and exhale as you lift your legs.

second position

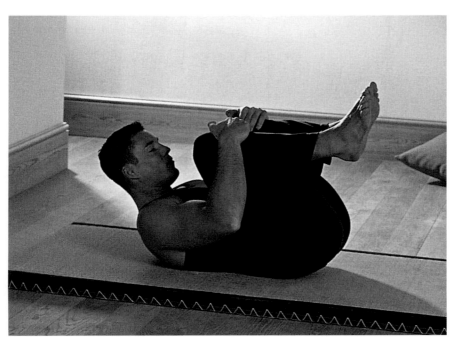

◁ Curl your head and shoulders off the floor, imagining curling up like a ball. Keep your neck soft: do not force your head forwards to your knees. Take care not to overgrip – keep your elbows open.

Checkpoints
- Curl up and down slowly
- Make sure your mat is thick enough to protect your back

Spine press

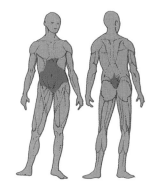

This movement mobilizes and stretches the lower spine. It is a good one to try whenever your lower back feels stiff, especially if you have been sitting for a long period, at your desk for example (and it can be done very discreetly). The curve of the spine should be very subtle. Take care not to over-curve your spine as you may "pinch" the muscles in the lower back. If it feels uncomfortable to curve your spine, or you have problems with your lower back, you may want to perform the second part of the movement only. When you tilt your pelvis, initiate the movement by imagining you are pressing your navel towards your spine. Avoid collapsing into the movement by lengthening your spine.

Purpose: To mobilize and stretch the lower back
Target muscles: Erector spinae and abdominals
Repetitions: Stretch twice; hold for 30 seconds each

Checkpoints
• Do not over-curve your spine
• Keep the abdominals hollowed
• Keep your head in alignment

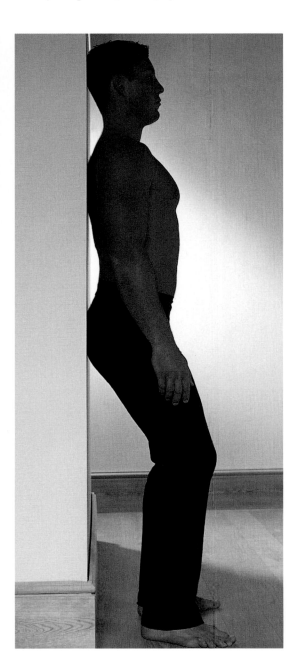

△ **1** Stand a short distance away from the wall, with your back against the wall, your knees bent and your arms by your sides. Lengthen up and glide your shoulder blades down your spine.

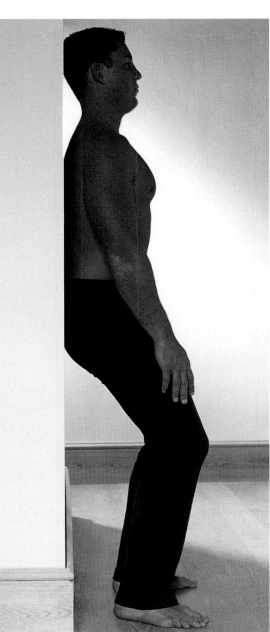

△ **2** Inhale, and as you exhale, push your spine flat against the wall by tilting your pelvis and contracting your abdominals. Keep your head in alignment. Try not to collapse into the movement: keep your abdominals hollowed.

Simple stretches

The following stretches are great for lengthening fatigued, tense muscles. The two upper-body stretches are great for opening up the chest; this is ideal if you have been sitting at a desk for a long period of time. On the first Chest Stretch, the wrist is also being slightly stretched. If this is uncomfortable, turn your hand round so that your fingertips point to the ceiling. In the Deep Chest and Back Stretch, slightly bend your knees if your legs are stretched beyond the comfort zone. When performing the gluteals stretch, be sure to keep your bottom on the floor or you will not stretch enough.

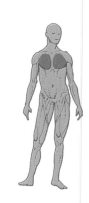

chest stretch

This feel-good stretch is great for relieving tightness in the chest and uses the wall for support. It can be done almost anywhere to relieve tightness in the chest.

Purpose: To stretch the chest
Target muscles: Pectorals
Repetitions: Stretch twice; hold for 30 seconds each

Checkpoints
• Keep your spine in neutral
• Feel the stretch in your chest
• Relax your shoulders

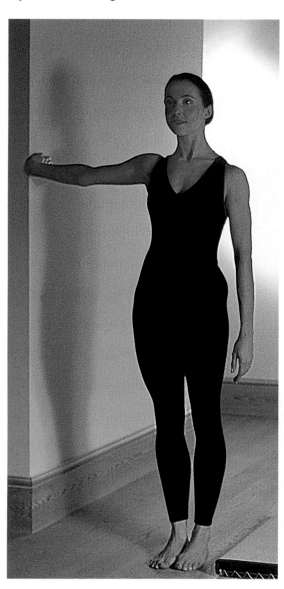

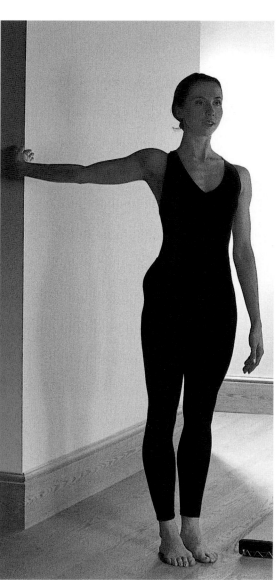

△ **1** Stand sideways to a wall. Extend one arm and place your hand flat on it. Keep your hand in line with your chest and your feet in line with your hips. Draw in your abdominals; your spine stays in neutral.

△ **2** Now turn your hips away from the wall, so that you feel a stretch in your chest. Relax your shoulders and enjoy the stretch. Change sides and repeat the movement.

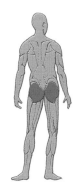

gluteals stretch

This stretch is reasonably easy to do and promotes a greater range of movement in the lower body. It is also a valuable stretch to do before many different sports that involve a lot of lower body work.

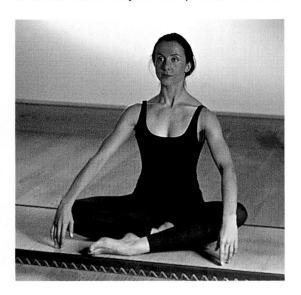

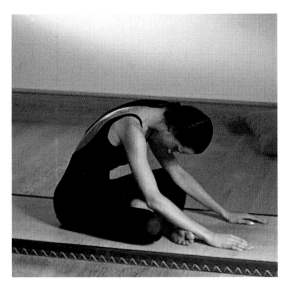

△ **1** Sit on the floor and position one leg in front of the other (the legs are not crossed). Relax your arms in front of you. Lengthen up through the spine, creating space between the vertebrae. Don't worry if your knees don't fall to the floor, just relax and let the knees fall into a natural position.

△ **2** Drop your chin towards your chest and curl down the spine while pushing the arms forwards and keeping your buttocks on the floor. Curl up again, switch the positions of the legs and repeat on the other side. Do not collapse into the movement; keep the abdominals pulled in throughout.

Purpose: To stretch the lower body
Target muscles: Gluteals
Repetitions: Stretch twice; hold for 30 seconds each

Checkpoints
• Keep your buttocks on the floor
• Replace the spine bone by bone
• Create length between the vertebrae

deep chest and back stretch

This stretch is ideal for easing tightness in the chest and back. Try to relax your shoulders and neck into the stretch. If this stretch is too intense, you can bend your knees.

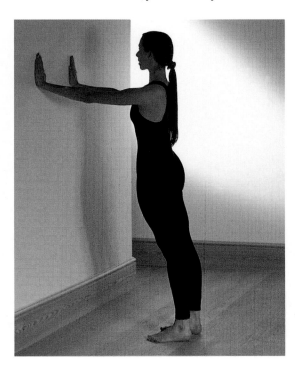

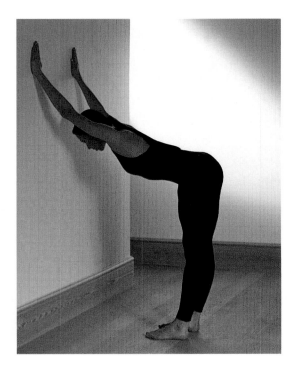

△ **1** Stand facing the wall with your feet together and place your hands flat on the wall level with your shoulders, just wider than shoulder-width apart. Lengthen up through the spine.

△ **2** Inhale, then as you exhale, lower your chest by bending from the hips, to feel a stretch in your chest and back. Keep your head in line with your spine. Keep the spine lengthened and the abdominals hollowed.

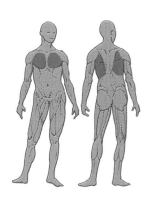

Purpose: To stretch the chest and shoulders
Target muscles: Pectorals and latissimus dorsi
Repetitions: Stretch twice; hold for 30 seconds each

Checkpoints
• Keep your head in line with your spine
• Keep your hips over your knees
• Bend the knees if necessary

▷

abdominal stretch

This is a very popular stretch that is similar to the "cobra" in yoga. It is very good for stretching the abdominals after all the hard work they have done. Take care not to throw your head back in this stretch. Keep facing the floor and lengthen up through the top of your head to avoid sinking into the shoulders. If you feel any pinching in your lower back, ease gently out of the stretch.

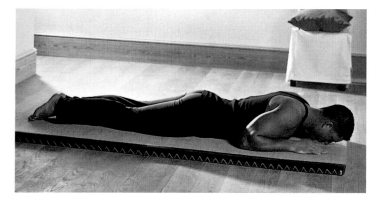

◁ **1** Drop your hips so that there is a straight line from your knees to your head. Glide your shoulder blades down your spine. Your fingertips should face forwards.

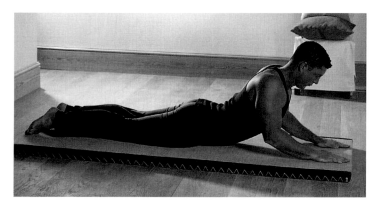

◁ **2** Inhale, and as you exhale, lift your upper body off the floor, resting the weight on your arms. Keep the abdominals hollowed and lifted, and take care not to over-curve the spine. Keep your hips on the floor. Do not sink into your neck, but lengthen up through your spine. Watch for tension in the neck. If you feel a pinch in your lower back, ease out of the stretch.

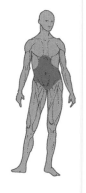

Purpose: To stretch the abdominals

Target muscles: Abdominals

Repetitions: Stretch twice; hold for 30 seconds each

Checkpoints

- Do not over-curve your spine
- Keep your head in line with your spine
- Keep your hips on the floor

hip flexor stretch

The hip flexors tend to be one of the tightest muscle groups, and when these muscles get overly tight they can cause discomfort and eventually imbalances. People involved in most sports benefit from this stretch, especially runners.

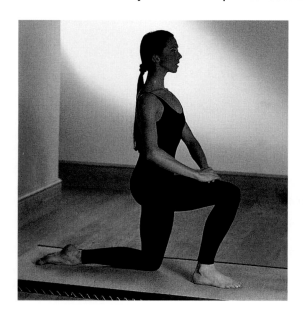

△ **1** Kneel down on the floor and take one step forwards, using your hands for support. If you need extra cushioning, place a pillow under the supporting knee.

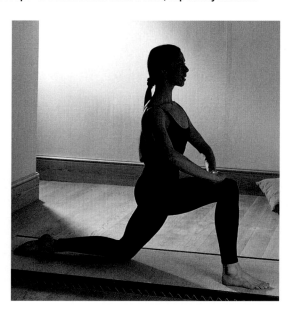

△ **2** Lunge carefully into the front leg, exhaling as you go forwards. Make sure your raised knee is directly over your foot. Lengthen up through the spine and keep the abdominals hollowed. You should feel this stretch at the top of the rear leg. Change legs and repeat.

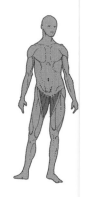

Purpose: To stretch the hip flexors

Target muscles: Hip flexors

Repetitions: Stretch twice; hold for 30 seconds each

Checkpoints

- Take care not to collapse into the stretch
- Lunge into the stretch
- Keep your head in alignment

waist lifts

This is a good movement to stretch and mobilize the spine. If it feels too intense or uncomfortable to have your arms overhead, then stretch with them by your side.

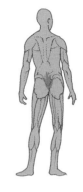

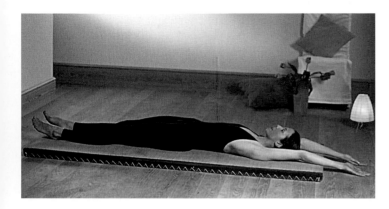

◁ **1** Lie on your back with your arms overhead or, if this is difficult, by your sides. Lengthen through your feet, spine and arms: visualize two cars pulling you in different directions. Draw the navel in to the spine.

Purpose: To stretch and mobilize the spine
Target muscles: Erector spinae
Repetitions: Stretch twice; hold for 30 seconds each

Checkpoints
- Ease out of the stretch if any pinching occurs
- Keep the abdominals strong
- Lengthen out the spine

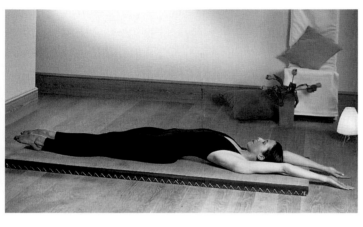

◁ **2** Carefully lift your waist. This is a very subtle movement; take care not to create a big curve in your spine. Keep the abdominals strong and the head in alignment. Watch for any gripping in your lower back. If you feel any pinching in your back, ease out of the stretch.

side stretch

This feels good at any time. No wonder cats and dogs are always stretching – it relieves the body of unwanted tension and liberates the spine and joints.

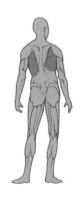

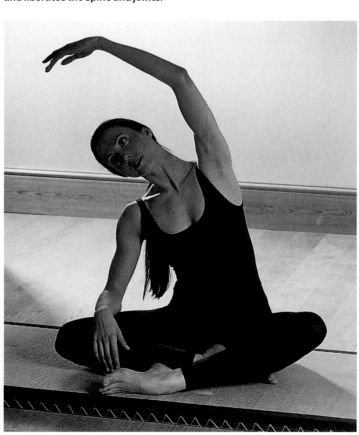

◁ Sit on the floor with one leg in front of the other (the legs are not crossed). Inhale as you prepare. Exhale as you raise one arm and lengthen up through the spine, then stretch into one side from a strong centre, taking care not to collapse into the stretch. Feel the stretch in your back. Pull the navel to the spine and keep your buttocks on the floor. If this leg positioning is uncomfortable, bend your legs and keep your feet flat on the floor.

Purpose: To stretch the back
Target muscles: The latissimus dorsi
Repetitions: Stretch twice on each side; hold for 30 seconds each

Checkpoints
- Keep your buttocks on the floor
- Lengthen up through the spine
- Don't let the abdominals sag

Sample programmes

To put together a programme that suits you, consult the chart on page 207, which shows the dominant muscles that are used. This will help you choose a selection of movements from each group to make a well-rounded programme. The majority of the exercises need to be repeated 10 times each (or, in the case of unilateral exercises, 10 times per side).

When putting together a programme, it is best to allow 5 minutes for each movement. A certain group of muscles may need more attention because of muscular imbalances or repetition of a certain activity. Also take into account the initial warm-up, final stretch and a relaxation period at the end. To get you started, two basic plans are suggested here.

Vary your programme from time to time so that you do not get bored. If you dislike an exercise or it does not feel right on a particular day, do a different movement that targets the same muscle groups. Always listen to your body. Most of the exercises have variations, so work your way progressively through the different levels of intensity.

The short programme

If you don't have time for an hour-long session, you can plan a mini programme lasting 25 minutes. However, try to base most sessions on the hour-long plan and use the short plan only when necessary (25 minutes is better than skipping the session entirely). You will obviously have to shorten the length of time spent on each exercise, as well as doing fewer of them: aim to achieve five to seven repetitions of each movement.

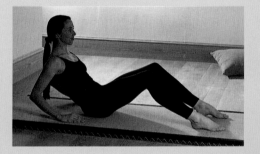

4

◁ **Rolling back**
3 minutes
(p.208)

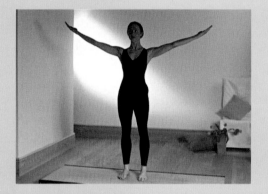

1

◁ **Warm-up**
8–10 minutes
ensures you are
warmed up
before you start
exercising (p.184).

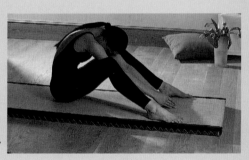

5

◁ **Spine stretch**
3 minutes
(p.228)

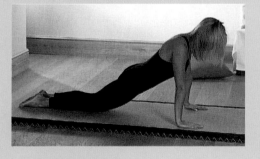

2

◁ **Push-ups**
3 minutes
(p.218)

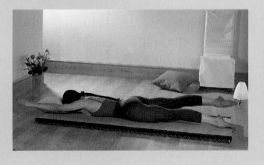

6

◁ **Hundred**
3 minutes
(p.210)

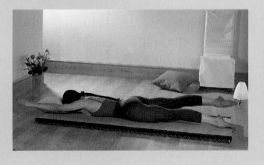

3

◁ **Swimming**
3 minutes
(p.211)

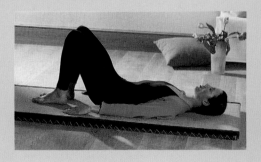

7

◁ **Relaxation**
Lie down and
relax for 2
minutes to finish
the session

The one-hour programme

This sample format includes some of the "core" movements; this would be a good programme to start with while you are adapting to these exercises. As with most Pilates programmes, the emphasis is on strengthening the torso. After a few weeks, you can change some of these movements for others; try always to do some movements from each of the different categories so that you are working on all parts of the body and developing strength, flexibility and mobility.

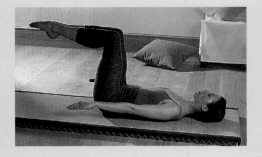

6

◁ **Hundred**
5 minutes
(p.210)

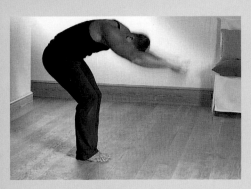

1

◁ **Warm-up**
8–10 minutes
ensures you are
warmed up
before you start
exercising (p.184).

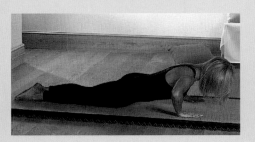

7

◁ **Spine stretch**
5 minutes
(p.228)

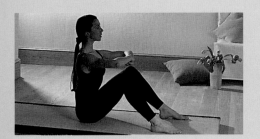

2

◁ **Spine twist**
5 minutes
(p.229)

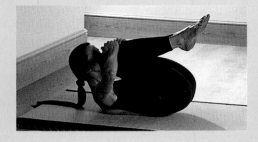

8

◁ **Push-ups**
5 minutes
(p.218)

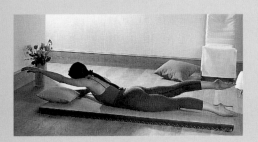

3

◁ **Swimming**
5 minutes
(p.211)

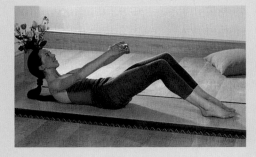

9

◁ **Rolling back**
5 minutes
(p.208)

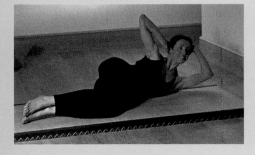

4

◁ **Side squeeze:
right side**
5 minutes
(p.216)

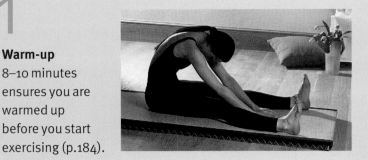

10

◁ **The roll-up**
5 minutes
(p.209)

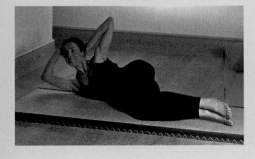

5

◁ **Side squeeze:
left side**
5 minutes
(p.216)

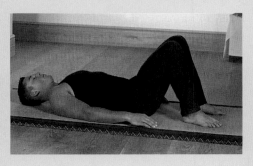

11

◁ **Relaxation**
Relax for
5 minutes to
finish the
session

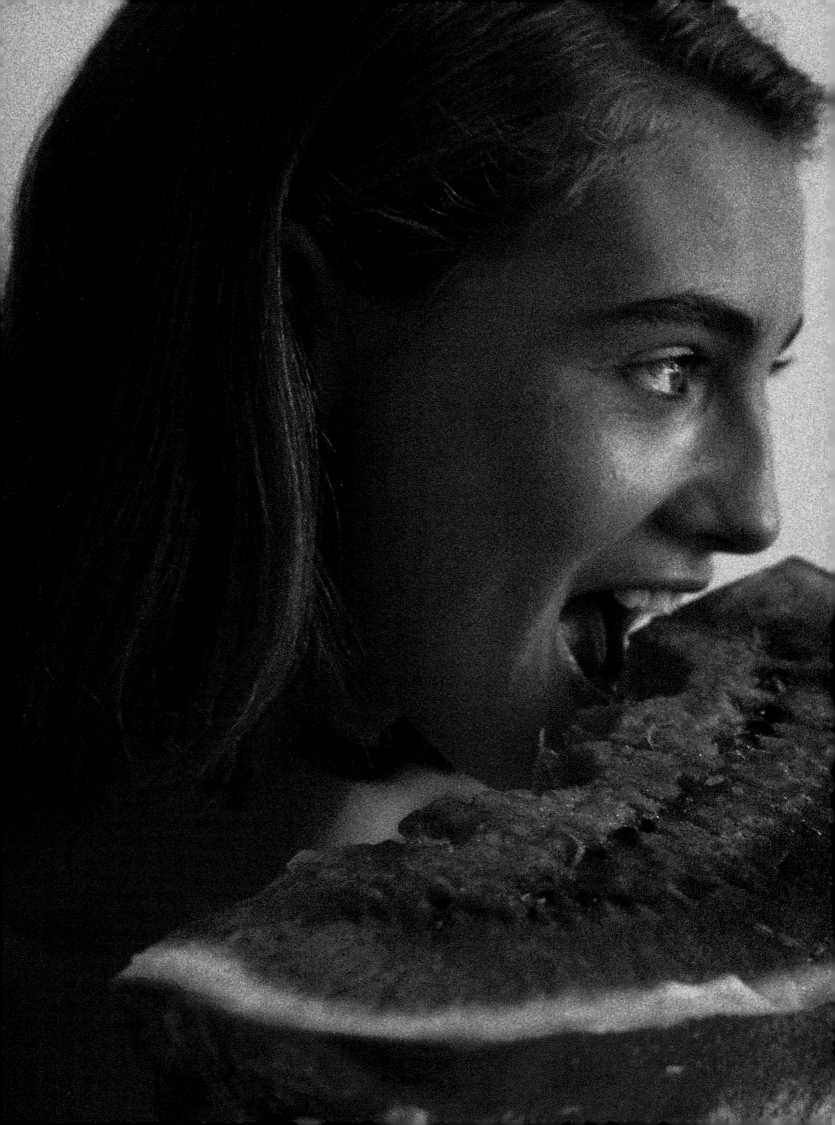

Healthy
eating

Developing healthy eating habits plays a huge part in how your body performs and how you feel about it. Eating foods that promote good health makes sense, and is surprisingly simple. So take advantage of the latest nutritional research to improve your diet, your health and your beauty.

A healthy balance

Balance is crucial to healthy eating, and understanding how to choose a healthy combination of foods is the first step towards improving your eating habits and lifestyle.

vital vitamins

Vitamins are crucial for a number of processes carried out by the body. Usually only a few milligrams are required each day but they are essential for good health. Most vitamins cannot be made by the body so they must be obtained from food.

Vitamins have a wide variety of functions in the body. Some vitamins play a part in enzyme activity. Enzymes are protein molecules and they are responsible for every aspect of metabolism, the energy we produce. Producing plenty of enzymes improves the processes of digestion, detoxification and immunity, and also helps to slow down the aging process.

Vitamins A, C and E are antioxidants which protect body cells from damage. If the body is under stress, vitamin C (ascorbic acid) is used more quickly. Smoking is a form of stress for the body, and smokers should be particularly careful to make sure that they eat fruit and vegetables containing vitamin C.

essential minerals

A wide variety of minerals is vital for good health, growth and body functioning. Some, such as calcium and iron, are needed in quite large amounts, and for some people there is a real risk of deficiency if they do not eat a healthy diet.

Calcium: A regular supply of calcium is vital because bone tissue is constantly being broken down and rebuilt. A calcium–rich diet is particularly important during adolescence, pregnancy, breastfeeding, the

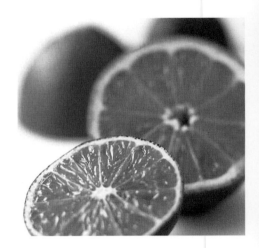

△ **Citrus fruits are a rich source of vitamin C. One orange a day provides an adult's daily requirement of vitamin C.**

menopause and old age. Smoking, lack of exercise, too much alcohol, high protein and high salt intakes all encourage calcium losses.

VITAMINS	BEST SOURCES	ROLE IN HEALTH
A (retinol in animal foods, beta-carotene in plant foods)	Milk, butter, cheese, egg yolks, margarine, carrots, apricots, squash, red (bell) peppers, broccoli, green leafy vegetables, mango and sweet potatoes.	Essential for vision, bone growth, and skin and tissue repair. Beta-carotene acts as an antioxidant and protects the immune system.
B1 (thiamin)	Wholegrain cereals, brewer's yeast, potatoes, nuts, pulses (legumes) and milk.	Essential for energy production, the nervous system, muscles and heart. Promotes growth and boosts mental ability.
B2 (riboflavin)	Cheese, eggs, milk, yogurt, fortified breakfast cereals, yeast extract, almonds and pumpkin seeds.	Essential for energy production and for the functioning of vitamin B6 and niacin as well as tissue repair.
Niacin (part of B complex)	Pulses, potatoes, fortified breakfast cereals, wheatgerm, peanuts, milk, cheese, eggs, peas, mushrooms, green leafy vegetables, figs and prunes.	Essential for healthy digestive system, skin and circulation. It is also needed for the release of energy.
B6 (piridoxine)	Eggs, wholemeal (whole-wheat) bread, breakfast cereals, nuts, bananas, and cruciferous vegetables such as broccoli and cabbage.	Essential for assimilating protein and fat, to make red blood cells, and for a healthy immune system.
B12 (cyanocobalamin)	Milk, eggs, fortified breakfast cereals, cheese and yeast extract.	Essential for formation of red blood cells, maintaining a healthy nervous system and increasing energy levels.
Folate (folic acid)	Green leafy vegetables, fortified breakfast cereals, bread, nuts, pulses, bananas and yeast extract.	Essential for cell division. Extra is needed pre-conception and during pregnancy to protect foetus against neural tube defects.
C (ascorbic acid)	Citrus fruits, melons, strawberries, tomatoes, broccoli, potatoes, peppers and green vegetables.	Essential for the absorption of iron, and for healthy skin, teeth and bones. An antioxidant that strengthens bones.
D (calciferol)	Sunlight, margarine, vegetable oils, eggs, cereals and butter.	Essential for bone and teeth formation. Helps the body to absorb calcium and phosphorus.
E (tocopherol)	Seeds, nuts, vegetable oils, eggs, wholemeal bread, green leafy vegetables, oats and cereals.	Essential for healthy skin, circulation and maintaining cells – an antioxidant.

▷ Not all fats are "bad" for you, but only small amounts are needed to stay healthy. Eat monounsaturated fats such as olive oil, and polyunsaturates such as sunflower oil, in preference to butter and other saturated fats.

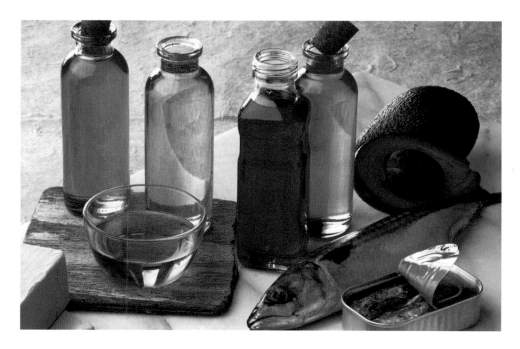

Iron: Only a fraction of the iron present in food is absorbed, although it is much more readily absorbed from red meat than from vegetable sources. Vitamin C also helps with absorption. Pregnant women, women who have heavy periods, and vegetarians should all be particularly careful about ensuring an adequate intake.

Trace elements: These include other essential minerals such as zinc, iodine, magnesium and potassium. Although important, they are needed in only minute quantities. They are found in a wide variety of foods and deficiency is very rare.

fats – good and bad

Eggs, butter, milk and meat are a good source of energy, but we tend to eat too much fat which is why many of us are overweight: fat produces fat. Cut down on fat in your diet but do not cut it out completely: eat less fatty red meat and more fish and poultry; grill (broil), bake or stir-fry (using polyunsaturated and monounsaturated oils); eat eggs in moderation; and use semi-skimmed (low-fat) or skimmed milk instead of full-fat (whole) milk. Use margarine, or switch to a reduced fat olive-oil spread instead of butter; if you like butter, reserve it for special occasions.

Saturated fats come mainly from animal products (milk, butter, cheese and meat) and in excess are thought to contribute to raised cholesterol levels.

Polyunsaturated fats are found in vegetable oils such as sunflower, safflower, corn and soya-bean oils; they are also found in some fish oils and some nuts, and are said to help lower cholesterol levels.

Mono-unsaturated fats are found in olive and rapeseed oils; they are also said to lower cholesterol levels.

MINERALS	BEST SOURCES	ROLE IN HEALTH
Calcium	Milk, cheese, yogurt, green leafy vegetables, sesame seeds, broccoli, dried figs, pulses, almonds, spinach and watercress.	Essential for building and maintaining bones and teeth, muscle function and the nervous system.
Iron	Red meat, egg yolks, fortified breakfast cereals, green leafy vegetables, dried apricots, prunes, pulses, wholegrains, tofu.	Essential for healthy blood and muscles.
Zinc	Peanuts, wholegrains sunflower and pumpkin seeds, pulses, milk, hard cheese and yogurt.	Essential for a healthy immune system, tissue formation, normal growth, wound healing and reproduction.
Sodium	Most of the salt we eat comes from processed foods such as crisps, cheese and canned foods. It is also found naturally in most foods.	Essential for nerve and muscle function and the regulation of body fluid.
Potassium	Bananas, milk, pulses, nuts, seeds, wholegrains, potatoes, fruits and vegetables.	Essential for water balance, normal blood pressure and nerve transmission.
Magnesium	Nuts, seeds, wholegrains, pulses, tofu, dried figs and apricots, and vegetables.	Essential for healthy muscles, bones and teeth, normal growth and nerves.
Phosphorous	Milk, cheese, yogurt, eggs, nuts, seeds, pulses and wholegrains.	Essential for healthy bones and teeth, energy production and the assimilation of nutrients.
Selenium	Avocados, lentils, milk, cheese, butter, brazil nuts and seaweed.	Essential for protecting against free radical damage and may protect against cancer.
Iodine	Seaweed and iodized salt.	Aids the production of hormones released by the thyroid gland.
Chloride	Table salt and foods that contain salt.	Regulates and maintains the balance of fluids in the body.
Manganese	Nuts, wholegrains, pulses, tofu and tea.	Essential component of various enzymes that are involved in energy production.

cereal grains

The seeds of cereal grasses, grains are packed with concentrated goodness and are an important source of complex carbohydrates, protein, vitamins and minerals. Grains are inexpensive and versatile.

Eat plenty of wholegrain foods such as brown rice, wholemeal bread, wholemeal flour and wholemeal pasta; they should form the bulk of a healthy diet.

fruit and vegetables

Make a habit of eating lots of fresh fruit and vegetables: these are rich in carbohydrates, vitamins and minerals. Nutritionists recommend that every day you should aim to eat at least five portions of fruit (one portion could be a medium apple or orange, a wine glass of fruit juice, two plums or kiwi fruit or one large slice of melon or pineapple) and vegetables (aim to eat two large spoonfuls of vegetables – fresh, frozen, or tinned – with your main meal). Fruit and vegetables contain

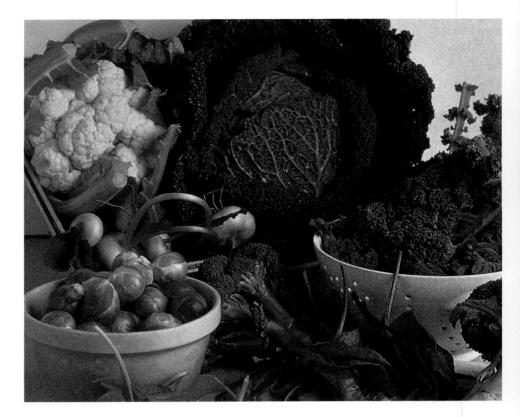

phytochemicals, the plant compounds that stimulate the body's enzyme defences against carcinogens (the substances that cause cancer). The best sources are broccoli, cabbages, kohlrabi, radishes, cauliflower, brussels sprouts, watercress, turnips, kale, pak choi (bok choy), mustard greens, spring greens (collards), chard and swede (rutabaga).

△ **One of the easiest ways to boost your intake of fibre, vitamins and minerals is to eat plenty of vegetables.**

sugary foods

Many of us tend to eat too much sugar so try cutting added sugar out of your diet completely for 21 days (your body will still

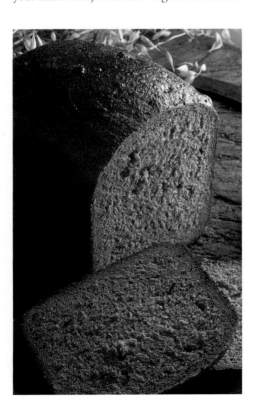

△ **Starchy carbohydrates should make up about 50 per cent of your daily diet.**

FACTS ON FIBRE

Fibre is important for a healthy diet. Your body cannot digest it, so, in rather basic terms, it goes in and comes out, taking other waste with it. Fibrous foods include bread, rice, cereals, vegetables, fruit and nuts. Aim for about 30g (just over 1oz) of fibre a day. These are some examples of good fibre sources:

good sources	average portion	grams of fibre
wholemeal pasta	75g/3oz (uncooked)	9
baked beans	115g/4oz	8
frozen peas	75g/3oz	8
bran flakes	50g/2oz	7
blackberries	90g/3½oz	6
raspberries	90g/3½oz	6
muesli	50g/2oz	4–5
baked jacket potato (with skin)	150g/5oz	3.5
banana	average fruit	3.5
brown rice	50g/2oz	3
cabbage	90g/3½oz	3
red kidney beans	40g/1½oz	3
wholemeal bread	1 large slice	3
high-fibre white bread	1 large slice	2
stewed prunes	6 fruit	2

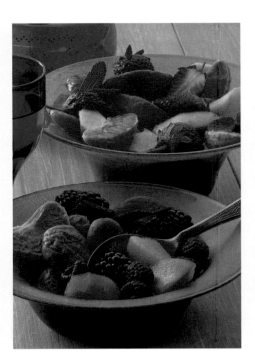

▽ **Fresh fruit makes a healthy, low-calorie snack that is filling as well as delicious.**

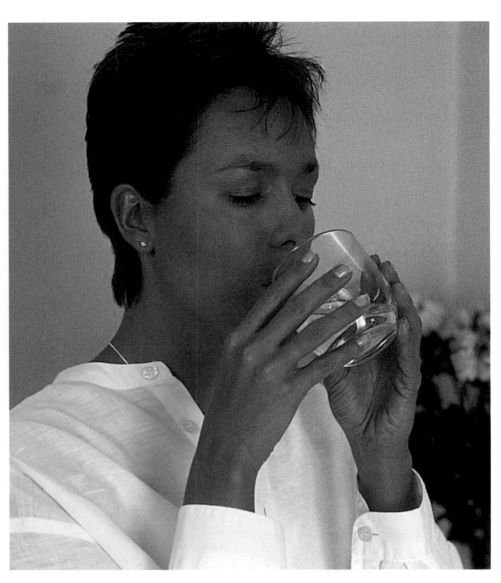

obtain it naturally from certain vegetables and fruit) and see how you feel. Even if you are not actively dieting you will probably find that you lose weight. Craving sugary foods when you are pre-menstrual is common, so try to eat little and often; snack on fruit with a high water content, such as watermelon and strawberries.

salty issues

It is generally a good idea to eat less salt as too much may lead to high blood pressure. There are some good low-sodium salts available, so use these instead if you do need to season food with salt. Do not buy salted butter, avoid processed and smoked cheeses, add just a little salt (or none at all) to cooking water, and avoid processed foods.

fluid intake

Drink plenty of water: your body loses 2–3 litres/3–5 pints of fluid every day, so drink no less than 1.5 litres/2¹/2 pints of water daily. Once you get into the swing of it, consciously drinking water is an easy habit to maintain. Just keep some to hand and sip it slowly throughout the day.

seeds, pulses and nuts

Pulses (legumes) are economical, easy to cook and good to eat. Low in fat and high in complex carbohydrates, vitamins and minerals, they are a valuable source of protein and good for diabetics, as they help to control sugar levels. Nuts are a good source of B complex vitamins and vitamin E, an antioxidant that has been associated with a lower risk of heart disease, stroke and certain cancers. They are a useful source of protein but are high in calories, so don't eat too many of them.

sea vegetables

Sea vegetables such as arame, laver and kombu are an excellent source of betacarotene, and contain some of the B complex vitamins. They are rich in minerals – calcium, magnesium, potassium, phosphorous and iron are all present – and are credited with boosting the immune system, reducing stress and helping the metabolism to function efficiently. Eating sea vegetables regularly can improve the hair and skin, and the iodine they contain improves thyroid function.

△ **As a rough guide you should aim to drink at least 8 glasses of water every day to keep your body properly hydrated.**

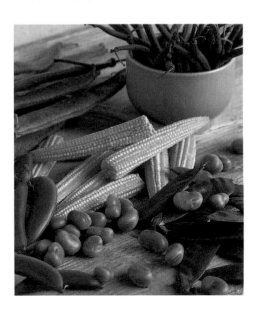

△ **It is worth remembering that thanks to super-efficient harvesting methods many frozen vegetables are more nutritious than fresh ones.**

Eating for health and beauty

What we eat has a profound effect on our health and wellbeing. There is ample evidence of a link between poor diet and poor health, and this will affect the way you look. Shining hair, clear skin and strong nails are synonymous with good health.

Specific foods can have a positive impact on our skin, hair, bodies and overall wellbeing when eaten as part of a sensible, well-balanced diet.

healthy hair and scalp

Aim for a balance of protein foods, including dairy produce, nuts and pulses (legumes). Your shopping list should include organic artichokes, sweet potatoes, carrots, spinach, broccoli, asparagus and beetroot (beet). Choose apricots, citrus fruits, kiwi fruit, berries and apples. Also eat plenty of oily fish and shellfish.

Dry hair and an itching, flaky scalp may be the result of zinc deficiency. Shellfish are good sources of zinc, as are red meat and pumpkin seeds. Essential fatty acids in vegetable oils, nuts and oily fish can also improve the condition of the scalp, while the minerals in sea vegetables, such as kombu and arame, help to make hair lustrous.

Vitamins A and B are important if hair is to be shiny and healthy. Eating liver once

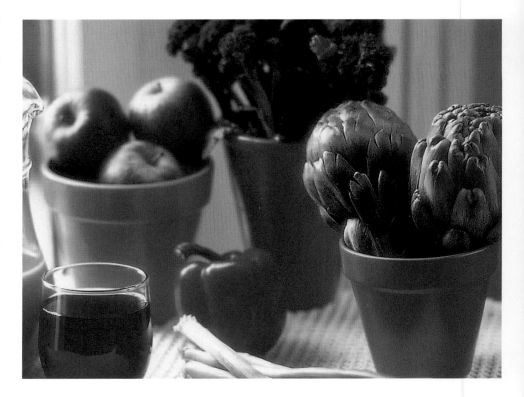

△ **Eating plenty of fresh fruit and vegetables is vital for maintaining a healthy immune system.**

a week is a great way of boosting your intake of vitamin A (retinol), provided that you are not pregnant. Fish liver oils are the richest source of retinol, but it can be obtained from eggs and full-cream (whole) milk. Also eat carrots, spinach, red (bell) peppers, sweet potatoes, peaches and dried apricots on a regular basis. These contain betacarotene, which the body converts to vitamin A.

improving your skin

The skin is the largest organ in the body, and is especially vulnerable to the effects of modern living. The most important thing you can do to improve the quality of your skin is to drink water – ideally six to eight large glasses every day.

Regular exercise and plenty of fresh air combined with a healthy diet will work wonders on your skin.

If you have a specific skin condition, such as eczema or acne, it is important to consult your doctor, but if you merely think your skin is looking a bit lifeless and could do with a lift, you may find the following advice helpful.

Eat fresh vegetables such as carrots, spinach, broccoli and sweet potatoes which deliver the antioxidant betacarotene. Citrus fruit, kiwi fruit, berries, avocados, vegetable oils, wholegrains, nuts, seeds and types of seafood provide the antioxidant vitamins C and E, selenium and zinc, which all help to transport nutrients to the skin and maintain collagen and elastin levels. Zinc-rich foods such as liver, pâté and eggs can improve conditions such as psoriasis and eczema. Apples are rich in pectin, which helps to cleanse the liver, and so aids skin detoxification.

Artichokes are good liver cleansers, too, along with asparagus and raw beetroot. Fish, meat and eggs provide B vitamins, which promote supple, glowing skin. Similar benefits can be gained from eating oily fish such as mackerel, salmon, tuna, sardines and herrings. The fatty acids these fish contain (also found in nuts, seeds and vegetable oils) soften and hydrate the skin.

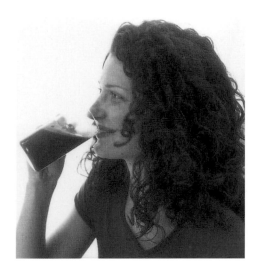

△ **A glass of carrot juice contains a valuable supply of antioxidants.**

▷ Healthy, shining hair not only feels and looks great, it also reflects good physical wellbeing and conscientious maintenance.

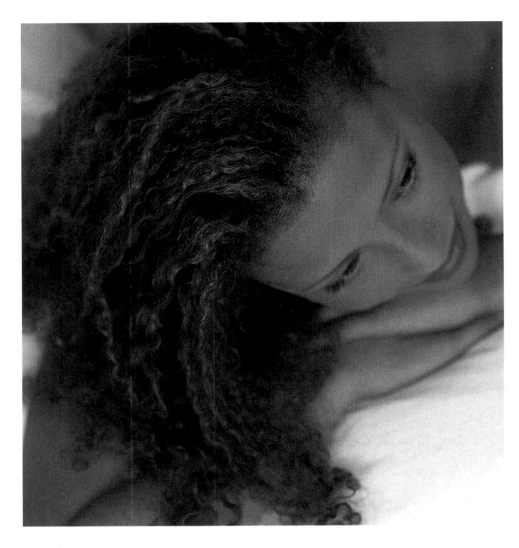

HEALTHY NAILS

• Drink plenty of water

• To strengthen nails, eat iron-rich foods such as liver, other red meat, fish, poultry, green leafy vegetables, dried apricots and wholegrain cereals. To optimize iron absorption, eat foods rich in vitamin C, such as tomatoes and potatoes.

• Dry brittle nails may indicate a zinc deficiency, and a meal of braised liver with onions and cherry tomatoes once a week may work wonders. Chickpeas and tofu are a good choice for vegetarians.

• Wide ridges may indicate a selenium deficiency which is closely associated with the function of vitamin E in the body. Good sources are meat, especially liver, fish and shellfish, chicken and wholegrain cereals.

maximizing nutritional value

To obtain the most nutritional value from your food, especially fruit and vegetables, it should be as fresh as possible, and preparation or cooking should ensure that as many nutrients as possible are retained.

• If you grow your own fruit and vegetables, or buy from a farm where the produce is picked or pulled as needed, freshness is guaranteed. If not, make sure your supplier has a rapid turnover.

• Transport produce home quickly. Remove any plastic wrapping. Store produce in a cool larder or in the refrigerator crisper.

• Avoid buying fresh produce from a supermarket or store that has installed fluorescent lighting over displays, as this can cause a chemical reaction, depleting nutrients in fruit and vegetables.

• Buy organic produce where possible, and avoid peeling if you can, since nutrients are concentrated just below the skin. Instead wash thoroughly. Prepared vegetables are convenient, but don't peel or slice produce until you are ready to use it, as the nutritional value diminishes rapidly after preparation.

• Try to eat the majority of your vegetables and fruit raw. Otherwise, use a steamer in preference to boiling because during this process soluble vitamins, such as thiamine, vitamin C and B vitamins leach into the water. If you must boil vegetables, use just a little water, and save the water to use in a soup or sauce.

• Buy nuts and seeds in small quantities.

Store them in airtight containers in a cool, dark place. Herbs, spices, pulses, flours and grains should be kept in the same way. Store oils in a cool, dark place to prevent oxidation.

▽ Strawberries are rich in B complex vitamins and vitamin C. They contain potassium, and have good skin-cleansing properties.

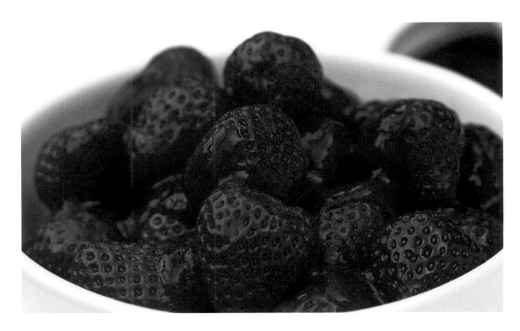

Eating for energy

How often do you feel tired and lethargic? Does your energy dip dramatically in the afternoons, making you feel dozy (even if you have not washed down a three-course lunch with a bottle of wine) and in need of 40 winks? If your life is regularly disrupted by fatigue and you want to take action, one of the wisest things to do is to look at your eating habits and, if necessary, change what you eat and how you eat it.

off to a good start

If you start the day with a substantial breakfast your body will get all the energy it needs early on. It is also true that those who fail to eat something sustaining for breakfast are more likely to snack mid-morning and this is unlikely to be a good nutritional choice. A bowl of muesli or porridge with fruit is a good slow-release option that will energize you to start your day.

changing your eating habits

You are most likely to succeed in changing your diet if you eat regularly, in moderation, and slowly – and savour every mouthful. Although the bonuses of eating in a balanced way do not come instantly, if you take stock now and concentrate on eating

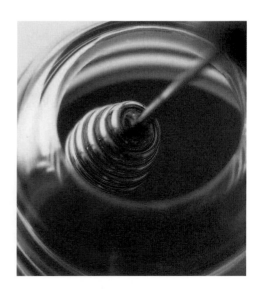

△ **Honey is a good source of natural sugar and is gently energizing.**

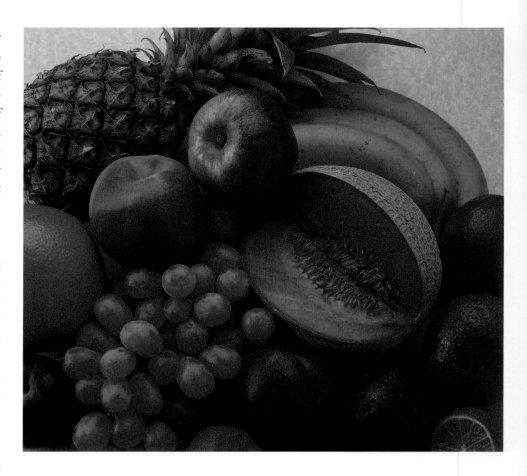

△ **Fruit is the ultimate convenience food. Packed with natural sugars it is ideal for giving you a boost when energy levels are low.**

the fresh foods suggested below, as well as avoiding high-fat, sugar-rich foods such as cakes, pastries and salty snacks, you will probably notice a marked difference in your energy levels within a couple of weeks.

If your energy levels take a dive because your blood sugar is low, don't reach for chocolate or a rich biscuit. The quick energy boost these give will be followed by a slump, and you may end up far more tired than you were at the start. Eat a wholemeal salad sandwich instead; the carbohydrate in the bread will give you a more efficient energy fix that will be more prolonged and even.

vitality foods for extra energy

A diet that makes you feel more energetic is based on natural, wholesome foods that are nutritious, rather than fatty and fast foods. If you want to boost your energy levels, stock up on fresh and dried fruits that are high in natural sugars, such as pears, kiwi

fruit and apricots, vegetables such as peas, spinach, cabbage, onions, oily fish, poultry, and red meats such as game and lean beef. Eat nuts, brown rice, seeds, pulses (legumes), wheatgerm, wholegrains, and foods that contain minerals such as magnesium, phosphorous, and zinc, and water-soluble vitamins B and C. Use cold-pressed oils such as grapeseed, olive, sesame, sunflower, hazelnut and walnut to dress salads; do not skip dairy foods but use milk and natural yogurt (preferably low-fat); replace sliced white loaves with bread made from wholemeal flour.

superfoods

Some foods are such a super-rich source of concentrated nutrients that they have earned themselves the title "superfoods".

▷ Fresh fruit and vegetable juices have a powerful effect on the body, stimulating the whole system, flushing out the digestive system and encouraging the elimination of toxins.

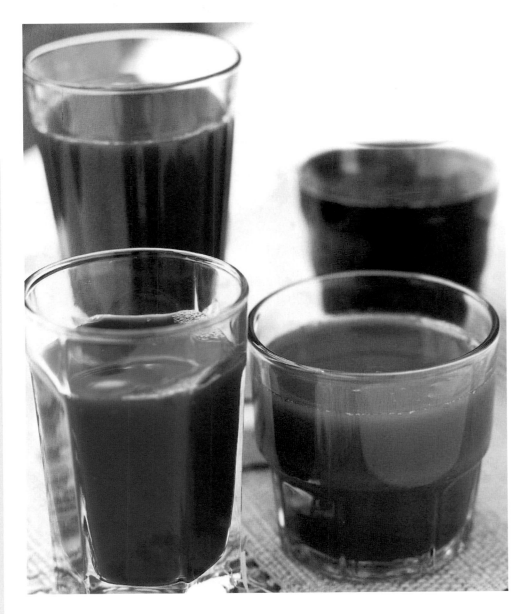

VITAMIN-PACKED JUICES

Drinking freshly made juices is a quick and easy way to increase your nutrient intake and boost your energy levels without placing the digestion under any strain. Here are some good juices to try:

• Apple, orange and carrot: packed with vitamin C and energizing fruit sugars to give you a lift.

• Papaya, melon and grapes: papaya is soothing to the stomach, and this juice can help the liver and kidneys.

• Carrot, beetroot (beet) and celery: a good juice to kickstart the system in the morning. Try using 90g/3¹/₂oz beetroot to three carrots and two celery sticks.

• Cabbage, fennel and apple: a cleansing juice with antibacterial properties. Use half a small red cabbage, half a fennel bulb, 2 apples and 15ml/1 tbsp lime juice.

• Grapefruit, orange and lemon: this refreshing juice is great for boosting the immune system. Use 1 pink grapefruit, 1 blood orange and 30ml/2 tbsp lemon juice.

ENERGY-BOOSTING SMOOTHIES

Homemade fruit juices and milk- or yogurt-based drinks are energy-boosting alternatives to commercially prepared drinks, and are easy to make. They are quick, low in fat, high-vitality and a great way of boosting your fruit intake. Choose sweet fruits such as mango, banana and apricots – these have a naturally high sugar content – then switch on the juicer or blender and drink them chilled. Here are two energizing smoothies to try:

• This smoothie is full of energizing natural sugars. Use 1 mango, 2 slices of pineapple, 1 banana, 150ml/¹/₄pint/²/₃cup semi-skimmed or skimmed (low-fat) milk or a small carton of natural (plain) low-fat yogurt and 2.5ml/¹/₂tsp honey (optional).

• For a more zesty energy-boosting smoothie use a handful of raspberries and strawberries, 2 apricots and 120ml/4fl oz/¹/₂cup milk or natural low-fat yoghurt.

Some, such as tofu, are old favourites, while others, such as quinoa, have only recently acquired widespread acclaim. Recent scientific research has discovered that plants contain thousands of different chemical compounds, and each of these compounds – known collectively as phytochemicals – has its own function. It is believed that some of them play a crucial role in preventing diseases such as cancer, heart disease, arthritis and hypertension.

To get the best from phytochemicals you need to eat at least five different types of fruit and vegetables daily, plus wholegrains, pulses, nuts and seeds. A number of phytochemicals also have antioxidant properties.

Antioxidants are vital for limiting damage to body cells by unstable molecules known as free radicals. The main antioxidant nutrients are vitamins A, C and E, and the minerals zinc and selenium. Good sources of antioxidants are: sweet potatoes, carrots, watercress, broccoli, peas, citrus fruit, watermelon, strawberries, and nuts and seeds.

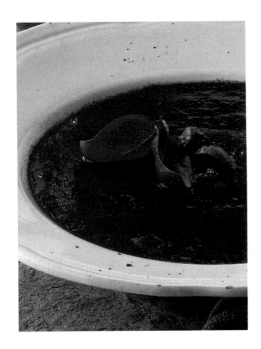

▷ Fresh tomato soup is packed with valuable antioxidant vitamins, while a sprinkle of basil aids digestion and calms the nervous system.

Eating for weight loss

People tackle weight loss in ways that suit their lifestyles. But the safest and best way to shift excess pounds is to combine regular exercise with a balanced calorie-controlled diet. What you eat when you are trying to take off weight should not be that different from a normal eating plan – except for the amount you consume. If you have only a small amount to lose and you cut your calorie intake by 1,000 from the recommended 2,300 calories per day, you will lose weight; if you are aiming to lose a significant amount, stick to 1,200 calories a day and you will get there. Your basic weight-loss ethos is less sugar and saturated fats, more fibre and starch; the calories you eat should come from foods that supply you with the right number of nutrients to keep your body functioning properly.

mind over matter

Quick weight loss is inspiring, but it is important to think ahead too; you need to retain your palate and eating habits and reassess your physical activity so that you can lose weight and stay slim. You cannot expect to achieve miracles in a few days, but

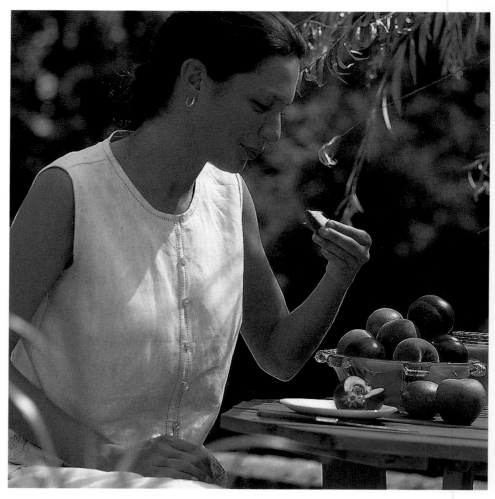

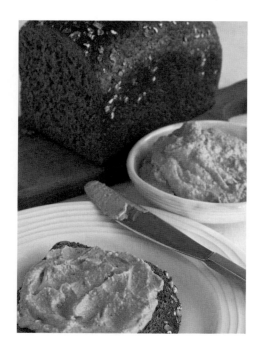

△ For an excellent high-fibre snack, hummus is delicious spread on wholegrain bread or toast.

you will see a difference within three or four weeks if you eat properly and exercise regularly. Losing weight successfully is like getting fitter: you need a horizon – or goal – ahead of you to help spur you on.

healthy weight loss

To lose weight you have to eat fewer calories than your body burns up every day, but the amount varies from person to person. The exact amount depends on your personal composition – how much fat your body has, your metabolism and how much you weigh to begin with. As a rule of thumb though, the heavier you are when you start slimming, the more weight you are likely to lose within 21 days or a month. When you lose weight it comes off all areas of your body, but it can take longer to shift from certain areas, such as your arms and legs.

△ **Fruit is the ideal snack when you are dieting. It is very low in fat and calories and provides vitamins and minerals as well as energizing natural sugar energy.**

This is where exercise is particularly helpful, because working on specific trouble spots will usually encourage the weight to come off more quickly.

weight gain and giving up smoking

You may put on a small amount of weight at first but if you are a smoker, stopping is the biggest leap you can make towards living a healthier lifestyle. If you think that kicking the smoking habit will make you pick at food all day, keep lots of raw vegetables and raisins on hand to munch on.

▷ Keeping a record of your measurements is one way of calculating weight loss. It may take longer to shift weight from certain areas, and this will also help you work out which areas you need to focus on when you exercise.

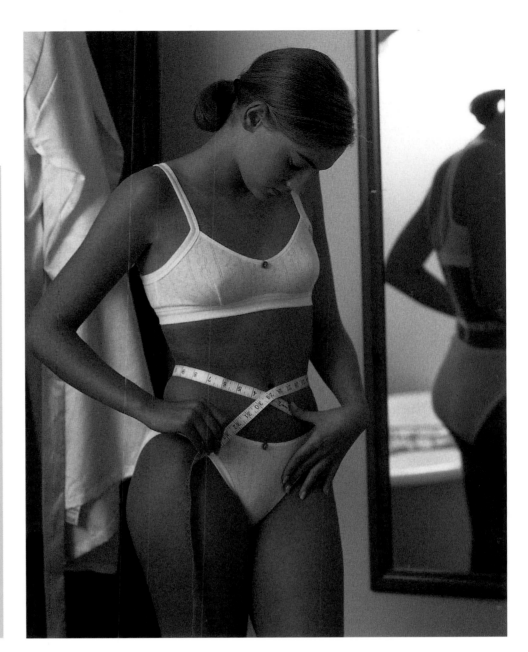

TIPS FOR WEIGHT LOSS

• If you can, it is better to eat more at the start of the day to give you energy and time to burn off the calories.

• Do not be tempted to skip meals. Skipping meals makes you crave and overeat at the next meal, and it slows down your metabolism, which ultimately hinders weight loss.

• Eat little and often to stop hunger pangs.

• Drink lots of water.

• If you want to snack, keep a supply of fruit, raw vegetables and raisins nearby.

• Don't be tempted to take slimming pills, diuretics or laxatives to speed up weight loss; they upset the body's natural equilibrium – something that can take considerable time to rebalance.

• Exercise regularly; extra activity uses up calories, and this is essential to weight loss.

• Don't give up if you lapse: it is quite normal to veer off track every so often, and as long as you get back on course as soon as you can, all your hard work will not be ruined.

eating out – and staying on course

The best way to solve the problem of dining out without lapsing – without drawing attention to yourself and still being able to enjoy yourself – is as follows:

• Order a salad starter.

• Skip bread or breadsticks, or eat a piece of bread without butter – if it's good bread it can be just as delicious.

• Drink one glass of wine, and lots of water.

• Choose a simple main course, something like grilled fish or chicken; avoid rich sauces and lots of butter.

• Choose a simple, low-fat dessert: a sorbet would be ideal.

• Finish with herbal tea (peppermint is refreshing and settles your stomach after eating); or, choose espresso or black coffee, not cappuccino.

gauging weight loss

You may choose to weigh yourself once a week first thing in the morning. Drawing up a goal chart to record any weight losses (and gains) may help to keep you inspired. Don't be tempted to weigh yourself too often because you are more likely to get discouraged; once a week is enough. Or, if you prefer, ignore the scales and just focus on how you feel by keeping a check on how your clothes feel. When tight clothes become more comfortable this is a sure sign that you are losing weight. Alternatively, you may prefer to keep a record of your measurements (bust, waist and hips) and see how they alter over the 21-day period. Do whatever works best for you, and when you have lost a little weight reward yourself with a treat such as new make-up, a manicure or a massage.

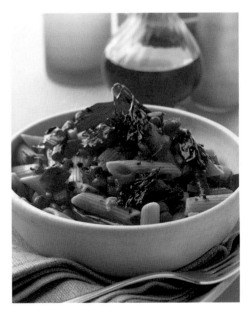

△ Nutritious, starchy foods such as pasta are not fattening if eaten with low fat sauces, and starchy foods stop you feeling hungry for longer.

Detoxing for health

A detox is thought to cleanse and rejuvenate your body, improve the circulation and metabolism, and strengthen the immune system. It can also improve the condition of your skin, hair and nails, and slow down the aging process. As well as the physical benefits, a detox can improve your ability to cope with stress, clear your mind and lift your mood.

Fast foods, sugary or salty snacks, alcohol, coffee and tea all contain toxins, which can build up in the body and cause us to feel lethargic and unhealthy. Even if you have a healthy lifestyle, you are still exposed to poisonous substances in the atmosphere. The air that we breathe contains chemicals, gases and dust particles, and it can pollute our land, water and food.

The body is a highly efficient machine, and it is constantly working to remove toxins from the circulation. However, an unhealthy diet, stress and late nights all put the body under pressure, and can affect how well its elimination systems work. Regular exercise supported by a healthy diet and a weekly detox massage regime will help improve your circulation, eliminate waste from the muscles and keep the detoxifying organs in good working order.

It is also vital that you drink plenty of water. We lose fluid through the natural processes of urination, defecation and sweat. This fluid needs to be replaced. To maintain good health and an efficient detox system we should drink at least 6–8 large glasses of water each day.

the art of detoxing

There are different approaches to detoxing. The most extreme method is fasting – which involves abstaining from all foods and drinking only water, herbal tea and juices over a short period.

Fasting has a tendency to slow the digestive system, so it can be counter-productive and is not recommended for most people. Your body is more likely to benefit from a gentle programme that does not place it under pressure. A detox is most effective if it is done over a day or two. During this time eat little and often, having only fibre-rich, healthy foods such as raw or lightly cooked fruits, vegetables and grains. Do several sessions of gentle exercise and rest as much as possible. Drink plenty of water to help flush toxins away. You can also drink fresh juices and herbal teas.

Massage can help to speed up the detox process, and brings a pleasurable, relaxing element to the day.

one-day mono-diet

A good introduction to detoxing, a one-day mono-diet is based on eating just one type of raw fruit or vegetable for a whole day. A one-day mono gives your digestive system a rest, allowing it to concentrate on eliminating stored toxins. You are unlikely to experience any dramatic side-effects but a mono-diet will have a noticeable positive effect on your health and wellbeing.

Raw fruit and vegetables have a powerful cleansing effect on the body and also supply plenty of vitamins, minerals and fibre. If possible, choose a day when you are not working, to make sure that you have time to rest, relax and sleep.

preparation

Choose just one of these fruits or vegetables:
- grapes
- apples
- pears
- pineapple
- papaya
- carrots
- cucumber
- celery

It is best to choose organic produce and you will need:
- 1–1.5kg/2–3lb of your chosen fruit or vegetable
- 2 litres/3$^{1/2}$ pints/8 cups still mineral water or filtered water
- herbal teas or fresh herbs to infuse

the days before detox

Prepare for your detox by cutting down on meat and dairy products, salt, wheat, tea, coffee and sugary foods. Avoid alcohol and cigarettes. The evening before, eat a light evening meal. A vegetable and bean soup or a stir-fry would be perfect. Have an aromatherapy bath and go to bed early.

detox day

Morning: Start your day with the juice of half a lemon in a cup of hot water. This

△ A cup of hot water and lemon juice will stimulate the liver and the gallbladder to kickstart the detoxing process.

HOW TO CUT DOWN TOXIN CONSUMPTION
- Buy organic foods whenever possible.
- Avoid drinking unfiltered tap water.
- Reduce intake of processed and packaged foods.
- Cut back on the amount of sweet, fatty and salty foods you eat.
- Always wash and peel non-organic fruit and vegetables.
- Cut down consumption of dairy products and meat. However, make sure that you eat other foods to obtain the calcium your body needs.
- Drink less tea, coffee and fizzy drinks.
- Read labels carefully to avoid artificial additives and genetically modified ingredients.

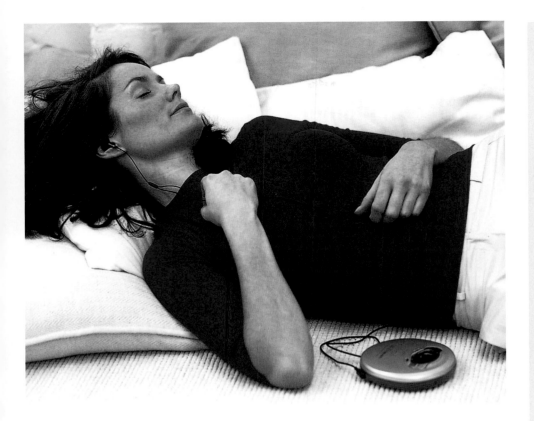

kickstarts the liver. Do some simple stretching exercises. Give yourself a dry skin brush to stimulate the circulation before you shower or bathe. For breakfast, prepare your chosen fruit or vegetable. Sip water at regular intervals throughout the day.

Late morning: Have a massage or try out some relaxation techniques. Eat some of your fruit or vegetable and drink plenty of water.

Lunch: Prepare and eat your fruit or vegetable. Drink plenty of water.

Afternoon: Try doing some gentle exercises, such as yoga, Pilates or body conditioning, or brisk walking, cycling or swimming. Follow this exercise with some of your fruit or vegetable and herbal tea.

Evening: Finish off your quota of fruit or vegetable. Meditate or practise a relaxation technique, such as visualization. Pamper yourself with a manicure or pedicure. Listen to some calming music. Have an Epsom salts bath to encourage the elimination of toxins through your skin. Pour 450g/1lb of salts into a warm bath. Go to bed early.

the day after

It is important to ease your body out of a detox gradually. Start the following day with a cup of hot water and lemon juice and some simple exercises. For the first few days keep to cleansing foods and simple recipes. Try not to over-exert yourself.

△ **You will benefit more from the detox if you take the day off so that you have time to rest, relax and sleep.**

lymphatic drainage massage

Lymphatic drainage massage is one of the most gentle forms of massage. It works on the lymph system, and since lymph vessels are close to the surface there is no need for heavy pressure. The lymphatic system of the body is a secondary circulation system which supports the work of the blood circulation. The lymphatic system has no heart to help pump the fluid around the vessels, and therefore it must rely on the activity of the muscles to aid movement.

Lymphatic massage involves using sweeping, squeezing movements along the skin. The action is always directed towards the nearest lymph node. The main nodes used when treating the foot are located in the hollow behind the knee. Lymphatic drainage massage is hugely beneficial in helping to eliminate waste and strengthen the body's immune system. It is a useful exercise to perform on your detox day.

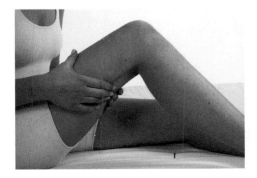

△ **1** To improve lymphatic drainage to the feet and legs, try a daily skin "brush" using your fingertips. Begin by working on the thigh. This clears the lymphatic channels ready to receive the lymph flood from the lower legs. Briskly brush all over the thigh from knee to top, three or four times.

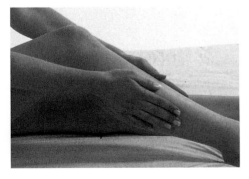

△ **2** Work on the lower leg in a similar way. Brush either side of the leg from ankle to knee, then treat the back of the leg. Follow this by brushing along the top of the foot, continuing up the front of the leg to the knee. Brush over each area twice more, making three times in total.

index

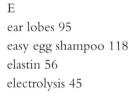

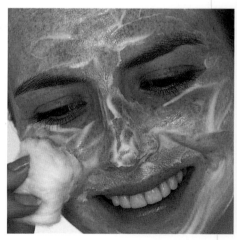

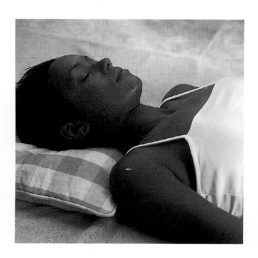

ACKNOWLEDGEMENTS

MAKE-UP AND HAIRSTYLING PRODUCTS

With many thanks to the following companies. **Beauty products** from The Body Shop, Boots, Bourjois, Crabtree & Evelyn, Cutex, Elancyl, L'Oréal, Rimmel and Sensiq. **Hair products** from Aveda, Bain de Terre, The Body Shop, Citre, Clynol, Daniel Gavin, Dome, Goldwell, John Frieda, Joico, KMS, Lamaur, Lazartigue, L'Oréal, Matrix Essentials, Neal's Yard Remedies, Nicky Clarke, Ore-an, Paul Mitchell, Phytologie, Poly, Redken, Revlon, Schwarzkopf, Silvikrin, St Ives, Trevor Sorbie, Wella and Vidal Sassoon and Zotos. **Electrical styling products** from Babyliss, Braun, Clairol, Carmen, Hair Tools, Philips, Rowenta and Vidal Sassoon. **Clothing and accessories** from Adrian Man, Bhs, Debenhams, Descamps, Empire, Fenwicks, Freemans, French Connection, Knickerbox, Marks & Spencer and Whistles.

HAIR PHOTOGRAPHY CREDITS

The Publishers are grateful for the following photographers and companies for permission to reproduce their photographs:

p105b: Silvikrin; p107tl: Braun; p107tm: Taylor Ferguson, Glasgow; p107tr: Antoinette Beenders at Trevor Sorbie, London for Denman, photography Simon Bottomley; p108bl and br: Regis; p109tr: Joseph and Jane Harling, Avon; p109ml: Paul Falltricks, Essex; p109mr: Regis; p109bl: Nicky Clarke, London; p109br: Essanelle Salons, Britain; p112l: Trevor Sorbie; p112r: L'Oréal; p114 all: Carlos Calico, Madrid; p114t: Silvikrin; p116: Daniel Galvin for L'Oréal, photography Iain Philpott; p120: Daniel Galvin, London; p122t: Bain de Terre Spa Therapy; p122bl & br: Daniel Galvin; p123tl: Bain de Terre Spa Therapy; p123br: Daniel Galvin; p124: Nicky Clarke; p125tl: Babyliss; p125tr: Yosh Toya, San Francisco, photography Gen; p125br: Daniel Galvin; p127tl: Daniel Galvin; p127tr: Wella, photography Mark Hill; p128: Clynol; p129tl: Terence Renati, London and Melbourne; p129tm: Patrick Cameron for Alan Paul, Wirral; p129tr: Regis; p130 bl: Richard M. F. Mendleson of David's Hair Designers, Maryland, USA; p130bm and br: Eugene at Xtension Masters, London; p131br: Macmillan, London; p131tr: Richard M. F. Mendleson; p135l: Sam Mcknight for Silvikrin; p135tr: Paul Falltrick, photography Iain Philpott; p135br: Jed Hamill of Graham Webb International for Clynol, photography Ian Hooton; p136tl & br: Regis, photography John Swannel; p136tm: Yosh Toya, photography Gen; p136bl and br: Regis, Europe, photography John Swannel; p137tr: Paul Fattrick, for Clynol, photography Alistair Hughes; p137tm: Yosh Toya, photography Gen; p137tr: Alan Edwards for L'Oréal. p137ml: Daniel Galvin; p137mr: Nicky Clarke, photography Paul Cox; p137bl: Frank Hession, Dublin, for L'Oréal; p137bm: Neville Daniel, London, photography Will White; p137br: Neville Daniel for Lamaur; p138tl: Charles Worthington, London for L'Oréal; p138tr: L'Oréal; p138bl: Trevor Sorbie, photography Mark Havrilliak; p138bml: Umberto Giannino, Kidderminster for L'Oréal; p138bmr: Stuart Kirby of Eaton-Hair Group, Portsmouth, for L'Oréal; p138bl: Anthony Mascolo, Toni & Guy, for L'Oréal; p139tl & tm: Yosh Toya, photography Gen; p139ml & mr: Regis, photography John Swannel; p139bl: Barbara Daley Hair Studio, Birmingham, for L'Oréal; p139bml: L'Oréal; p139bmr & br: Mod Hair, France, for Schwarzkopf; p140tl: Steven Carey, London; p140bl & r: Neville Daniel, for Lamaur; p141tl: Daniel Galvin; p141tm & tr: Nicky Clarke; p141ml & mr: Silvikrin; p141bl: John Frieda, London and New York; p141bm & br: Daniel Galvin; p142tl: Adam Lyons, Grays, for L'Oréal; p142tm: Taylor Ferguson; p142tr: Paul Falltricks, for Clynol, photography Alistair Hughes; p142b (all): Taylor Ferguson; p143tl: Zotos International; p143tm: Steven Carey, photography Alistair Hughes; p143tr: Schwarzkopf; p143bl: Regis, photography Mark York; p143bml: Steven Carey, photography Alistair Hughes; p143bmr: Partners, London; p143br: Keith Harris for Braun; p146bl: Silvikrin; p146tr: Clynol; p147tr: Babyliss; p148br: Babyliss; p149tr: Silvikrin.